Digital Twins and Healthcare:

Trends, Techniques, and Challenges

Loveleen Gaur
Amity University, India

Noor Zaman Jhanjhi
Taylor's University, Malaysia

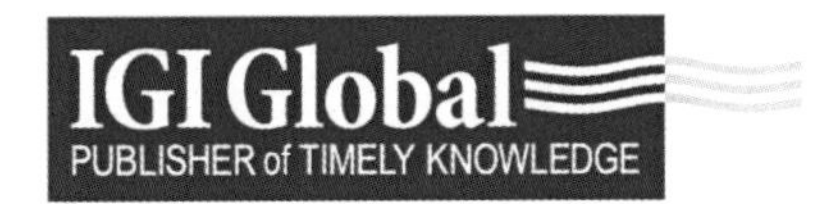

A volume in the Advances in Medical Technologies and Clinical Practice (AMTCP) Book Series

Published in the United States of America by
IGI Global
Medical Information Science Reference (an imprint of IGI Global)
701 E. Chocolate Avenue
Hershey PA, USA 17033
Tel: 717-533-8845
Fax: 717-533-8661
E-mail: cust@igi-global.com
Web site: http://www.igi-global.com

Library of Congress Cataloging-in-Publication Data

Names: Gaur, Loveleen, editor. | Zaman Jhanjhi, Noor, DATE- editor.
Title: Digital twins and healthcare : trends, techniques, and challenges / Loveleen Gaur and Noor Zaman Jhanjhi, editor.
Description: Hershey, PA : Medical Information Science Reference, [2023] | Includes bibliographical references and index. | Summary: "Digital twins are digital representations of human physiology built on computer models and this book highlights uses of digital twins in healthcare to revolutionize clinical processes and hospital management by enhancing medical care with digital tracking and advancing modelling of the human body"-- Provided by publisher.
Identifiers: LCCN 2022023244 (print) | LCCN 2022023245 (ebook) | ISBN 9781668459256 (hardcover) | ISBN 9781668459263 (ebook)
Subjects: MESH: Physiological Phenomena--physiology | Patient-Specific Modeling | Algorithms | Image Interpretation, Computer-Assisted | Health Services for the Aged
Classification: LCC RA971.6 (print) | LCC RA971.6 (ebook) | NLM QT 26.5 | DDC 362.10285--dc23/eng/20220727
LC record available at https://lccn.loc.gov/2022023244
LC ebook record available at https://lccn.loc.gov/2022023245

This book is published in the IGI Global book series Advances in Medical Technologies and Clinical Practice (AMTCP) (ISSN: 2327-9354; eISSN: 2327-9370)

British Cataloguing in Publication Data
A Cataloguing in Publication record for this book is available from the British Library.

For electronic access to this publication, please contact: eresources@igi-global.com.

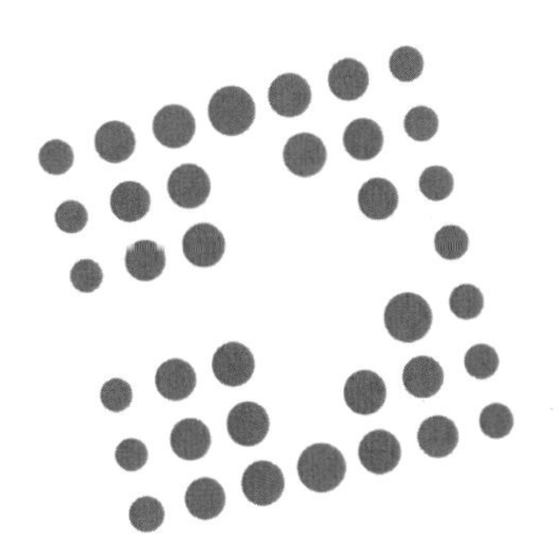

Advances in Medical Technologies and Clinical Practice (AMTCP) Book Series

Srikanta Patnaik
SOA University, India
Priti Das
S.C.B. Medical College, India

ISSN:2327-9354
EISSN:2327-9370

Mission

Medical technological innovation continues to provide avenues of research for faster and safer diagnosis and treatments for patients. Practitioners must stay up to date with these latest advancements to provide the best care for nursing and clinical practices.

The **Advances in Medical Technologies and Clinical Practice (AMTCP) Book Series** brings together the most recent research on the latest technology used in areas of nursing informatics, clinical technology, biomedicine, diagnostic technologies, and more. Researchers, students, and practitioners in this field will benefit from this fundamental coverage on the use of technology in clinical practices.

Coverage

- Diagnostic Technologies
- Biomedical Applications
- Nursing Informatics
- Medical Imaging
- Clinical High-Performance Computing
- Medical Informatics
- Nutrition
- Neural Engineering
- E-Health
- Biomechanics

IGI Global is currently accepting manuscripts for publication within this series. To submit a proposal for a volume in this series, please contact our Acquisition Editors at Acquisitions@igi-global.com or visit: http://www.igi-global.com/publish/.

The Advances in Medical Technologies and Clinical Practice (AMTCP) Book Series (ISSN 2327-9354) is published by IGI Global, 701 E. Chocolate Avenue, Hershey, PA 17033-1240, USA, www.igi-global.com. This series is composed of titles available for purchase individually; each title is edited to be contextually exclusive from any other title within the series. For pricing and ordering information please visit http://www.igi-global.com/book-series/advances-medical-technologies-clinical-practice/73682. Postmaster: Send all address changes to above address.

Titles in this Series

For a list of additional titles in this series, please visit: www.igi-global.com/book-series/advances-medical-technologies-clinical-practice/73682

Diverse Perspectives and State-of-the-Art Approaches to the Utilization of Data-Driven Clinical Decision Support Systems
Thomas M. Connolly (DS Partnership, UK) Petros Papadopoulos (University of Strathclyde, UK) and Mario Soflano (Glasgow Caledonian University, UK)
Medical Information Science Reference • © 2023 • 380pp • H/C (ISBN: 9781668450925) • US $345.00

Using Multimedia Systems, Tools, and Technologies for Smart Healthcare Services
Amit Kumar Tyagi (National Institute of Fashion Technology, New Delhi, India)
Medical Information Science Reference • © 2023 • 353pp • H/C (ISBN: 9781668457412) • US $380.00

The Internet of Medical Things (IoMT) and Telemedicine Frameworks and Applications
Rajiv Pandey (Amity University, Lucknow, India) Amrit Gupta (MRH, Sanjay Gandhi Postgraduate Institute of Medical Sciences, Lucknow, India) and Agnivesh Pandey (D.A-V. College, Chhatrapati Shahu Ji Maharaj University, Kanpur, India)
Medical Information Science Reference • © 2023 • 340pp • H/C (ISBN: 9781668435335) • US $380.00

Machine Learning and AI Techniques in Interactive Medical Image Analysis
Lipismita Panigrahi (GITAM University (Deemed), India) Sandeep Biswal (O.P. Jindal University, India) Akash Kumar Bhoi (KIET Group of Institutions, India & Sikkim Manipal University, India) Akhtar Kalam (Victoria University, Australia) and Paolo Barsocchi (Institute of Information Science and Technologies, Italy)
Medical Information Science Reference • © 2023 • 226pp • H/C (ISBN: 9781668446713) • US $380.00

Exploring the Convergence of Computer and Medical Science Through Cloud Healthcare
Ricardo Queirós (ESMAD, Polytechnic Institute of Porto, Portugal) Bruno Cunha (PORTIC, Polytechnic Institute of Porto, Portugal) and Xavier Fonseca (PORTIC, Polytechnic Institute of Porto, Portugal)
Medical Information Science Reference • © 2023 • 287pp • H/C (ISBN: 9781668452608) • US $435.00

AI-Enabled Multiple-Criteria Decision-Making Approaches for Healthcare Management
Sandeep Kautish (Lord Buddha Education Foundation, Nepal) and Gaurav Dhiman (Government Bikram College of Commerce, India & Lebanese American University, Lebanon)
Medical Information Science Reference • © 2022 • 274pp • H/C (ISBN: 9781668444054) • US $420.00

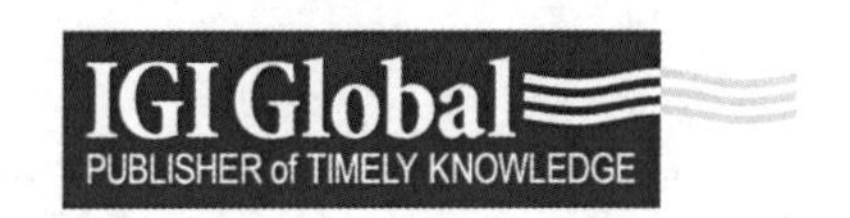

701 East Chocolate Avenue, Hershey, PA 17033, USA
Tel: 717-533-8845 x100 • Fax: 717-533-8661
E-Mail: cust@igi-global.com • www.igi-global.com

Table of Contents

Detailed Table of Contents

A digital twin (DT) is a virtual representation of a physical object or activity that acts as its real-time digital equivalent. The authors evaluated the structure of research in the same field, and to do so, the authors used the techniques of bibliometric analysis using VOSviewer. This study scrutinizes the dynamics of scientific publications devoted to understanding DT application in the healthcare sector all over the world over the years. The documents were extracted from the database of Scopus. The evolution of the concept of DT is studied from documents, including research articles, conference papers, and book chapters, which helped forecast future research trends.

The ability of IoT technology to simplify the adoption of artificial intelligence is precious to consumer product companies. The robustness of consumer companies' IoT initiatives will determine whether they benefit from the rise of IoT. A well-thought-out IoT strategy and execution will improve supply chain efficiency and align products with modern, post-COVID consumer behaviour. It must be noted that the network is not only restricted to computers but also has a web of devices of various sizes and kinds, including medical instruments and industrial systems. Expert analysts put forward the inherent capabilities of IoT devices to not only communicate and exchange information but also create a starting point for new, fresh revenue sources, ignite the business foundation and business models and enhance the techniques of services that propel numerous industries and sectors.

Machine learning and deep learning are branches of artificial intelligence consisting of statistical, probabilistic, and optimisation techniques that allow machines to learn from previous observations recorded by humans. These machine learning algorithms, when combined with other technologies, can be used to perform very intuitive yet awkward human-like tasks. Using these algorithms, humans can enable computers to learn about certain things like recognising an object in an image. Prognosis is an important clinical skill, particularly for cancer patients' clinicians, neurooncologists. One of the biggest challenge for AI in prognosis is to verify and validate its models. Unlike diagnosis, the prognosis models are centered on predictive data that usually addresses the patient and not the disease. Prognosis models were developed to aid in the decision-making of patients' treatment.AI can have bigger impact in the health care domain with more healthcare providers using AI to make the first diagnosis and prognosis more accurate and interpretable with the available patient data for better therapy.

Machine learning is a branch of artificial intelligence (AI) and computer science which focuses on the use of data and algorithms to imitate the way that humans learn, gradually improving its accuracy. Machine learning is a significant part of the developing field of information science. Using factual strategies, calculations are prepared to make characterizations or forecasts, revealing key experiences inside information mining projects. These bits of knowledge thusly drive decision making inside applications and organizations, preferably affecting key development measurements. As large information proceeds to extend and develop, the market interest for information researchers will increment, expecting them to aid the recognizable proof of the most significant business questions and accordingly the information to respond to them.

With the massive digital innovation and adaptions, healthcare is also changing quickly to digital health care. The term 'digital twin' refers to a wide-reaching concept that comprises the structure via amalgamating many technologies and functionalities for digital transformation in the healthcare sector. The digital twin (DT) will enable the healthcare industry to reform, enhance, and optimize comprehensive and complicated clinical trials. This chapter will feature digital twin broadly, using the 4P Medicine framework for a sustainable medical solution. DT will enable personalized, predictive, participative, and preventive medical solutions for patients of today to an improved state of patient of tomorrow by incorporating pre-specified covariate modifications.

With the fast growth of big data, IoT, industrial internet, and intelligent control technology, digital twins are extensively employed as a novel form of technology in many aspects of life. Digital twins have emerged as the ideal connection between the real world of manufacturing and the digital virtual world, as well as an effective technological way of realizing the interaction and cooperation of the real and information worlds. Digital twins rely on knowledge mechanisms, digitization, and other technologies to build digital models. They use IoT and other technologies to convert data and information in the physical world into general data. Its necessity is mainly reflected in the massive data processing and system self-optimization in the digital twin ecosystem, so that the digital twin ecosystem is orderly and intelligent cloud travel, and it is the central brain of the digital twin ecosystem. The rapidly expanding digital twin market indicates that this technology is already in use across many industries and is demanded to rise at an estimated USD 48.2 billion in 2026.

The "digital twin" concept creates a virtual portrayal, with the actual and virtual worlds being in perfect sync. The digitization process of a product's whole life cycle, from design to maintenance, will provide the organization with a predictive analysis of problems. Using digital representations' maximum effect of predicting issues in the development of technology would be to deliver caution in advance, avoid any disruption to the new opportunities, and design an upgraded technology. Indeed, these will have a greater impact on transmitting outstanding consumer feelings both inside and outside the company. Emerging trends of Industry 4.0, such as AI, ML, DL, and IoT play a crucial part in the creation of virtual twins, mainly used in the manufacturing, industrial IoT, and automotive industries.

In the past decades, medical image technologies have been rapidly growing. The x-rays, ultrasound (US), MRI scan, and CT scan are the pulmonary techniques to examine human diseases, and CT techniques have more resolution images than other techniques. HRCT is another advanced technology derived from the CT family and working in 3D to capture the images. High-resolution computed tomography techniques are used to examine all humankind's problems like heart, brain, breast, lung, kidney, etc. The diagnosis accuracy depends on expert doctors, radiologists, or pathologists, and wrong judgment leads to wrong treatment or diagnosis. To overcome this, a computer-based technology is introduced instead of manual operation because of its higher efficiency, accuracy, and achieved by transfer learning methods.

A digital twin refers to a virtual model of a process, product, or service. It is a bridge between the physical world and digital world. Due to its obvious benefits, more organizations are adopting it, particularly in medicines and healthcare. The big data can be collected through wearable sensors, GPS, images, and IoT, and analysed with AI and machine learning that can be very helpful in various aspects of health sector. The GIS improves data capture and integration, leads to better real-time visualisation, offers detailed analysis and automation of future projections, and facilitates communication and cooperation. Digital twins are very helpful in personalised healthcare, monitoring the treatment. There are, however, many challenges associated with the digital data of patients, such as digitization of health records, security of data, and real-time analysis and predication to provide efficient and economical healthcare services.

Assistive technology for the elderly was the focus of the literature review that would help support the elderly's healthcare. This chapter discusses the potential of assistive technology in general to offer a cost-effective way of assisting healthcare services for the elderly; no systematic research on the expenses of these technologies for this population has been carried out. Throughout the process of evaluation, evidence of significance is considered. This chapter explains the methods and conclusions of the literature review. As a result of this chapter, the elderly will have better access to health care.

In the domain of information retrieval, there exists a number of models which are used for different sorts of applications. The extraction of multimedia is one of the types which specifically deals with the handling of multimedia data with different types of tools and techniques. This chapter provides a complete insight into the audio, video, and text semantic descriptions about the multimedia data with the following objectives: i) methods ii) data summarization iii) data categorization and its media descriptions. Upon considering this organization, the entire chapter has been dealt with a case study depicting feature extraction, merging, filtering, and data validation.

The purpose of this study is to investigate the preventive strategies to reduce musculoskeletal disorders of nursing personnel. The findings of this study stated that there are three key themes of strategies to handle the research puzzle. Physical facilities such as lifts, equipment, electric beds, footwear, and other equipment provide physical infrastructure to deal with the issue. Moreover, the findings revealed that the physical facilities alone may not be effective in the long run. The second theme focuses on guidelines, procedures, or principles such as education, staffing, no lift policy, a healthy lifestyle, the culture of safety, training on manual handling, workflow management, need analysis, and stories which provide the supportive structure in addressing the issue. We argue that physical facilities, procedures, guidelines, and principles alone may not work effectively in reducing the musculoskeletal disorders of nurses and there should be a simultaneous implementation of themes one and two. We introduce the Musculoskeletal Prevention Model to deal with the research issue.

Data in medical data warehouses are often used in data analytics and online analytical processing tools. OLAP techniques do not process enterprise data for hidden or unknown intelligence. The data analytics process takes data from a medical data warehouse as input and identifies the hidden patterns; i.e., data analytics process extracts hidden predictive information from the medical data warehouse through the deep neural networks tools. In this work, the authors attempt to identify the hidden patterns in context to healthcare data analytics case analytics using deep neural networks for medical applications. The authors have experimented with the deep network algorithms for the healthcare data set used through controlled learning that is to be carried out with the medical data set.

The pragmatic model works in an open ecosystem with entrance to GPS knowledge. The proposal has four phases. Tier 1 is the legendary implicit model produced during upfront architecture. It maintains decision-making at the idea conception and preparatory study. Tier 2 is a digital counterpart. It is proficient in including enforcement, wellness, and livelihood data from the mechanical twin. It is an instantiation of the universal arrangement. It introduces group updates and maintains high-level determination. It creates the conceptual scheme, technology blueprint, preceding scheme, and construction. It has the vehicle interface library of the Modelica device. It has a vehicle with a power split. The chassis prototype has a single stage with mass-and speed-dependent resistance features. Tier 3 is the adaptive digital twin. Tier 4 has unsupervised automation ability. The approach improves the system by 7.75% in user experience and 40.6% in performance using the recommendation library compared to the previous contribution.

Over the last few years, the world has witnessed a fast-paced digital transformation in many aspects of human life in healthcare owing to the coronavirus (COVID-19) pandemic. Business and service providers had to adapt to digital changes quickly to overcome containment challenges and survive in an ever-changing world. Healthcare-related data collection, preservation, and analysis using digital technologies are helping pandemic mitigation strategies. With the rapid development of virtual systems integration methods and data acquisition techniques, digital twin (DT) technology is ushering in a new dawn for modern healthcare services and information systems. However, IoT-based information systems are vulnerable to privacy and security-related issues. This chapter presents an information system framework that consists of IoT with blockchain technology to mitigate vulnerability issues using lightweight cryptography.

Preface

The world has witnessed the upsurge in digital transformation technologies recently and that have stimulated digital twin model development – simulating fusion of transformational technologies such as IoT, Cloud, AI, and AR/VR. Several industry verticals including industrial, aerospace, and automotive have been implementing digital twin to enhance and augment their operations. By observing the remarkable advantages, it extends to transform patient care; the Healthcare industry has also seen great potential in it.

The healthcare industry is starting to adopt digital twins to improve personalized medicine, healthcare organization performance, and new medicine and devices. These digital twins can create useful models based on information from wearable devices, omics, and patient records to connect the dots across processes that span patients, doctors, and healthcare organizations as well as drug and device manufacturers. In 2002, Dr. Michael Grieves coined the term Digital Twin. It is a virtual representation of physical assets, processes, people, or places. It shows the visualization of complex assets and processes and helps businesses to improve their performance. Digital Twin can perform bi-directional automated data flow between the physical object and digital representation.

Digital twins are digital representations of human physiology built on computer models. The use of digital twins in healthcare is revolutionizing clinical processes and hospital management by enhancing medical care with digital tracking and advancing modelling of the human body. These tools are of great help to researchers in studying diseases, new drugs, and medical devices. The digital twins begin the digital prototype and continues to live alongside its physical twin. The digital twin is continually monitoring and analysing the state of its physical counterpart to optimise performance through the activation of self-optimization and self-healing processes possible through AI. The interaction between digital twins and physical twin is based on a "closed-loop," based on data flow between the cyber and physical worlds. In healthcare, digital twins gets data from its physical counterpart synchronises itself with it, employs AI algorithms to detect anomalies, and then provides the physical twin self-healing or optimization activities. The goal of extending digital twin technology to humans through the development of human digital twin, which are digital models of humans customised for every patient, is to enable clinicians to monitor the patient's health. Human digital twin differs from the industry digital twin generated and used in Industry 4.0; specialists are expected to update the digital twin regularly with physical twin health status.

In the chapter 1 with title "Digital Twin and Healthcare: Research Agenda and Bibliometric Analysis," the authors used the techniques of bibliometric analysis using VOSviewer. This study scrutinizes the dynamics of scientific publications devoted to understanding DT application in the healthcare sector all over the world over the years. The documents were extracted from the database of Scopus. The evolution of the concept of DT is studied from documents, including research articles, conference papers, and book chapters, which helped forecast future research trends.

In the chapter 2 with the title "The Role of the IoT and Digital Twin in the Healthcare Digitalization Process: IoT and Digital Twin in the Healthcare Digitalization Process," discusses the ability of IoT technology to simplify the adoption of artificial intelligence is precious to consumer product companies. The robustness of consumer companies' IoT initiatives will determine whether they benefit from the rise of IoT. A well-thought-out IoT strategy and execution will improve supply chain efficiency and align products with modern, post-COVID consumer behaviour.

Chapter 3, "A Comprehensive Study on Algorithms and Applications of Artificial Intelligence in Diagnosis and Prognosis: AI for Healthcare," discusses Prognosis, which is an important clinical skill, particularly for cancer patients' clinicians, neuro-oncology. One of the biggest challenges for AI in prognosis is to verify and validate its models. Unlike diagnosis, the prognosis models are centered on predictive data that usually addresses the patient and not the disease. Prognosis models were developed to aid in the decision-making of patients' treatment.AI can have bigger impact in the health care domain with more healthcare providers using AI to make the first diagnosis and prognosis more accurate and interpretable with the available patient data for better therapy.

Chapter 4, "Appositeness of Digital Twins in Healthcare," discusses the use of factual strategies, calculations are prepared to make characterizations or forecasts, revealing key experiences inside information mining projects. These bits of knowledge thusly drive decision making inside applications and organizations, preferably affecting key development measurements. As large information proceeds to extend and develop, the market interest for information researchers will increment, expecting them to aid the recognizable proof of the most significant business questions and accordingly the information to respond to them.

Chapter 5, "Digital Twin in Healthcare Present and Future Scope," will feature Digital Twin broadly using the 4P Medicine framework for a sustainable medical solution. DT will enable Personalized, Predictive, Participative and Preventive medical solutions for patients of today to an improved state of patient of tomorrow by incorporating pre-specified covariate modifications.

Chapter 6, "Digital Twins Enabling Technologies, Including Artificial Intelligence, Sensors, Cloud and Edge Computing," discusses the fast growth of big data, IoT, industrial internet and intelligent control technology, digital twins are extensively employed as a novel form of technology in many aspects of life. Digital twins have emerged as the ideal connection between the real world of manufacturing and the digital virtual world, as well as an effective technological way of realizing the interaction and cooperation of the real and information worlds. Digital twins rely on knowledge mechanisms, digitization and other technologies to build digital models. They use IoT and other technologies to convert data and information in the physical world into general data. Its necessity is mainly reflected in the massive data processing and system self-optimization in the digital twin ecosystem, so that the digital twin ecosystem is orderly and intelligent cloud travel, and it is the central brain of the digital twin ecosystem. The rapidly expanding digital twin market indicates that this technology is already in use across many industries and demand to rise at an estimated USD 48.2 billion in 2026.

Chapter 7, "Use Cases for Digital Twin: Use Cases helpful for Digital Twins," make use of digital representations maximum effect of predicting issues in the development of technology would be to deliver caution in advance, avoid any disruption to the new opportunities, and design an upgraded technology. Indeed, these will have a greater impact on transmitting outstanding consumer feelings both inside and outside the company. Emerging trends of Industry 4.0, such as AI, ML, DL, and IoT play a crucial part in the creation of virtual twins, mainly used in the manufacturing, industrial IoT, and automotive industries.

Chapter 8, "An Advanced Lung Disease Diagnosis Using Transfer Learning Method for High-Resolution Computed Tomography (HRCT) Images: High-Resolution Computed Tomography," discusses medical image technologies development. The x-rays, ultrasound (US), MRI scan and CT scan are the pulmonary techniques to examine human diseases, and CT techniques have more resolution images than other techniques. HRCT is another advanced technology derived from the CT family and working in 3D to capture the images. High-Resolution Computed Tomography techniques are used to examine all humankind's problems like heart, brain, breast, lung, kidney, etc. The diagnosis accuracy depends on expert doctors, radiologists or pathologists and wrong judgment leads to wrong treatment or diagnosis. To overcome this, a computer-based technology is introduced instead of manual operation because of its more efficiency, accuracy and achieved by transfer learning methods.

Chapter 9, "Geospatial Information Based Digital Twins for Healthcare," focuses on the big data which is collected through wearable sensors, GPS, images, and IoT, and analysed with AI, and machine learning that can be very helpful in various aspects of health sector. The GIS improves data capture and integration, leads to better real-time visualisation, offers detailed analysis and automation of future projections, and facilitates communication and cooperation. Digital twins are very helpful in personalised healthcare, monitoring the treatment. There are however many challenges associated with the digital data of patients, such as digitization of health records, security of data and real-time analysis and predication to provide efficient and economical healthcare services.

Chapter 10, "Healthcare for the Elderly With Digital Twins," focuses on assistive technology for the elderly was the focus of the literature review that would help support the elderly's healthcare. This chapter discusses the potential of assistive technology in general to offer a cost-effective way of assisting healthcare services for the elderly; no systematic research on the expenses of these technologies for this population has been carried out. Throughout the process of evaluation, evidence of significance is considered. This chapter explains the methods and conclusions of the literature review. As a result of this chapter, the elderly will have better access to health care.

Chapter 11, "Healthcare Multimedia Data Analysis Algorithms, Tools and Applications," provides a complete insight into the audio, video, text semantic descriptions about the multimedia data with the following objectives, i) methods ii) data summarization iii) data categorization and its media descriptions. Upon considering this organization, the entire chapter has been dealt with a case study depicting feature extraction, merging, filtering, and data validation.

Chapter 12, "Preventive Strategies to Reduce Musculoskeletal Disorders of Nursing Personnel; A Systematic Review: Musculoskeletal Disorders of Nursing Personnel," focuses on to investigate the preventive strategies to reduce musculoskeletal disorders of nursing personnel. The findings of this study stated that there are three key themes of strategies to handle the research puzzle. Physical facilities such as lifts, equipment, electric beds, footwear, and other equipment provide physical infrastructure to deal with the issue. Moreover, the findings revealed that the physical facilities alone may not be effective in the long run. The second theme focuses on guidelines, procedures, or principles such as education, staffing, no lift policy, a healthy lifestyle, the culture of safety, training on manual handling, workflow management, need analysis, and stories which provide the supportive structure in addressing the issue. We argue that physical facilities, procedures, guidelines, and principles alone may not work effectively in reducing the musculoskeletal disorders of nurses and there should be a simultaneous implementation of themes one and two. We introduce the Musculoskeletal Prevention Model to deal with the research issue.

Chapter 13, "Review on Knowledge-Centric Healthcare Data Analytics Case Using Deep Neural Network for Medical Data Warehousing Application," attempts to identify the hidden patterns in context to healthcare data analytics case analytics using deep Neural Networks for medical applications. We have experimented with the deep network algorithms for the healthcare data set used through controlled learning that is to be carried out with the medical data set.

Chapter 14, "Smart System Engineering: Digital Twin," focuses on the pragmatic model works in an open ecosystem with entrance to GPS knowledge. The proposal has four phases. Tier 1 is the legendary implicit model produced during upfront architecture. It maintains decision-making at the idea conception and preparatory study. Tier 2 is a digital counterpart in which the pragmatic composition. It is proficient in including enforcement, wellness, and livelihood data from the mechanical twin. It is an instantiation of the universal arrangement. It introduces group updates and maintains high-level determination. It creates the conceptual scheme, technology blueprint, preceding scheme, and construction. It has the Vehicle Interface Library of the Modelica device. It has a vehicle with a power split. The chassis prototype has a single stage with mass-and speed-dependent resistance features. Tier 3 is the Adaptive Digital Twin. Tier 4 has unsupervised automation ability. The approach improves the system by 7.75% user experience and 40.6% performance using the recommendation library compared to the previous contribution.

Chapter 15, "Security Solutions for IoT Applications with Cryptography and Blockchain in Healthcare Industry," describes an information system framework that consists of IoT with blockchain technology to mitigate vulnerability issues.

According to the reports, the global healthcare digital twins market size was valued at USD 462.6 million in 2021 and is expected to expand at a compound annual growth rate (CAGR) of 25.6% from 2022 to 2030. Digital Twins and Healthcare: Trends, Techniques, and Challenges facilitates the advancement and knowledge dissemination in methodologies and applications of digital twins in the healthcare and medicine fields. This book raises interest and awareness of the uses of digital twins in healthcare in the research community. The book has covered topics such as deep neural network, edge computing, and transfer learning method, this premier reference source is an essential resource for hospital administrators, pharmacists, medical professionals, IT consultants, students and educators of higher education, librarians, and researchers.

Loveleen Gaur
Amity University, India & Taylor's University, Malaysia & University of the South Pacific, Fiji

Noor Zaman Jhanjhi
Taylor's University, Malaysia

Chapter 1
Digital Twin and Healthcare Research Agenda and Bibliometric Analysis

Loveleen Gaur
https://orcid.org/0000-0002-0885-1550
Amity University, India & Taylor's University, Malaysia & University of the South Pacific, Fiji

Jyoti Rana
https://orcid.org/0000-0001-7474-3702
Amity University, India

Noor Zaman Jhanjhi
https://orcid.org/0000-0001-8116-4733
Taylor's University, Malaysia

ABSTRACT

A digital twin (DT) is a virtual representation of a physical object or activity that acts as its real-time digital equivalent. The authors evaluated the structure of research in the same field, and to do so, the authors used the techniques of bibliometric analysis using VOSviewer. This study scrutinizes the dynamics of scientific publications devoted to understanding DT application in the healthcare sector all over the world over the years. The documents were extracted from the database of Scopus. The evolution of the concept of DT is studied from documents, including research articles, conference papers, and book chapters, which helped forecast future research trends.

INTRODUCTION

Integrating Internet connectivity into everyday objects and technologies has substantially impacted human relationships and communications (Ramu et al., 2020). Devices may now communicate and interact via the internet and handle data remotely. IoT (Gaur et al., 2017; Gaur et al., 2021)is a term used to de-

DOI: 10.4018/978-1-6684-5925-6.ch001

scribe a phenomenon that is transforming how people interact with physical items and the environment. Home, health, transportation, and environmental monitoring devices are among the most recent Internet of Things innovations. Health and wellness apps that use wearable devices, in particular, have emerged as a rapidly growing sector of intelligent apps that are becoming increasingly popular. This emerging trend is expected to act as a quick and valuable resource for obtaining consumer data, which will then be used to provide healthy lifestyle recommendations. The rationale of the study is to determine the use of digital technologies like DT in their emergence and application in healthcare.

Additionally, the synergistic effect of ubiquitous connectivity, widespread sensor technologies, advances in AI, cloud computing, etc., has accelerated the spread of industrially diffused DT technology to aviation, manufacturing, and healthcare (Maddikunta et al., 2020). The DT begins the digital prototype and continues to live alongside its physical twin (PT). The DT is continually monitoring and analysing the state of its physical counterpart to optimise performance through the activation of self-optimization and self-healing processes possible through AI. The interaction between DT and PT is based on a "closed-loop," based on data flow between the cyber and physical worlds. In healthcare, DT gets data from its PT, synchronises itself with it, employs AI algorithms to detect anomalies, and then provides the PT self-healing or optimization activities. The goal of extending DT technology to humans through the development of human DTs, which are digital models (Liu et al., 2022) of humans customised for every patient, enables clinicians to monitor the patient's health. Human DTs differ from the industry DTs generated and used in Industry 4.0; specialists are expected to update the DT regularly with PT's health status.

DT In Sports

According to research, having a healthy coach-athlete relationship improves the athlete's ability to respond to stress and improves their overall performance. A negative coaching experience, for the same reason, can have a detrimental impact on an athlete's motivation and ability to perform well. Work is being done to teach professional coaches, but it is also being done to help these experts understand how to communicate more effectively with those not involved in sports. However, not everyone has the luxury of working with a skilled professional who can assist them in improving their physical condition or overcoming specific physical limits. People who cannot attend a coaching session due to financial constraints might benefit from Smart Coaching, which can serve as a helpful tool, if not a substitute for qualified specialists, in this situation (Thiong et al., 2022). Innovative coaching is beneficial not just to athletes but also to the elderly. Several organisations, including the World Health Organization, have designated 2020–2030 as the decade of healthy aging (Mozumder et al., 2022). One of the main recommendations in their report on aging and health is to "guarantee a sustainable and appropriately trained health workforce," with "supply a sustainable and appropriately trained health workforce" being one of the principal recommendations.

Smart Coaching is derived from other domains such as e-learning. E-learning is described as "learning supported by digital electronic tools and media" or "learning aided by digital electronic tools and media." In other words, the DT's Smart Coaching component can be viewed as a subset of e-learning. Students are increasingly acclimating to learning in a digital environment (Xing et al., 2022). They are enthusiastic about e-learning, and it is projected that by 2025, online education will be widely available, particularly following the COVID-19 phase. The extensive usage of digital learning in today's population will contribute to the acceptance of DT Coaching as a technology. Sports leagues, teams, and player associations can develop a new roadmap by utilising virtual copies to analyse performance, quickly test solutions, and make real-time modifications in the field. As digital twins grow in popularity, the authors are confident that everyone participating in sports will benefit from having more information sources available to them shortly.

Governance officials or executives should not overlook the importance of ethical issues in collecting, managing, and using data. To develop DT, sensitive information must be gathered. If any information about the project is leaked, it will put a stumbling block to achieving its objectives and negatively impact its overall reputation. To stimulate (Khan et al., 2022) innovation, data availability must be made more widely available. Openness is advantageous for bringing on academic researchers, start-ups, businesses, and universities who would be delighted to obtain these datasets to test and develop innovative twins. Leagues with an eye on the future must advocate for such policies immediately.

DT in Aviation to Healthcare- History/Evolution of DT

DT is a real-time digital equivalent of a virtual depiction of a physical object or activity. Even though the concept had been around for a long, NASA came up with the first realistic definition of the DT in 2010 to better spacecraft physical model simulation. NASA began developing mirrored systems in the 1970s to monitor inaccessible physical regions (for example, spacecraft in orbit) to discover answers (Zhong et al., 2022) to unexpected difficulties by utilising the mirror to evaluate prospective solutions. The replicated environment was constructed by engineers at NASA's Houston and Kennedy Space Center and used to save astronauts during the Apollo 13 mission (mirrored system). Engineers used the simulated environment (Sahal et al.,2022) to create and test several solutions after the air tanks exploded. They successfully invented an improvised air purifier that acted as a temporary solution. It was constructed using materials already aboard the spaceship, owing to engineering instructions transmitted from Earth to the astronauts. Engineers on Earth were able to achieve this by simulating different scenarios, which allowed them to uncover a way to bring the crew of Apollo 13 back to Earth alive. Although DT systems effectively bridge the gap between real and virtual environments, they lack the features essential for the intelligent interaction between the two. These qualities distinguish DTs, virtual twins who live alongside and are synchronised with their physical twin (PT). With a seamless link and constant touch with their PT and the external world, (Garg et al., 2022) DTs can duplicate the conditions of the PT continuously, assisting them in improving their performance. The figure 1 below highlight the domains of using DT.

Dynamical systems models are commonly used in aviation to improve aircraft performance and minimise failure costs by anticipating damages and implementing self-healing actions to prevent them from occurring. The first application of DT in healthcare was for predictive maintenance of medical devices and tools to optimize the performance of predictions and outputs, for example, the examination speed and energy consumption of devices to optimize the hospital cycle.

DT in Healthcare

When it comes to manufacturing, DT is used for damage prediction and self-healing mechanisms, which are made possible by virtualizing manufacturing machines. Digital technologies are becoming more common (Alrashed et al., 2022) in healthcare due to their success in the aviation and manufacturing industries. The first applications adopted in healthcare were predictive maintenance of medical devices

Figure 1. Represented the domains of application of DT

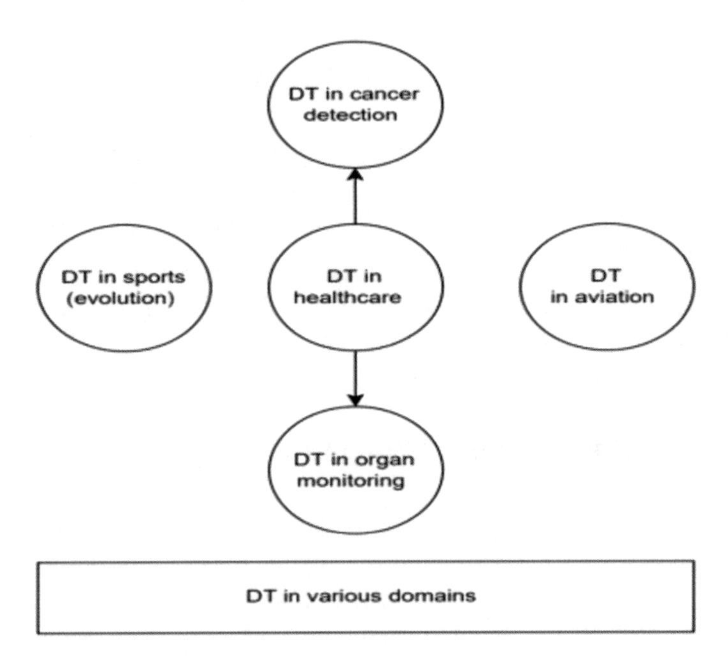

and optimization of their performance in terms of examination speed and energy consumption, (Zhang et al., 2022) followed by subsequent applications that effectively optimized the hospital lifecycle.

For building the human-DT, DT technology is being researched in the medical and clinical domains. An automated DT enables a detailed and real-time continuous inspection of the human health status, predicting illness and providing the best prevention and treatment options by taking into account the PT's medical history and current activities like location and time. Human DT is significant because (Ahmadi et al., 2021) would facilitate the transition from the current "one-size-fits-all" treatment method. Patients are treated following some "norm" or "Standard of Care" to "personalised medicine," in which treatments are tailored (Volkov et al.,2021) to the individual's "physical asset," defined by all of the person's structural, physical, biological, and historical characteristics.

The development of computer models like the "AnyBody Modeling System, "1 which allows researchers to simulate the human body (Elayan et al., 2021) working in connection with its surroundings, has evolved from research dedicated to the production of human DTs. The AnyBody model will enable users to run complicated simulations and calculate individual muscle forces, joint contact forces and moments, metabolism, elastic energy in tendons, and antagonistic muscle action.

DT and Organ Monitoring

The development of DTs for monitoring organ states or functions in patients is expected to rise clinicians' in silico forecasts significantly. The DT of the heart is developed for monitoring myocardial conditions (Dillenseger et al., 2021), and the DT of the airway system, specifically designed for monitoring asthmatic symptoms, are examples of DTs for monitoring the needs of patients' organs. Due to the availability of low-cost storage and easy access to and sharing of medical examinations (mainly pictures) from various modalities and sources (source machine types). Although DTs have found widespread success in multiple disciplines, the DTs produced in healthcare (Wu et al., 2021) differ significantly from those developed in industry, owing to two factors. First, human DTs, for example, should be built on top of AI algorithms and should be utilised extensively. The second reason is that humans lack embedded sensors, which means medical data describing their (Firouzi et al., 2021) current health status can only be received through medical examinations; as a result, a seamless connection between people and their DT is impossible to achieve (Zheng et al., 2021).

BLEND OF DT TECHNOLOGIES IN HEALTHCARE

In healthcare systems, digital representations of healthcare data, such as hospital environment, lab findings, human physiology, and so on, are created using computer models. According to surveys, 66% of healthcare executives (Voigt et al., 2021) anticipate a rise in DT investment during the next three years. DT is gaining popularity because it enhances healthcare organization performance, finds areas for improvement, customizes and personalizes medicine and diagnostics, and allows for the development of novel pharmaceuticals and technologies.

THE USE OF DT IN CANCER DETECTION

DT is helping transform significant diseases like cancer. The digital representation of cancer patients is developed in real-time on clinical data with computing modeling and simulation techniques. Cancer patient digital twins (CPDTs) make treatment predictions and personalized health care decisions.

When CPDTs are used to their potential, they reflect a patient's molecular, physiological, and behavioral characteristics as they change over *i* learning" loop to assist patients in making better decisions. According to the researchers' findings and individual patient predictions, CPDTs will provide policymakers with insights into the most promising cancer therapies, guiding investment and resource allocation and assisting healthcare systems in responding more effectively to public health emergencies in real-time. While CPDTs have the potential to transform how cancer and other complicated diseases are treated and managed, the authors noted that before they can be adopted, the scientific community must overcome data gathering, modeling, and integration problems, as well as ethical considerations. To avoid reinforcing pre-existing preconceptions, the team determined that data (Gupta et al., 2021) would need to be collected from diverse populations and adhered to FAIR principles (Findability, Accessibility, Interoperability, and Reusability).

MEDICAL DIGITAL TWIN (MDT)

A medical digital twin (MDT) is a virtual representation of a person used in medical treatments. MDT uses cutting-edge technology like the IoT, AI, and big data to predict a person's health and offer clinical recommendations. The security of medical DT depends on a complete understanding of their architecture and the implementation of the new vulnerability-tolerant method. MDT systematically employs (Lu et al., 2021) haptic-AR navigation and deep learning algorithms to create virtual replicas and cyber–human interaction. In real-world MDT circumstances, a unique solution that is both vulnerabilities tolerance and cyber-resilient must be implemented. One of the MDT's pro-to kinds can acquire many real-world datasets.

APPLICATIONS OF DT IN HEALTH CARE

Using Software As A Medical Device To Assist In The Diagnosis And Treatment Of Patients

According to the business, the diagnostic procedure will be aided by the patient's DT feed from various health data sources, including imaging records, in-person measurements, test results, and genetic data. Using available clinical data, the patient model will replicate the patient's current health status, and statistical models will be used to infer the patient's missing parameters. Examples include (De Maeyer et al., 2021) the use of cardiovascular imaging in conjunction with computational fluid dynamics, allowing for the non-invasive characterisation of flow fields and diagnostic measures.

Designing And Optimising Medical Equipment – Medical Technology

Two worlds come together in this place. On the one hand, we have the DT of the patient, which contains the patient's characteristics. On the other hand, we have the digital twin of the medical device, which includes the device's design. We can use both models to investigate what occurs when a specific gadget is implanted into a particular patient and compare the results. This is particularly true for (Boată et al., 2021) groups that cannot be examined in clinical settings without causing harm, such as patients with rare diseases or children with developmental disabilities. DT is highly advantageous in medicine, particularly for optimization tasks such as optimising a device's operation through hundreds of simulations with various scenarios and patients. Additionally, as 3D printing technology advances, patient digital twins may enable the personalization of medical devices by producing one-of-a-kind designs for each patient.

Drug Development And Dose Optimization Are Both Accomplished In Clinical Trials

We can computationally treat a DT with numerous different therapies to discover the ideal one or ones for the current situation. It does not have to be limited to already accessible drugs. We may create a digital cohort of actual patients with diverse genotypes who share ailments and test potential new medicines to discover which one has the best chance of success and the correct dosage for each (Meraghni et al., 2021) patient. If the first shoot is enhanced, the number of clinical studies required in the future will be reduced. While a genuine clinical trial would need thousands of patients to watch only a few of these cases, a virtual clinical trial will illuminate processes that would take years to see in vivo or estimate the risk of rare occurrences.

SURGERY SIMULATION – RISK ASSESSMENT IN THE OPERATING THEATRE

Surgeons are trained to treat each patient individually. Throughout the surgical process, a patient's demands are considered from the current stage to the optimal end. Personalization is essential for increasing intervention success while lowering the patient's risk of adverse outcomes. Digital twins will assist by modeling an invasive clinical procedure to forecast the result before the treatment is chosen (Canzoneri et al.,2021). It starts with the choice of medical equipment and ends with determining surgical variables (magnitude, angle, shape).

TECHNOLOGY'S BENEFITS IN HEALTHCARE

Digital twins can potentially improve the healthcare industry's data-driven decision-making processes significantly. By connecting digital twins to their real-world counterparts at the edge, businesses may better understand the state of physical assets, adjust to changes, improve operations, and add value to systems (Wickramasinghe et al., 2021).

Make The Most Use Of The Resources You Have

Data from the hospital and the surrounding environment, both historical and real-time, aid in creating digital twins of hospital operations. Past data, such as COVID-19 cases and traffic accidents, and the surrounding environment, can assist hospital administration in identifying bed shortages, optimising staff schedules, and helping operating rooms. This data improves resource efficiency (Erol et al., 2020) and optimises hospital and personnel operations while lowering the institution's expenditures. According to a review study, integrating digital twins to ensure the seamless coordination of several functions enabled a hospital to significantly reduce the time necessary to treat stroke patients by up to 30%.

Risk Prevention And Mitigation

DT can be used to evaluate changes in system performance (such as personnel levels or operation room vacancy, as well as device maintenance) in a controlled environment, enabling the implementation of data-driven strategic (Gaur et al., 2021) decisions in a complicated and delicate issue.

Diagnosis On A Case-By-Case Basis

Individuals can track persistent diseases and, as a result, their priorities and interactions with doctors through DT. They may collect and use meaningful data (e.g., blood pressure, oxygen levels, and so on) on an individual basis, thanks to DT. As a result, such tailored data is used to construct clinical trial and laboratory research datasets (Gaur et al., 2021). By focusing only on the individual, physicians avoid developing treatments based on huge samples of individuals. Rather than that, they employ (Sharma et al., 2022) tailored simulations to monitor each patient's response to numerous medicines, thereby increasing the precision of the treatment plan. Despite increased (Gaur et al., 2021) interest in the increasing effort into customized treatment, there is no digital twin application for actual patients.

DISADVANTAGES OF TECHNOLOGY IN HEALTHCARE

Cybersecurity Threats In The Healthcare Industry

When it comes to cybersecurity risk, it is not just about exposing private information or paying ransoms in response to data breaches. Changed data offer significant risks, and the ramifications of data change can be catastrophic. The data they use must be genuine and reliable for patients and healthcare professionals who rely on data to make treatment decisions. When data is lost or corrupted, it might result (Beard et al., 2017) in an inaccurate diagnosis or treatment plan and other adverse repercussions. It exemplifies one of the primary disadvantages of the IoT in healthcare. If the appropriate security procedures are not in place, access to patients' connected medical equipment may modify its functionality (Fuller et al., 2020) . Ultimately, the worst-case scenario results in a significant gadget breakdown in critical conditions, culminating in death.

Lack of Empathy

Engaging with networked medical devices and computers eliminates the human element of treatment, leading to a lack of empathy for the patient (Liu et al., 2019). Using technology as a care interface, particularly for the elderly and most vulnerable patients, can produce frustration and disappointment, (Bruynseels et al., 2018) leading to poorly understood treatment plans and patients who do not follow their treatment regimens, among other issues.

Frustration Due To A Lack Of Effective Implementation Of Technology

As AI and machine learning (ML) (Laamarti et al., 2020) become more prevalent, educating healthcare practitioners on these technologies' limits. Numerous ML models are trained on historical data and do not scale well when operational and learned data are drastically out of sync. As with AI/ML systems, over-reliance on them may lead to clinicians becoming complacent, failing to cross-check (Jimenez et al., 2020) or examine alternatives to the system's predictions.

Adoption Is Limited

The use of DT technology in the clinical setting is still in its early stages. Enhancing the influence of technology on digital simulations, critical clinical operations (Sharma et al., 2007), and overall medical care should be a top objective for healthcare facilities (such as hospitals and labs). DT is prohibitively expensive in the healthcare system (Gaur et al., 2021). This technology will become a privilege reserved for those with more financial resources, increasing unfairness in the healthcare system.

The Quality Of The Data Is Not Assured

In digital twins, an artificial intelligence system is used. Learn from the biological information that is already available; yet, because commercial companies obtain the data, the quality of the data may be questionable. As a result, analysing and representing data becomes complicated. It harms the models' reliability in diagnosis and treatment operations (Gaur et al., 2021).

BIBLIOMETRIC ANALYSIS OF DT IN HEALTHCARE

We evaluated the structure of research in the same field, and to do so; the authors used the techniques of bibliometric analysis using VOSviewer1.6.16.0. The documents were extracted from the database of Scopus. The evolution of the concept of DT is studied from records, including research articles, conference papers, and book chapters, which helped forecast future research trends. This chapter provides direction that reflects the evolution of DT in healthcare (Mahbub et al., 2022) and future lines of research that require attention. This study scrutinizes the dynamics of scientific publications devoted to understanding DT application in the healthcare sector all over the world over the years. The authors undertake a bibliometric analysis to determine the current status of existing research conducted on the keyword "Digital Twin" and "Healthcare" over the years. The research objective is to analyze the pool of scientific publications from the Scopus database using Vosviewer and undertake a bibliometric analysis. This study aims to determine the prominent authors, studies, and countries in the DT and healthcare sector domain. In this investigation, the authors selected VOSviewer because it can create maps with thousands of things and display maps (Ramakrishnan and Gaur, 2019) with over ten thousand items. Zooming, scrolling and searching are available in VOSviewer, enabling detailed examination of large maps.

Design/Methodology/Approach For Bibliometric Analyses

The research employed a publication search by article title, abstract, and keywords to collect the data set. The selected publications were visualized using the software VOSviewer 1.6.16.0 and Scopus and database tools based on the conceptual and whole articles reading. A popular and rigorous method, Bibliometric analysis can examine and interpret scientific material (Ramakrishnan and Gaur, 2016) . We can elucidate the evolution of a field while also offering light on the field's emerging regions. However, its applications in business research are still in their infancy, and many are underdeveloped. The data was extracted from the Scopus database on 21 April 2022. Figure 2 below provides the data cleaning process opted by the authors (Gaur et al., 2022) .

Year-Wise Publication

Figure 3 below denotes the year-wise publication of documents on the usage of DT in healthcare to improve the patient's diagnosis and treatment. The data was collected as on 21 April 2022, hence the year 2022 publication are included for 4 months there it denotes 11 publiation.

Prominent Most Cited Authors

To determine the most cited author, the author used the minimum number of documents an author has, like 2, and the minimum (Santosh and Gaur, 2022; Santosh and Gaur, 2021; Afaq et al., 2021; Santosh & Gaur, 2021) citation as 20. And out of 331, only 14 authors could meet the threshold. Table 1 below shows the same.

Figure 2. Represented the pre-processing data stage

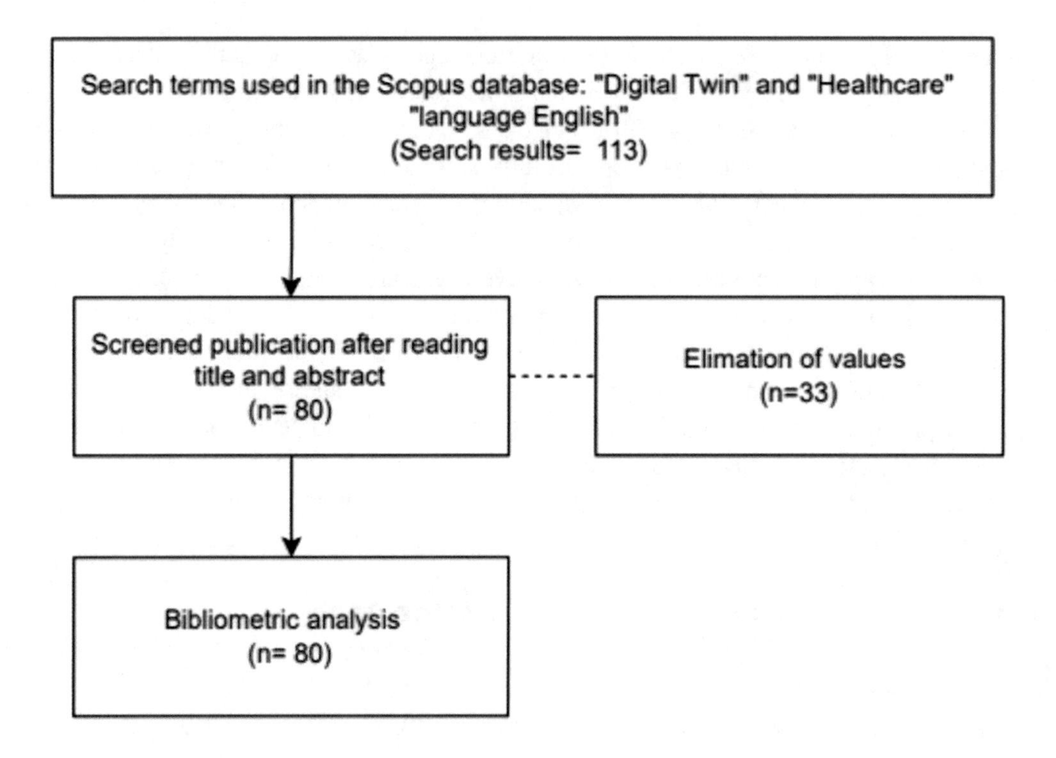

Figure 3. Represents the year wise publication trend

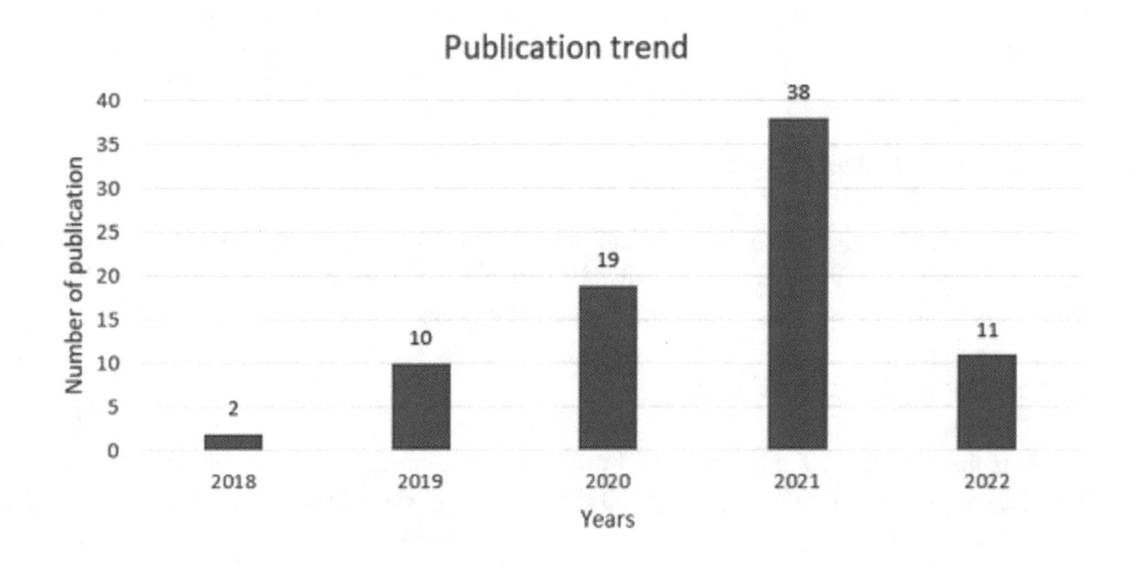

Table 1. Represents the most cited authors

Top Authors	Documents	Ciations
Faisal Arafsha	2	36
Fedwa Laamarti	2	36
Jacob D. Hochhalter	2	29
Patrick E. Leser	2	29
William P. Leser	2	29
Hamid Jahankhani	2	26
Jaime Ibarra Jimenez	2	26
Stefan Kendziers	2	26
Katja Akgun	2	20
Anja Dillenseger	2	20
Rocco Haase	2	20
Hernan Inojosa	2	20
Isabel Voigt	2	20
Tjalf Ziemssen	2	20

Prominent Countries

To determine the most cited countries, the author used the minimum number of documents an author has, like 2, and minimise citation to 20. And out of 59, only 79 countries could meet the threshold. Table 2 below represents the same.

Table 2. Represents the top most cited countries

Top countries	Documents	Ciations
United States	11	72
Italy	10	23
United Kingdom	10	231
Germany	9	42
Canada	7	189
India	7	33
China	6	138
Netherlands	4	128
Belgium	2	20

Most Cited Document

To determine the most cited documents, the author used the minimum number (Kaswan et al., 2021) of citations a document has like 20, and it met the threshold out of the 80 documents. The list of top-cited research papers published is shown in Table 3.

Table 3. Represents the topmost cited research articles

References	Title	citations
(Fuller *et al.*,2020)	Digital Twin: Enabling Technologies, Challenges, and Open Research	186
(Bruynseels *et al.*,2018)	Digital Twins in health care: Ethical implications of an emerging engineering paradigm	124
(Liu *et al.*,2019)	A Novel Cloud-Based Framework for the Elderly Healthcare Services Using Digital Twin	116
(Laamarti *et al.*,2020)	An ISO/IEEE 11073 Standardized Digital Twin Framework for Health and Well-Being in Smart Cities	25
(Jimenez *et al.*,2020)	Health Care in the Cyberspace: Medical Cyber-Physical System and Digital Twin Challenges	23
(Elayan *et al.*, 2021)	Digital Twin for Intelligent Context-Aware IoT Healthcare Systems	22

Keyword Analysis

The author's keyword analysis of 317 keywords shows the keywords repeated twice or more in the dataset. Forty-five keywords met the threshold, forming different clusters and themes, denoted in Figure 4 and Table 4 (Ramakrishnan and Gaur, 2020; Gaur et al., 2022; Saeed et al., 2022; Bhandari et al., 2022).

Table 4 denotes the themes and representation of topics and clusters in different colors indicating similarity in the topics. Cluster 1 of red color represents the DT in digital healthcare. Cluster 2 of green color depicts the green AI and digital transformation trends. Cluster 3 in blue denotes DT technologies. In yellow, cluster 4 predicts resilience and healthcare. In 5 cluster shows IoT and medical, cluster 6 shows stimulation personalized medicine, and the last cluster 7 shows Covid and e-health.

CONCLUSION

Our findings suggest that publishing prominent authors, countries, and affiliations implement DT in healthcare. The authors listed the top ten articles based on the documents' citations and conducted keyword analysis based on the occurrence of a keyword in the database. Further studies should be conducted to gain deeper insights into the emerging use of DT in healthcare from the patients' willingness to adopt new technologies like AI, DT, and deep learning models.This chapter adds on the readers' knowledge about the utilization of novel technologies like DT in healthcare to improve the patients and help practitioners in early diagnostics and take preventive measures. Within a hospital, the use of digital twin technology aids in predicting problems such as cardiopulmonary and respiratory arrest, assisting the hospital organization in better preventative maintenance while delivering individualized health care costs. Creates individualized treatment regimens for each patient.

Figure 4. Represents the keyword analysis

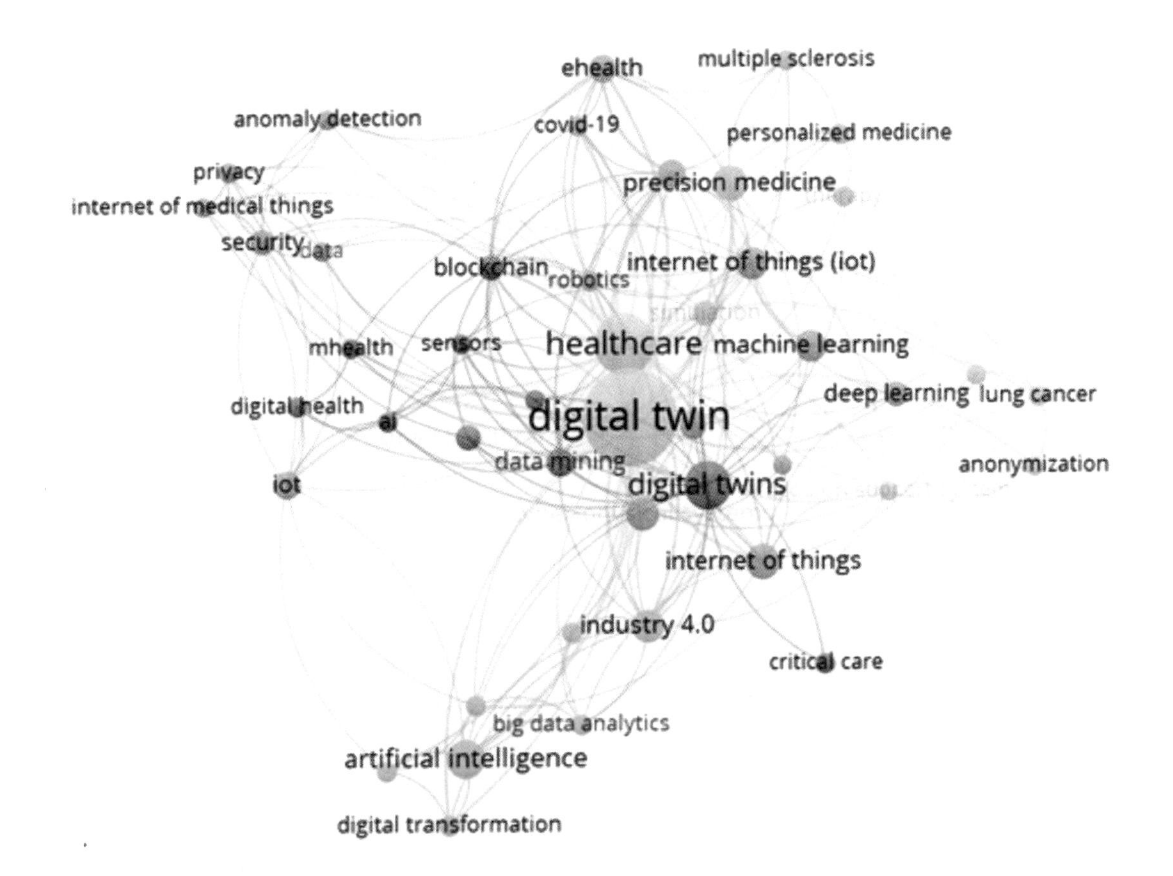

Table 4. Represents the keyword analysis

Topics	Occurances
Cluster 1 (10 items) Red, Digital twin, and digital health	
Digital twins	11
Data mining	4
Blockchain	3
Smart healthcare	3
Prediction	2
Mhealth	2
Sensors	2
AI	2
Critical care	2
Digital health	2
Cluster 2 (7 items) Green AI and digital transformation	
Artificial intelligence	7

continues on following page

Table 4. Continued

Topics	Occurances
Big data analytics	2
Smart cities	2
Industry 4.0	5
Edge computing	2
Digital transformation	2
Data analytics	2
Cluster 3 (6 items) Blue technologies and DT	
Internet of things	6
Cyber-physical systems	5
Machine learning	5
Digital twin (dt)	4
Deep learning	3
Cloud computing	2
Cluster 4 (6 items) Yellow cyber resilience and healthcare	
Digital twin	44
Healthcare	18
Cyber resilience	2
Decision support system	2
Lung cancer	2
Anonymization	2
Cluster 5 (6 items) Purple IoT and medicial	
Iot	4
Security	3
Privacy	2
Data	2
Internet of medical things	2
Anomaly detection	2
Cluster 6 (5 items) Light Blue stimulation personalized medicine	
Precision medicine	6
Simulation	3
Multiple sclerosis	2
Personalized medicine	2
Therapy	2
Cluster 7 (4 items) Orange Covid and e- health	
Ehealth	4
Big data	4
Covid-19	2
Robotics	2

REFERENCES

Afaq, A., Gaur, L., Singh, G., & Dhir, A. (2021). COVID-19: transforming air passengers' behaviour and reshaping their expectations towards the airline industry. Tourism Recreation Research., https://doi.org/10.1080/02508281.2021.2008211.

Ahmadi, H., Nag, A., Khar, Z., Sayrafian, K., & Rahardja, S. (2021). Networked Twins and Twins of Networks: An Overview on the Relationship between Digital Twins and 6G. *IEEE Communications Standards Magazine, 5* (4), pp. 154-160. doi:10.1109/MCOMSTD.0001.2000041

Alrashed, S., Min-Allah, N., Ali, I., & Mehmood, R. (2022). COVID-19 outbreak and the role of digital twin. *Multimedia Tools and Applications*. doi:10.100711042-021-11664-8

Beard, J. R.,, Officer, A.,, de Carvalho, I. A.,, Sadana, R.,, Pot, A.M.,, Michel, J.-P.,, Lloyd-Sherlock, P.,, & Epping-Jordan, J. E., Peeters, G. M. E. E., & Mahanani, W. R. (2016). The world report on ageing and health:A policy framework for healthy ageing. *Lancet*, *387*, 2145–2154.

Bhandari, M., Parajuli, P., Chapagain, P., & Gaur, L. (2022). Evaluating Performance of Adam Optimization by Proposing Energy Index. In K. Santosh, R. Hegadi, & U. Pal (Eds.), Recent Trends in Image Processing and Pattern Recognition. RTIP2R 2021. Communications in Computer and Information Science (Vol. 1576). Springer. https://doi.org/10.1007/978-3-031-07005-1_15.

Biswas, M., Chaki, S., Ahammed, F., Anis, A., Ferdous, J., Siddika, A. M., & Gaur, L. (2022). Prototype development of an assistive smart-stick for the visually challenged persons. *Proceedings of 2nd International Conference on Innovative Practices in Technology and Management*, (pp. 477-482). Science Open. doi:10.1109/ICIPTM54933.2022.9754183

Biswas, M., Kaiser, M. S., Mahmud, M., Al Mamun, S., Hossain, M. S., & Rahman, M. A. (2021). An XAI Based Autism Detection: The Context Behind the Detection. In M. Mahmud, M. S. Kaiser, S. Vassanelli, Q. Dai, & N. Zhong (Eds.), Lecture Notes in Computer Science: Vol. 12960. Brain Informatics. BI 2021. Springer. https://doi.org/10.1007/978-3-030-86993-9_40.

Biswas, M., Tania, M. H., Kaiser, M. S., Kabir, R., Mahmud, M., & Kemal, A. A. (2021). ACCU3RATE: A mobile health application rating scale based on user reviews. *PLoS One*, *16*(12), e0258050.

Boată, A., Angelescu, R., & Dobrescu, R. (2021). Using digital twins in health care. UPB Scientific Bulletin, Series C, *Electrical Engineering and Computer Science*, *83*(4), 53–62.

Bruynseels, K., Santoni de Sio, F., & Van den Hoven, J. (2018). Digital twins in health care: Ethical implications of an emerging engineering paradigm. *Frontiers in Genetics*, 31.

Canzoneri, M., De Luca, A., & Harttung, J. (2021). Digital Twins: A General Overview of the Biopharma Industry. *Advances in biochemical engineering/biotechnology*, *177*, pp. 167-184. doi:10.1007/10_2020_157

De Maeyer, C., & Markopoulos, P. (2021). Future outlook on the materialisation, expectations and implementation of Digital Twins in healthcare. *34th British Human Computer Interaction Conference Interaction Conference,* (pp. 180-191). Science Open. doi:10.14236/ewic/HCI2021.18

Dillenseger, A., Weidemann, M. L., Trentzsch, K., Inojosa, H., Haase, R., Schriefer, D., Voigt, I., Scholz, M., Akgün, K., & Ziemssen, T. (2021). Digital biomarkers in multiple sclerosis. *Brain Sciences, 11*(11), 1519. doi:10.3390/brainsci11111519

Elayan, H., Aloqaily, M., & Guizani, M. (2021). Digital Twin for Intelligent Context-Aware IoT Healthcare Systems. *IEEE Internet of Things Journal, 8*(23), pp. 16749-16757. doi:10.1109/JIOT.2021.3051158

Erol, T., Mendi, A. F., & Dogan, D. (2020). The Digital Twin Revolution in Healthcare. *4th International Symposium on Multidisciplinary Studies and Innovative Technologies, Proceedings*. Science Open. doi:10.1109/ISMSIT50672.2020.9255249

Firouzi, F., Farahani, B., Daneshmand, M., Grise, K., Song, J., Saracco, R., Wang, L.L., Lo, K., Angelov, P., Soares, E., Loh, P.-S., Talebpour, Z., Moradi, R., Goodarzi, M., Ashraf, H., Talebpour, M., Talebpour, A., Romeo, L., Das, R., Heidari, H., Pasquale, D., Moody, J., Woods, C., Huang, E.S., Barnaghi, P., Sarrafzadeh, M., Li, R., Beck, K.L., Isayev, O., Sung, N., & Luo, A. (2021). Harnessing the Power of Smart and Connected Health to Tackle COVID-19: IoT, AI, Robotics, and Blockchain for a Better World. *IEEE Internet of Things Journal, 8* (16), pp. 12826-12846. doi:10.1109/JIOT.2021.3073904

Fuller, A., Fan, Z., Day, C., & Barlow, C. (2020). Digital twin: Enabling technologies, challenges and open research. *IEEE Access: Practical Innovations, Open Solutions, 8*, 108952–108971.

Garg, H., Sharma, B., Shekhar, S., & Agarwal, R. (2022). Spoofing detection system for e-health digital twin using EfficientNet Convolution Neural Network. *Multimedia Tools and Applications*. doi:10.100711042-021-11578-5

Gaur, L., Afaq, A., Singh, G., & Dwivedi, Y. K. (2021). Role of artificial intelligence and robotics to foster the touchless travel during a pandemic: A review and research agenda. *International Journal of Contemporary Hospitality Management, 33*(11), 4079–4098. https://doi.org/10.1108/IJCHM-11-2020-1246

Gaur, L., Afaq, A., Solanki, A., Singh, G., & Sharma, S., Jhanjhi, N.Z, My, H. T., & Le, D. N. (2021). Capitalizing on big data and revolutionary 5G technology: Extracting and visualizing ratings and reviews of global chain hotels. *Computers & Electrical Engineering, 95*, 107374. doi:10.1016/j.compeleceng.2021.107374

Gaur, L., Bhandari, M., Razdan, T., Mallik, S., & Zhao, Z. (2022). Explanation-driven deep learning model for prediction of brain tumour status using MRI image data. *Frontiers in Genetics, 13*. doi:10.3389/fgene.2022.822666

Gaur, L., Bhatia, U., & Bakshi, S. (2022). Cloud driven framework for skin cancer detection using deep CNN. *Proceedings of 2nd International Conference on Innovative Practices in Technology and Management,* (pp. 460-464). Science Open. doi:10.1109/ICIPTM54933.2022.9754216

Gaur, L., Bhatia, U., Jhanjhi, N. Z., Muhammad, G., & Masud, M. (2021). Medical image-based detection of COVID-19 using deep convolution neural networks. *Multimedia Systems*, 1–10. doi:10.100700530-021-00794-6

Gaur, L., Singh, G., & Ramakrishnan, R. (2017). Understanding Consumer Preferences using IoT Smart-Mirrors. *Pertanika Journal of Science & Technology, 25*(3).

Gaur, L., Singh, G., Solanki, A., Jhanjhi, N. Z., Bhatia, U., Sharma, S., & Kim, W. (2021). Disposition of youth in predicting sustainable development goals using the neuro-fuzzy and random forest algorithms. *Human-Centric Computing and Information Sciences, 11*. doi doi:10.22967/HCIS.2021.11.024

Gaur, L., Solanki, A., Wamba, S. F., & Jhanjhi, N. Z. (2021). Advanced AI Techniques and Applications in Bioinformatics (1st ed.). CRC Press. https://doi.org/10.1201/9781003126164.

Gupta, D., Kayode, O., Bhatt, S., & Gupta, M. (2021). Tosun, AS Hierarchical Federated Learning based Anomaly Detection using Digital Twins for Smart Healthcare. Proceedings - 2021 IEEE 7th International Conference on Collaboration and Internet Terms and conditions Privacy policy. *Computing, CIC*, 16–25. IEEE. doi:10.1109/CIC52973.2021.00013

Jimenez, J. I., Jahankhani, H., & Kendzierskyj, S. (2020). Health care in the cyberspace: Medical cyber-physical system and digital twin challenges. In *Digital twin technologies and smart cities* (pp. 79–92). Springer.

Khan, S., Arslan, T., & Ratnarajah, T. (2022). Digital Twin Perspective of Fourth Industrial and Healthcare Revolution. *IEEE Access, 10*, 25732-25754. doi:10.1109/ACCESS.2022.3156062

Laamarti, F., Badawi, H. F., Ding, Y., Arafsha, F., Hafidh, B., & El Saddik, A. (2020). An ISO/IEEE 11073 standardized digital twin framework for health and well-being in smart cities. *IEEE Access: Practical Innovations, Open Solutions*, *8*, 105950–105961.

Liu, Y., Zhang, L., Yang, Y., Zhou, L., Ren, L., Wang, F., Liu, R., Pang, Z., & Deen, M. J. (2019). A novel cloud-based framework for the elderly healthcare services using digital twin. *IEEE Access: Practical Innovations, Open Solutions*, *7*, 49088–49101.

Liu, Y.K., Ong, S.K., Nee, A.Y.C. (2022). State-of-the-art survey on digital twin implementations. *Advances in Manufacturing, 10*(1), . doi:10.1007/s40436-021-00375-w

Loveleen, G., Mohan, B., Shikhar, BS, Nz, J., Shorfuzzaman, M. & Masud, M. (2022). Explanation-driven HCI Model to Examine the Mini-Mental State for Alzheimer's Disease. *ACM Transactions on Multimedia Computing, Communications, and Applications (TOMM)*. doi:10.1145/3527174

Lu, Q., Ye, Z., Fang, Z., Meng, J., Pitt, M., Lin, J., Xie, X., & Chen, L.(2021). Creating an Inter-Hospital Resilient Network for Pandemic Response Based on Blockchain and Dynamic Digital Twins *Proceedings - Winter Simulation Conference*. doi:10.1109/WSC52266.2021.9715517

Maddikunta, P.K.R., & Pham, Q.-V., B, P., Deepa, N., Dev, K., Gadekallu, T.R., Ruby, R., & Liyanage, M. (2022). Industry 5.0: A survey on enabling technologies and potential applications. *Journal of Industrial Information Integration, 26*, art. no. 100257. doi:10.1016/j.jii.2021.100257

Mahbub, M. K., Biswas, M., Gaur, L., Alenezi, F., & Santosh, K. C. (2022). Deep features to detect pulmonary abnormalities in chest X-rays due to infectious diseaseX: Covid-19, pneumonia, and tuberculosis. *Information Sciences, 592*, 389–401. doi:10.1016/j.ins.2022.01.062

Meraghni, S., Benaggoune, K., Al Masry, Z., Terrissa, L.S., Devalland, C., & Zerhouni, N. (2021). Towards Digital Twins Driven Breast Cancer Detection. *Lecture Notes in Networks and Systems, 285*, pp. 87-99. doi:10.1007/978-3-030-80129-8_7

Mozumder, M. A. I., Sheeraz, M. M., Athar, A., Aich, S., & Kim, H.-C. (2022). Overview: Technology Roadmap of the Future Trend of Metaverse based on IoT, Blockchain, AI Technique, and Medical Domain Metaverse Activity. *International Conference on Advanced Communication Technology, ICACT,* (pp. 256-261). doi:10.23919/ICACT53585.2022.9728808

Ramakrishnan, R., & Gaur, L. (2016). Application of Internet of Things (IoT) for smart process manufacturing in Indian packaging industry. In *Information Systems Design and Intelligent Applications* (pp. 339–346). Springer.

Ramakrishnan, R., & Gaur, L. (2019). *Internet of Things: Approach and Applicability in Manufacturing*. CRC Press.

Ramakrishnan, R., Gaur, L., & Singh, G. (2016). Feasibility and efficacy of BLE beacon IoT devices in inventory management at the shop floor. *Iranian Journal of Electrical and Computer Engineering*, *6*(5), 2362–2368. doi:10.11591/ijece.v6i5.10807

Ramu, S. P., Boopalan, P., Pham, Q.-V., Maddikunta, P. K. R., Huynh-The, T., Alazab, M., Nguyen, T. T., & Gadekallu, T. R. (2022). Federated learning enabled digital twins for smart cities: Concepts, recent advances, and future directions. *Sustainable Cities and Society*, *79*, 103663. doi:10.1016/j.scs.2021.103663

Rana, J., Gaur, L., Singh, G., Awan, U., & Rasheed, M. I. (2021). Reinforcing customer journey through artificial intelligence: a review and research agenda. *International Journal of Emerging Markets*. doi:10.1108/IJOEM-08-2021-1214

Saeed, S., Jhanjhi, N. Z., Naqvi, M., Humyun, M., Ahmad, M., & Gaur, L. (2022). *Optimized Breast Cancer Premature Detection Method With Computational Segmentation: A Systematic Review Mapping*. Approaches and Applications of Deep Learning in Virtual Medical Care.

Sahal, R., Alsamhi, S. H., Brown, K. N., O'Shea, D., & Alouffi, B. (2022). Blockchain-Based Digital Twins Collaboration for Smart Pandemic Alerting: Decentralized COVID-19 Pandemic Alerting Use Case (2022). *Computational Intelligence and Neuroscience*, 7786441. doi:10.1155/2022/7786441

Santosh, K., & Gaur, L. (2021). Introduction to AI in Public Health. In Artificial Intelligence and Machine Learning in Public Healthcare. SpringerBriefs in Applied Sciences and Technology. Springer. https://doi.org/10.1007/978-981-16-6768-8_1.

Santosh, K., & Gaur, L. (2021). AI in Precision Medicine. In Artificial Intelligence and Machine Learning in Public Healthcare. SpringerBriefs in Applied Sciences and Technology. Springer. https://doi.org/10.1007/978-981-16-6768-8_5.

Sharma, C., & Gupta, G. (2021). Innovation insight for healthcare provider digital twins: A review. Mobile Health: Advances in Research and Applications, pp. 97-128.

Sharma, D. K., Gaur, L., & Okunbor, D. (2007). Image compression and feature extraction with neural network. In Allied Academies International Conference. Academy of Management Information and Decision Sciences, *11*(1), 33. Jordan Whitney Enterprises, Inc .

Sharma, S., Singh, G., Gaur, L., & Sharma, R. (2022). Does psychological distance and religiosity influence fraudulent customer behaviour? *International Journal of Consumer Studies*. Advance online publication. doi:10.1111/ijcs.12773

Singh, G., Gaur, L., & Ramakrishnan, R. (2017). Internet of things – technology adoption model in india. *Pertanika Journal of Science & Technology*, *25*(3), 835–846.

Thiong'o, G.M., & Rutka, J.T. (2022). Digital Twin Technology: The Future of Predicting Neurological Complications of Pediatric Cancers and Their Treatment. *Frontiers in Oncology*, *11*, 781499

Voigt, I., Inojosa, H., Dillenseger, A., Haase, R., Akgün, K., & Ziemssen, T. (2021). Digital Twins for Multiple Sclerosis. *Frontiers in Immunology*, *12*, 669811. doi:10.3389/fimmu.2021.669811

Volkov, I., Radchenko, G., & Tchernykh, A. (2021). Digital Twins, Internet of Things and Mobile Medicine: A Review of Current Platforms to Support Smart Healthcare. *Programming and Computer Software*, *47* (8), pp. 578-590. doi:10.1134/S0361768821080284

Wickramasinghe, N., Jayaraman, P. P., Zelcer, J., Forkan, A. R. M., Ulapane, N., Kaul, R., & Vaughan, S. (2021). A Vision for Leveraging the Concept of Digital Twins to Support the Provision of Personalised Cancer Care. *Internet Computing*. doi:10.1109/MIC.2021.3065381

Wu, Y., Zhang, K., & Zhang, Y. (2021). Digital Twin Networks: A Survey. *IEEE Internet of Things Journal, 8* (18), pp. 13789-13804. doi:10.1109/JIOT.2021.3079510

Xie, S., Zhu, S., & Dai, J. (2021). Feasibility study of intelligent healthcare based on digital twin and data mining. *Proceedings - 2021 International Conference on Computer Information Science and Artificial Intelligence*, (pp. 906-911). IEEE. doi:10.1109/CISAI54367.2021.00182

Xing, X., Del Ser, J., Wu, Y., Li, Y., Xia, J., Lei, X., Firmin, D., Gatehouse, P., & Yang, G. (2022). HDL: Hybrid Deep Learning for the Synthesis of Myocardial Velocity Maps in Digital Twins for Cardiac Analysis. *IEEE Journal of Biomedical and Health Informatics*. doi:10.1109/JBHI.2022.3158897

Zhang, J., & Tai, Y. (2022). Secure medical digital twin via human-centric interaction and cyber vulnerability resilience. *Connection Science*, *34*(1), 895–910. doi:10.1080/09540091.2021.2013443

Zheng, Y., Lu, R., Guan, Y., Zhang, S., & Shao, J. (2021). Towards Private Similarity Query based Healthcare Monitoring over Digital Twin Cloud Platform. *IEEE/ACM 29th International Symposium on Quality of Service*. doi:10.1109/IWQOS52092.2021.9521351

Zhong, X., Babaie Sarijaloo, F., Prakash, A., Park, J., Huang, C., Barwise, A., Herasevich, V., Gajic, O., Pickering, B., & Dong, Y. (2022). A multidisciplinary approach to the development of digital twin models of critical care delivery in intensive care units. *International Journal of Production Research*. doi:10.1080/00207543.2021.2022235

Chapter 2
The Role of the IoT and Digital Twin in the Healthcare Digitalization Process:
IoT and Digital Twin in the Healthcare Digitalization Process

Imdad Ali Shah
School of Computer Science SC, Taylor's University, Malaysia

Quratulain Sial
Aga Khan University Hospital, Karachi (AKUH), Pakistan

Noor Zaman Jhanjhi
School of Computing Science and Engineering SCE, Taylor's University, Malaysia

Loveleen Gaur
https://orcid.org/0000-0002-0885-1550
Amity University, India & Taylor's University, Malaysia & University of the South Pacific, Fiji

ABSTRACT

The ability of IoT technology to simplify the adoption of artificial intelligence is precious to consumer product companies. The robustness of consumer companies' IoT initiatives will determine whether they benefit from the rise of IoT. A well-thought-out IoT strategy and execution will improve supply chain efficiency and align products with modern, post-COVID consumer behaviour. It must be noted that the network is not only restricted to computers but also has a web of devices of various sizes and kinds, including medical instruments and industrial systems. Expert analysts put forward the inherent capabilities of IoT devices to not only communicate and exchange information but also create a starting point for new, fresh revenue sources, ignite the business foundation and business models and enhance the techniques of services that propel numerous industries and sectors.

DOI: 10.4018/978-1-6684-5925-6.ch002

INTRODUCTION

Hospitals are one of the most challenging systems to manage and represent one of the most complicated systems among all work and organisation competitions. This is because things in daily life that are uncertain or highly variable interact (Evans, 2021). It shows up in different ways inside the hospital, such as clinical variability, flow variability, and professional variability.

Since it is the hospital's responsibility to offer medical care and activities centred on the prevention and treatment of diseases, the alleviation of pain, diagnostic procedures, and other such things, the data entry for patients frequently needs to be done in real-time. As a direct result of this, there is a gap between the actual data and the registered data, and the registered data are the ones that are typically employed when conducting performance analysis (Biesinger, 2019; Qi, 2021). Constantly developing technology has enabled the creation of new sensors that can detect data in real-time (Quirk & Lanni, 2020). The operating room is one of the essential areas in the hospital, and how it is managed affects many other aspects of the hospital's operations, such as the assignment of beds, the creation of surgery waiting lists, the recruitment of staff, and so on.

As a result, one of the most common themes in many scientific disciplines, including engineering, health, economics, and management, is maximising and improving OR efficiency. Repetitive and manual operations are fundamental problems leading to errors and time waste (Ferreira, 2019). In reality, the medical team must record the different times corresponding to the numerous phases the patient must go through for the surgery to be effective because these actions frequently occur in the operating room. The crew often creates these processes at the end of each shift or whenever they have some free time. Of course, this could result in errors and inaccuracies caused by people (Singh, 2021). Industry 4.0 marked the introduction of digital twin technology into our daily lives in the production and engineering sectors. More recently, investigations in the area of health have demonstrated its transformative potential (Erol & Mendi, 2020). A digital replica that enables modelling the condition of a physical asset or system is called a "digital twin." In the healthcare industry, significant advances have been made in creating digital twins of patients and medical equipment and the shows Digital Twince architecture in fig 1.

Transferring the patient's bodily traits and physical changes to the digital world creates the patient's digital twin. One of the most crucial aspects of medicine is providing innovative and conclusive solutions for accurate diagnosis and adherence to patient-appropriate treatment methods. The use of technology is also evident in research in the fields of pharmaceuticals and customised medicine. Qualified studies that will serve as a roadmap for future research are highlighted in this study, which considers the fantastic potential of Digital Twin technology in the health field Dahmen 2018. Transferring the patient's bodily traits and physical changes to the digital world creates the patient's digital twin. One of the most crucial aspects of medicine is providing innovative and conclusive solutions for accurate diagnosis and adherence to patient-appropriate treatment methods Sharma 2021, Autiosalo 2019. The use of technology is also evident in research in the fields of pharmaceuticals and customised medicine. This study highlights qualified studies that can be used as a guide for future research. It also looks at the fantastic potential of Digital Twin technology in health.

Figure 1. Shows Digital Twince architecture Botín-Sanabria 2022

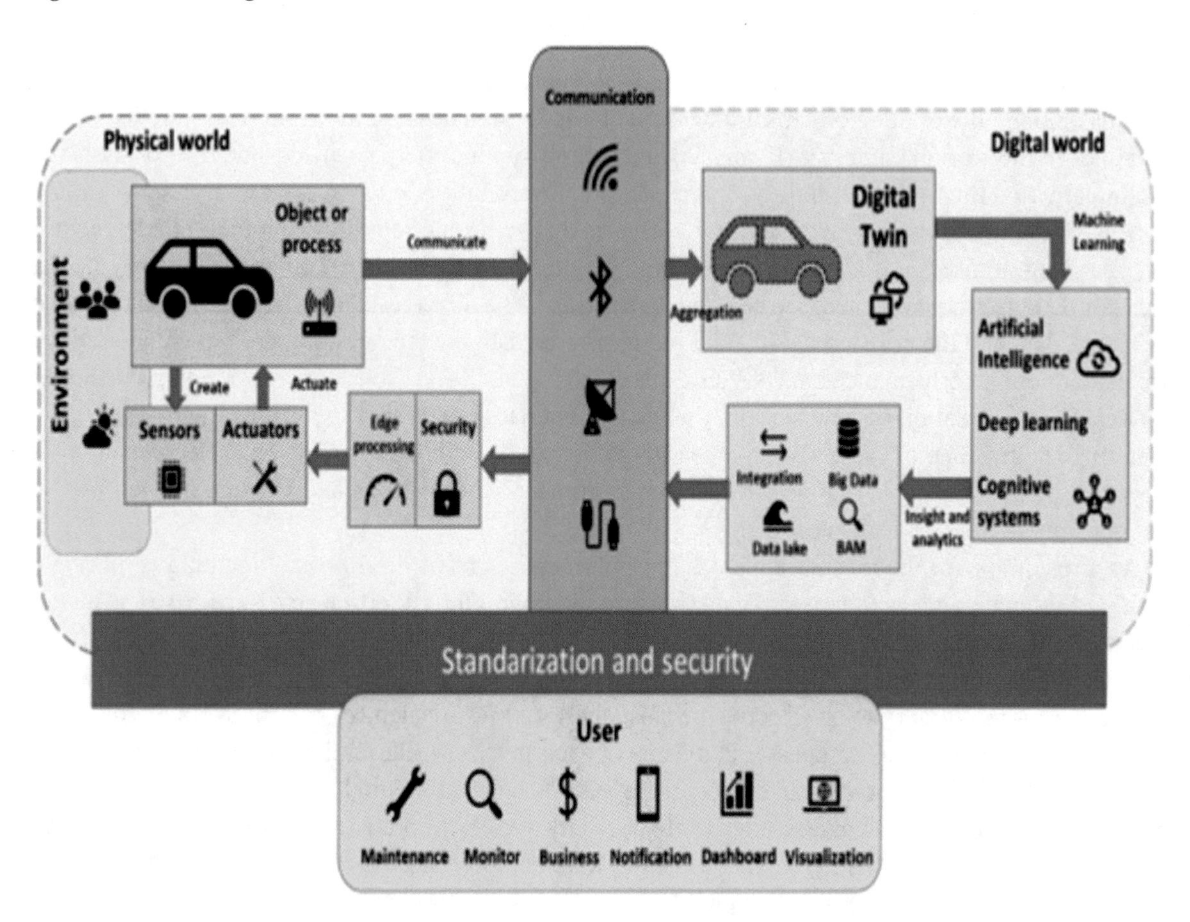

LITERATURE REVIEW

The industrial and business sectors are entirely transformed by our digital era. Following the COVID-19 pandemic, which caused most of their activities to be interrupted, it became clear that those who had selected a digital transformation plan and had begun its execution fared better than those who hadn't (Lim, 2020). The advantage of the digitally transformed company was its ability to connect (Ran, 2019). Digital technology, tools, and techniques that these organisations have applied to accomplish the digitization goal were listed by McKinsey (Sharma, 2018). A crucial prerequisite for integrating and deploying all these technologies in the digitization process is the availability of a dependable, high-performance, high-speed network connection using cutting-edge networking technology Rathore 2021. Additionally, it would enable users to command and initiate operations in the physical system via these interfaces without physically being there. The term "Digital Twin" refers to this style of deployment. Further complicating matters, the phrase "digital twin" is frequently used to refer to a particular strategy or approach rather than a particular artefact. The phrase "digital twin," in the manufacturing sector tends to refer to a particular manufacturing and testing approach rather than specifically to a given class of high-quality, dynamic representations (Tao, 2018). According to this view, the phrase refers to a process or an approach rather than a specific artefact (Stojanovic 2018; Mandolla, 2019). Different bioinformatics applications for in silico therapy will be automatically counted as part of the digital twin paradigm, even if they do not create a digital twin (Tao, 2018). As a result, determining the status of the digital transition takes time and effort.

Several of our interviewees' conversations automatically veered towards these applications, even though they don't currently reveal digital twins as such. Full view of patients, instead focusing on a select few factors important for a specific type of diagnostic (Quirk, 2020; Briggs, 2020). Further complicating matters, the phrase "digital twin" is frequently used to refer to a particular strategy or approach rather than a particular artefact. The phrase "digital twin" in manufacturing refers to a particular manufacturing and testing approach rather tha" a given cla"s of high-quality, dynamic representations.

However, this gradual transition is incredibly complicated. Respondents typically found it challenging to predict the future of the digital twin, but this may be an inherited effect of the title "digital twin" itself. Given that our respondents do not consider themselves taking part in a widespread shift towards the digital twin, at least not in their day-to-day work, we could infer that our broad cross-sectoral perspective on the issue surprised them a little. In several fields, the future of digital twins is uncertain (Ivanov, 2020; Wright, 2020) The generalisation of already developed applications comes first. There will be fewer restrictions on what can be copied and simulated in the future than a few decades ago when computer simulation of the human body was restricted to specific organs or functions. As a result, the industry of "digital twins" is quickly evolving from a specialised project centred, for example, on a certain organ or physiological function, to an accepted method of diagnosis and treatment. Additionally, the digital twin's quality has improved (Dembski, 2020; Zhou, 2019). There was agreement that a digital twin will continue to advance as a diagnostic and therapeutic tool, although occasionally, it is questioned if the social and financial expenses required for this advancement are worthwhile given the advantages. Despite this, there were clear differences among respondents regarding the areas that will bring about this development. People who work with models frequently concentrate on future, better models, whereas people who work with data-gathering tools (sensors) frequently concentrate on future, better tools. However, it was implied or expressly accepted that "excellent data and good modelling" are interdependent.

The upgraded digital twin will not only enhance treatment but also function as a better "filtering mechanism," which would help reduce the burden of the disease. Respondents offered contrasting predictions for the industry in which digital twins will advance quickly. Some believe that certain professions, like cardiology, have the "benefit" of significantly increasing the demand for data and real-time optimization. However, oncology has the advantage of collecting data much more quickly since patients diagnosed with cancer are less likely to consider their comfort or privacy. "Data protection is something for healthy individuals," one participant said in a stark imitation of this (Haiyuan, 2021; Haiyuan, 2021). Keeping with the comparison, organ-level reproductions and implants offer the benefit that the conclusions they draw and their potential uses are not necessarily restricted to particular illnesses or therapies. Because of these different benefits, predicting where the digital twin will "strike" hardest in the coming decades is tough.

DIGITAL TWIN TECHNOLOGY

The DT's five-dimensional framework comprises the physical entity, virtual model, links, DT data, and service (Tao, 2019). These dimensions create DT's structural model. The physical thing could be a prod-

Figure 2. The digital twin's structural model and technical makeup Schrotter, G. 2021

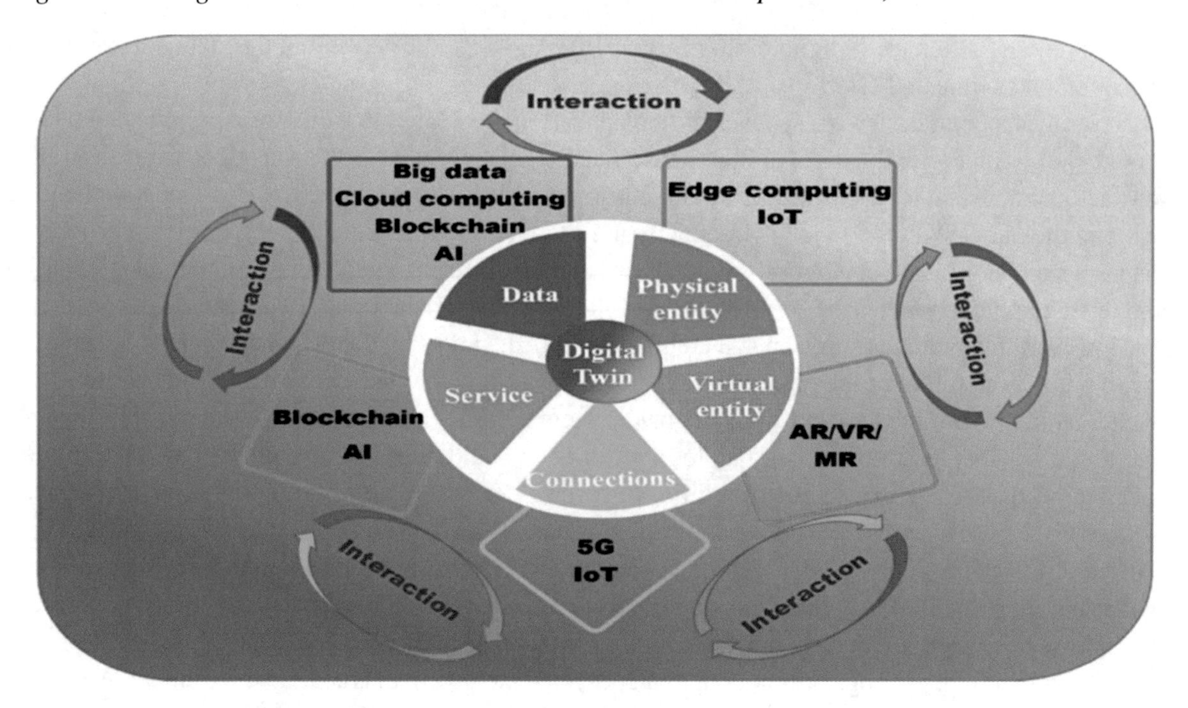

uct, a system, or even a city; it can perform specified tasks while gathering data via sensors (Guevara, 2019). A digital model is a physical object. It displays physical properties, geometries, and behaviours in the virtual environment. The virtual model comprises the actual entity's variables and capabilities. In addition to human-robot interaction and collaboration, human-computer interaction technologies should be examined (Bentley Systems Incorporated, 2021). Blockchain can safeguard twin data from alteration and assure DT's data security Tagliabue, L 2020. DT's service model includes a real and virtual entities. Calibrating the model's parameters and maintaining its performance increases its authenticity (Conejos, 2020). AI can analyse, fuse, and deeply learn twin data by matching the best algorithms. Data value, timeliness, and accuracy may improve the digital twin's structural model and technical makeup in fig 2.

A continuous digital twin generated using a System Dynamics methodology was created with Powersim, a product of Powersim Software AS. It replicates the patient's actions, from entering the operating room to leaving. The nine states (T1-T9) are represented by the states in this model, which uses a top-down method (White, 2021). Each state is dependent on the previous state. As a result, the flow is enabled once the last event's duration has passed, and the patient can go to the next state (Schrotter, 2021). A circumstance that enables the patient to move across the arrows from one state to another causes the state shift. The database that houses the information gathered from the buttons feeds the Digital Twin, which simulates surgical procedures (Raes, 2021). This technique makes it feasible to know the anticipated wait time and the likelihood of receiving service at a specific moment. This is helpful for both patients, who can learn how long they will have to wait for their surgery, and even for nurses and surgeons, who can plan their operations more efficiently.

The beginnings of the digital twin concept may be traced back to NASA's Apollo programme, which sought to develop physical replicas of its systems on Earth that matched those in space. This occurred in the 1960s. They evaluated the behaviour and functionality of their systems by simulating numerous scenarios, testing them under various settings, and testing various cases (Prasad, 2012). Later, Michael Grieves developed the idea of digital twins for the manufacturing sector in the early 2000s by building digital twins of plants to track operations, anticipate breakdowns, and boost production (Beil, 2020; Nativi, 2020; Lee, 2020). The idea received increased prominence and importance after being included in Gartner's list of the top 10 key technology trends for 2017 Nativi, S., and being implemented by multiple industry titans like Siemens (Marcucci, 2020; Russell, 2020), where the connection between digital and physical systems conveying data and managing information was defined as the essential component of digital twins. With this knowledge, a digital twin can provide all the information needed about the physical system in real-time, making it the ideal target for digital twins. (Sakdirat, 2021) Intelligent manufacturing has received much attention in recent years thanks to the introduction of Industry 4.0. There have been attempts made by governments to explore digitalization, and numerous studies have been carried out on digital systems which are capable of remote company management. The digital twin (DT) is a virtual replica that represents the status of a physical entity or system. More and more businesses are turning to it to improve their management and production efficiency.

Professor Michael Grieves was the one who first presented the idea of the DT in 2002, and he did so to characterise product life cycle management (Yitmen, 2021; Godager, 2020). Defined a "digital twin" as "a virtual instance of a physical system (twin) that is continually updated with the latter's performance, maintenance, and health status data throughout the physical system's life cycle." This definition of a digital twin can be found in the article "A Digital Twin Is a Virtual Instance of a Physical System."These copies can interact in real-time with in-depth information and physical space generally hidden from view (Carvalho, 2020). In addition, artificial intelligence (AI) can identify potential needs for machine maintenance before machine faults occur by utilising deep learning.

DIGITAL TWIN APPLICATIONS

Many areas have adopted digital twins for the many benefits outlined above and their tremendous potential for properly reflecting physical systems. Several of these domains include:

Manufacturing

The fourth industrial revolution, often known as Industry 4.0, is the advancement now occurring in the manufacturing sector. In an Industry 4.0 report (Gutierrez-Franco, 2021), all of which can be delivered by digital twins was described as the autonomous integration of nine technologies. These technologies include industrial IoT, simulation, augmented reality, cloud services, big data and analytics, additive manufacturing, horizontal and vertical system integration, and sophisticated robotics. Industrial and manufacturing systems that use digital twins can make digital copies of their factories and production lines. This allows it to manage, monitor, and improve all processes in real-time without stopping the production stream.

Healthcare

Healthcare is one of the most important fields to deploy digital twins. With the development of wearable technologies that sense and gather data on human vitals, it is now possible to create digital twins of people who can predict potential health complications and take preventative action, such as calling an ambulance to the patient's location or alerting their healthcare provider to any concerning circumstances (Pan, 2021). The digital twin can also train future surgeons by replicating how the human body works. Additionally, as suggested by the authors, digital twins can be employed in more challenging situations like remote surgery. In the same sense, the writers realizedd how crucial it is to have a network that connects the digital and virtual twins for this application case to be realized (Erol, 2020). Second, a neural network is trained to predict unknown blood pressure waveforms using readily available waveforms (Laubenbacher, 2021; Laamarti, 2019). Finally, the inverse model's waveform was analysed by another neural network to determine disease severity. Another alternative uses offline and online methods. Use high-fidelity simulation and training data to build an offline Motion capture, and IK technologies provide real-time body position and pose.

- *Medicine Digital Twin*

Precision medicine requires personalization and patient-centric modelling. With the fast expansion and development of several activation technologies, DT in medicine has great promise. IoT devices are cheaper and easier to implement, increasing network connectivity (Laaki, 2019). DT Healthcare is a unique medical simulation method that uses interdisciplinary, multiphysics and multiscale models to provide robust, precise, and effective medical services. AI and other cutting-edge technologies may effectively discover the disease's origin, define the therapy goal, and provide individualised and exact treatment (Pedersen, 2021; He, 2021). Several exploratory investigations have laid the groundwork for medical DT use.

- *Orthopaedics*

Unity3D software was used to create a 3D virtual reality system to record the lumbar spine's real-time biomechanical performance, which could improve spine treatment planning. We predicted real-time intradiscal pressure and facet contact force using the DT construction method and dynamically connected physical and digital spaces, an overview of Digital Twin and Orthopaedics in fig 3.

Aubert built the DT of a patient's fracture and modelled four stabilisation strategies to maximise surgical trauma procedures and postoperative decision-making (Sujatha, 2012). The amount of bone measured the risk of repeated fractures stressed above the local yield strength and by the strains between the broken pieces.

- *Cardiovascular Disease*

DT can create digital heart models and accurately treat cardiovascular illnesses. Philips created the customised DT model using pre-surgery CT pictures of the heart (Latif, 2020). Surgeons can use real-time 3D locations to find and choose equipment (Muzafar, 2020). Deep learning derives inverse aortic blood pressure waveforms from easy-to-access arteries like the radial or carotid. Using inverse analysis, an active DT can monitor and prevent medical issues from worsening. This biological approach could make it less important to use complicated and invasive diagnostic tools and more important to use non-invasive or minimally invasive methods of testing. (Jung 2022; Shah, 2022) used clinical cavity pressure

Figure 3. Overview Digital Twin and Orthopaedics Dahmen, U. 2018

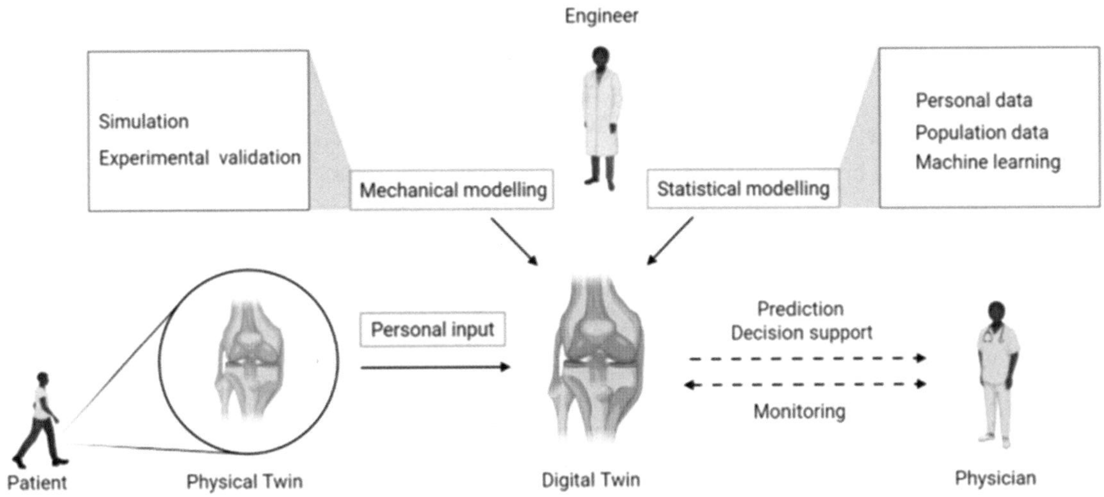

data from people with aortic coarctation to calibrate a ustomized 3D electromechanics model and make a high-fidelity cellular scale model.

- *Pharmacy*

In 2014, Dassault Systèmes and the FDA approved the SIMULIA Living Heart, the first digital investigation of organ–drug interactions (Shah, 2021; Shah, 2022). Medical researchers or instructors validated this DT model of human hearts. This method allows doctors and pharmaceutical engineers to see how complex cardiac tissue structure and movement are, allowing for more effective treatment.

Takeda Pharmaceuticals uses DT technology to produce breakthrough treatments worldwide. DT models shorten pharmaceutical procedures and forecast biochemical reaction input–output realistically (Shah, 2022). Atos and Siemens developed physical DT models for the pharmaceutical industry to boost efficiency and productivity. IoT, AI, and other sophisticated technologies support it.

DISCUSSION

Both natural and artificial variability has an impact on the healthcare sector. The inherent component of health care delivery leads to the random nature of the natural variability. Every patient is unique due to age, co-morbidities, therapy response, and other natural variations. Artificial variability is not random and is frequently associated with flaws or bad organisational decisions. Litvak's assertion that "the unfamiliarity with a new technology may be addressed by education and certification" is an example of artificial variability. In other words, whereas natural variability can only be observed and measured, the manager can concentrate on the subject and eliminate manufactured variability (Singh, 2020). Where ANOVA analysis shows high noise through SSE, it effectively illustrates these general ideas. A drawback of the study is that only one surgical specialisation, not only one kind of surgery, was chosen for the sample size and the surgical procedures that were chosen. There is still a need to investigate methods that enable doctors to organize surgical activity better while avoiding the influence of artificial unpredictability. The definition of a digital twin was most recently applied to the healthcare industry by Karakra et al. They employed IoT devices specifically for real-time data captioning (Shah, 2022). This data is used to fuel the discrete event simulation model that FlexSim, created by FlexSim Software Products, Inc., implements. The authors' method replicates the effectiveness of the services, allowing the decision-maker to modify the schedule of operations. Starting from this context, the authors decided to advance the use of real-time simulation, creating a daily tool accessible to the surgical decision-maker. This suggests that it may be possible to get a recommendation from the model for better resource allocation. For instance, the model might be able to forecast, based on a data warehouse of comparable operations, the anticipated time of the surgical act's conclusion (T4), allowing the decision-maker to plan how to proceed optimally in light of the total amount of time available for operations in a single day. The immediate result is better resource management.

In 2014, Dassault Systèmes and the FDA approved the SIMULIA Living Heart, the first digital investigation of organ–drug interactions (Shah, 2022; Kiran, 2021). Medical researchers or instructors validated this DT model of human hearts. This method allows doctors and pharmaceutical engineers to see how complex cardiac tissue structure and movement are, allowing for more effective treatment. Takeda Pharmaceuticals uses DT technology to produce breakthrough treatments worldwide. DT models shorten pharmaceutical procedures and forecast biochemical reaction input–output realistically. Atos and Siemens developed physical DT models for the pharmaceutical industry to boost efficiency and productivity. IoT, AI, and other sophisticated technologies support it.

The DT is supposed to revolutionise medicine by quantifying health and sickness. It can aid hospital management, design, and patient care. Before scheduling and executing changes like bed scheduling and treatment options, the DT can predict and assess situations in a virtual environment, reducing risks and expenses. It can also verify treatment procedures and medications using the model to optimise the treatment plan and achieve early disease diagnosis or prevention. Hospital staff cannot plan surgeries without the DT. Numerous risk factors for maternal health and infant mortality are avoidable (Umrani, 2021;Shah, 2022; Shah, 2022; Jhanjhi, 2022). Preconception care that is timely and appropriate can improve everyone's general health, promote better pregnancies for women, and considerably minimise negative mother-and-baby outcomes at the population level. Although the preconception stage is the focus of this article, many other factors are directly related to lifetime health, such as leading a healthy lifestyle, eating better, exercising, maintaining good mental health, and so on.

BOOK CHAPTER CONTRIBUTION AND DISCUSSION

For consumer goods manufacturers, the ability of IoT technology to simplify AI adoption is priceless. Whether consumer companies profit from the rise of IoT will depend on how strong their IoT projects are. The effectiveness of the supply chain will increase with a well-executed IoT strategy, and products will be more in line with contemporary, post-COVID consumer behaviour. It should be highlighted that the network includes devices of all sizes and types, including industrial and medical systems, and is not just limited to computers. The inherent abilities of IoT devices to not only communicate but also exchange information have been highlighted by expert analysts. These abilities also serve as a springboard for brand-new revenue streams, ignite the business foundation and business models, and improve the techniques of services that drive numerous industries and sectors. One of the biggest obstacles to developing the DT and the clinical translation is collecting data, such as geometry, performance, sensor, etc. Electronic health data and information are currently dispersed and challenging to combine. Unstructured data necessitates manual labour and lacks automated processing tools. The DT has found a lot of use in industry as a virtual replica that simulates the state of a real entity. The DT can help medical practitioners virtually simulate various scenarios before making actual adjustments, lowering risks and saving money. In the future, DT technology could help clinicians make accurate diagnoses, create the right treatment plans, and predict how the treatment will affect the patient.

CONCLUSION AND FUTURE WORK

The ability of IoT technology to simplify the adoption of artificial intelligence is precious to consumer product companies. The robustness of consumer companies' IoT initiatives will determine whether they benefit from the rise of IoT. A well-thought-out IoT strategy and execution will improve supply chain efficiency and align products with modern, post-COVID consumer behaviour. It must be noted that the network is not only restricted to computers but also has a web of devices of various sizes and kinds, including medical instruments and industrial systems. Expert analysts put forward the inherent capabilities of IoT devices to not only communicate and exchange information but also create a starting point for new, fresh revenue sources, ignite the business foundation and business models and enhance the techniques of services that propel numerous industries and sectors. A digital twin is a representation of service in digital form. This technology can be used to repeat processes to gather information and estimate how they will perform in adding to tangible assets.

Risks related to society and ethics exist in DT healthcare as well. The primary factor that makes DT potentially harmful is privacy, which is the most crucial. Additionally, the high expense of DT healthcare may result in unfairness and inequality, exacerbating the socioeconomic divide already present. Emerging technology is viewed as more adaptable in its early stages because foundational research and clinical trials have not yet been completed, and its societal consequences are relatively manageable. The key to developing and accepting DT technology is educating patients and the general public about its uses and potential. Undoubtedly, those in good health are more concerned about data privacy than those with terminal cancer.

REFERENCES

Autiosalo, J., Vepsalainen, J., Viitala, R., & Tammi, K. (2019). A Feature-Based Framework for Structuring Industrial Digital Twins. *IEEE Access, 8*, 1193–1208. [CrossRef]

Amir Latif, R. M., Hussain, K., Jhanjhi, N. Z., Nayyar, A., & Rizwan, O. (2020). A remix IDE: Smart contract-based framework for the healthcare sector by using Blockchain technology. *Multimedia Tools and Applications*, 1–24. https://ieeexplore.ieee.org/abstract/document/9214512

Ao, F., Zhang, M., Liu, Y., & Nee, A. Y. (2018). Digital twin driven prognostics and health management for complex equipment. *CIRP Annals*, *67*(1), 169–172. doi:10.1016/j.cirp.2018.04.055

Beil, C., & Kolbe, T. H. (2020). Combined Modelling of Multiple Transportation Infrastructure Within 3D City Models and its Implementation in CityGML 3.0. [CrossRef]. *ISPRS Ann. Photogramm. Remote Sens. Spatial Inf. Sci., 6*, 29–36. doi:10.5194/isprs-annals-VI-4-W1-2020-29-2020

Bentley Systems Incorporated. (2021). Discover OpenCities Planner–Connect The Data, People, Workflows, and Ideas Necessary to Support Today's Infrastructure Projects. *Report P-18.* https://www.bentley.com/es/products/brands/ opencities-planner.

Biesinger, F., & Weyrich, M. (2019). The Facets of Digital Twins in Production and the Automotive Industry. In *23rd International Conference on Mechatronics Technology (ICMT)*, Salerno, Italy. 10.1109/ICMECT.2019.8932101

Botín-Sanabria, D. M., Mihaita, A. S., Peimbert-García, R. E., Ramírez-Moreno, M. A., Ramírez-Mendoza, R. A., & Lozoya-Santos, J. D. J. (2022). Digital twin technology challenges and applications: A comprehensive review. *Remote Sensing, 14*(6), 1335. doi:10.3390/rs14061335

Briggs, B., & Buchholz, S. (2020). Deloitte Tech Trends 2020. *Insights, 2020*, 1–130.

Campos-Ferreira, A., Lozoya-Santos, J. J., Vargas-Martínez, A., Mendoza, R., & Morales-Menéndez, R. (2019). Digital Twin Applications: A review. In *Memorias del Congreso Nacional de Control Automático*, (pp. 606–611). Asociación de México de Control Automático.

Carvalho, A., Melo, P., Oliveira, M., & Barros, R. The 4-corner model as a synchromodal and digital twin enabler in the transportation sector. In Proceedings of the 2020 IEEE International Conference on Engineering, Technology and Innovation (ICE/ITMC), (pp. 15–17). IEEE. [CrossRef] 10.1109/ICE/ITMC49519.2020.9198592

Conejos, P., Martínez, F., Hervas, M., & Alonso, J. C. (2020). Building and Exploiting a Digital Twin for the Managmenet of Drinking Water Distribution Networks. [CrossRef]. *Urban Water Journal, 17*(8), 704–713. doi:10.1080/1573062X.2020.1771382

Dembski, F., Wossner, U., Letzgus, M., Ruddat, M., & Yamu, C. (2020). Urban Digital Twins for Smart Cities and Citizens: The Case Study of Herrenberg, Germany. [CrossRef]. *Sustainability, 12*(6), 2307. doi:10.3390u12062307

Dahmen, U., & Rossmann, J. (2018). Experimentable Digital Twins for a Modeling and Simulation-based Engineering Approach. In *Proceedings International Systems Engineering Symposium (ISSE).* IEEE. 10.1109/SysEng.2018.8544383

Erol, T., Mendi, A. F., & Doğan, D. (2020, October). The digital twin revolution in healthcare. *2020 4th International Symposium on Multidisciplinary Studies and Innovative Technologies (ISMSIT)* (pp. 1-7). IEEE. https://ieeexplore.ieee.org/abstract/document/9255249

Erol, T., Mendi, A. F., & Doğan, D. (2020, October). The digital twin revolution in healthcare. *2020 4th International Symposium on Multidisciplinary Studies and Innovative Technologies (ISMSIT)* (pp. 1-7). IEEE. https://ieeexplore.ieee.org/abstract/document/9255249

Evans, S., Savian, C., Burns, A., & Cooper, C. (2019). Digital Twins for the Built Environment: An Introduction to the Opportunities, Benefits, Challenges and Risks. *Built Environmental News*. https://www.theiet.org/impact-society/ sectors/built-environ ment/built-environment-news/digital-twins-for-the-built-envi
ronment/.

Godager, B.; Onstein, E.; Huang, L. (2021). *The Concept of Enterprise BIM: Current Research Practice and Future Trends*. IEEE

Guevara, N., Diaz, C., Sguerra, M., Martinez, M., Agudelo, O., Suarez, J., Rodriguez, A., Acuña, G., & Garcia, A. (2019). Towards the design and implementation of a Smart City in Bogotá, Colombia. Rev. Fac. DeIng. [CrossRef]. *Univ. Antioq.*, *93*(93), 41–45. doi:10.17533/udea.redin.20190407

Gutierrez-Franco, E., Mejia-Argueta, C., & Rabelo, L. (2021). Data-Driven Methodology to Support Long-Lasting Logistics and Decision Making for Urban Last-Mile Operations. [CrossRef]. *Sustainability*, *13*(11), 6230. doi:10.3390u13116230

Haiyuan, Y., Dachuan, W., Mengcha, S., & Qi, Y. (2021). Application of Digital Twins in Port System. [CrossRef]. *Journal of Physics: Conference Series*, •••, 1846.

He, X., Qiu, Y., Lai, X., Li, Z., Shu, L., Sun, W., & Song, X. (2021). Towards a shape-performance integrated digital twin for lumbar spine analysis. *Digital Twin.*, *1*, 8. doi:10.12688/digitaltwin.17478.1

Ivanov, S., Nikolskaya, K., Radchenko, G., Sokolinsky, L., & Zymbler, M. Digital Twin of City: Concept Overview. In *Proceedings of the 2020 Global Smart Industry Conference (GloSIC)*, Chelyabinsk, Russia, 17–19 November 2020. 10.1109/GloSIC50886.2020.9267879

Jung, A., Gsell, M. A. F., Augustin, C. M., & Plank, G. (2022). An integrated workflow for building digital twins of cardiac electromechanics-a multi-fidelity approach for personalising active mechanics. *Mathematics*, *10*(5), 823. doi:10.3390/math10050823 PMID:35295404

Kiran, S. R. A., Rajper, S., Shaikh, R. A., Shah, I. A., & Danwar, S. H. (2021). Categorization of CVE Based on Vulnerability Software By Using Machine Learning Techniques. *International Journal (Toronto, Ont.)*, *10*(3).

Lee, S., Jain, S., Zhang, Y., Liu, J., & Son, Y. J. A Multi-Paradigm Simulation for the Implementation of Digital Twins in Surveillance Applications. In *Proceedings of the 2020 IISE Annual Conference*, New Orleans, LA, USA, 30 May–2 June 2020.

Laubenbacher, R., Sluka, J., & Glazier, J. (2021). Using digital twins in viral infection. [CrossRef]. *Science*, *371*(6534), 1105–1106. doi:10.1126cience.abf3370 PMID:33707255

Laamarti, F.; Badawi, H.; Ding, Y.; Arafsha, F.; Hafidh, B.; El Saddik, A. An ISO/IEEE 11073 Standardized Digital Twin Framework for Health and Well-Being in Smart Cities. IEEE Access 2020, 8, 105950–105961. [CrossRef]

Laaki, H.; Miche, Y.; Tammi, K. Prototyping a Digital Twin for Real Time Remote Control Over Mobile Networks: Application of Remote Surgery. IEEE Access 2019, 7, 20325–20336. [CrossRef]

Lim, K., Zheng, P., & Chen, C. (2020). A state-of-the-art survey of Digital Twin: Techniques, engineering product lifecycle management and business innovation perspectives. [CrossRef]. *Journal of Intelligent Manufacturing*, *31*(6), 1313–1337. doi:10.100710845-019-01512-w

Mandolla, C., Petruzzelli, A. M., Percoco, G., & Urbinati, A. (2019). Building a digital twin for additive manufacturing through the exploitation of blockchain: A case analysis of the aircraft industry. *Computers in Industry*, *109*, 134–152. doi:10.1016/j.compind.2019.04.011

Marcucci, E., Gatta, V., Le-Pira, M., Hansson, L., & Brathen, S. (2020). Digital Twins: A Critical Discussion on Their Potential for Supporting Policy-Making and Planning in Urban Logistics. *Sustainability*, *12*(24), 623. doi:10.3390u122410623

Muzafar, S., & Jhanjhi, N. Z. (2020). Success stories of ICT implementation in Saudi Arabia. In *Employing Recent Technologies for Improved Digital Governance* (pp. 151–163). IGI Global. https://www.igi-global.com/chapter/success-stories-of-ict-implementation-in-saudi-arabia/245980 doi:10.4018/978-1-7998-1851-9.ch008

Nativi, S., Mazzetti, P., & Craglia, M. (2021). Digital Ecosystems for Developing Digital Twins of the Earth: The Destination Earth Case. *Remote Sensing*, *13*(11), 2119. doi:10.3390/rs13112119

Pan, S., Zhou, W., Piramuthu, S., Giannikas, V., & Chen, C. (2021). Smart city for sustainable urban freight logistics. Int. J. Prod. Res. 2021, 59, 2079–2089. [CrossRef] 51. Shengli, W. Is Human Digital Twin possible? *Comput. Methods Programs Biomed. Update*, *1*, 100014.

Pedersen, A., Brup, M., Brink-Kjaer, A., Christiansen, L., & Mikkelsen, P. (2021). Living and Prototyping Digital Twins for Urban Water Systems: Towards Multi-Purpose Value Creation Using Models and Sensors. *Water (Basel)*, *13*(5), 592. doi:10.3390/w13050592

Prasad, R. B., & Groop, L. (2019). Precision medicine in type 2 diabetes. *Journal of Internal Medicine*, *285*(1), 40–48. doi:10.1111/joim.12859 PMID:30403316

Quirk, D., Lanni, J., & Chauhan, N. (2020). Digital twins: Answering the hard questions. *ASHRAE Journal*, *62*, 22–25.

Qi, Q., Tao, F., Hu, T., Anwer, H., Liu, A., Wei, Y., Wang, L., & Nee, A. (2021). Enabling technologies and tools for digital twin. *Journal of Manufacturing Systems*, *53*, 3–21. doi:10.1016/j.jmsy.2019.10.001

Quirk, D., Lanni, J., & Chauhan, N. (2020). *Digital Twins: Details of Implementation: Part 2. AHRAE J.*, *62*, 20–24.

Ran, Y., Lin, P., Zhou, X., & Wen, Y. (2019). A Survey of Predictive Maintenance: Systems, Purposes and Approaches. *Comput. Sci. Eng.* http://xxx.lanl.gov/abs/1912.07383.

Rathore, M.; Shah, S.; Shukla, D.; Bentafat, E.; Bakiras, S. (2021). The Role of AI, Machine Learning, and Big Data in Digital Twinning: A Systematic Literature Review, Challenges, and Opportunities. IEEE.

Raes, L., Michiels, P., Adolphi, T., Tampere, C., Dalianis, T., Mcaleer, S., & Kogut, P. (2021). DUET: A Framework for Building Secure and Trusted Digital Twins of Smart Cities. *IEEE Internet Computing*.

Sharma, M., & George, J. P. (2018). *Digital Twin in the Automotive Industry: Driving Physical-Digital Convergence; TCS White Papers*. Tata Consultancy Services Limited.

Sharma, A., Kosasih, E., Zhang, J., Brintrup, A., & Calinescu, A. (2021). Digital Twins: State of the Art Theory and Practice, Challenges, and Open Research Questions. arXiv 2021, arXiv:2011.02833.

Juarez, M., Botti, V., & Giret, A. (2021). Digital Twins: Review and Challenges. *Journal of Computing and Information Science in Engineering*, *21*, 030802.

Schrotter, G., & Hurzeler, C. (2021). The Digital Twin of the City of Zurich for Urban Planning. *J. Photogramm. Remote Sens. Geoinf. Sci.*, *88*, 99–112.

Sakdirat, K., Rungskunroch, P., & Welsh, J. (2019). A Digital-Twin Evaluation of Net Zero Energy Building for Existing Buildings. *Sustainability*, *11*, 159.

Sujatha, R., Chatterjee, J. M., Jhanjhi, N. Z., & Brohi, S. N. (2021). Performance of deep learning vs machine learning in plant leaf disease detection. *Microprocessors and Microsystems*, *80*, 103615. doi:10.1016/j.micpro.2020.103615

Shah, I. A., Wassan, S., & Usmani, M. H. (2022). E-Government Security and Privacy Issues: Challenges and Preventive Approaches. In Cybersecurity Measures for E-Government Frameworks (pp. 61-76). IGI Global.

Shah, I. A., & Rajper, S., & Zaman-Jhanjhi, N. (2021). Using ML and Data-Mining Techniques in Automatic Vulnerability Software Discovery. *International Journal (Toronto, Ont.)*, *10*(3).

Shah, I. A. (2022). Cybersecurity Issues and Challenges for E-Government During COVID-19: A Review. *Cybersecurity Measures for E-Government Frameworks*, 187-222.

Shah, I. A., Jhanjhi, N. Z., Amsaad, F., & Razaque, A. (2022). The Role of Cutting-Edge Technologies in Industry 4.0. In *Cyber Security Applications for Industry 4.0* (pp. 97–109). Chapman and Hall/CRC. doi:10.1201/9781003203087-4

Shah, I. A., Jhanjhi, N. Z., Humayun, M., & Ghosh, U. (2022). Health Care Digital Revolution During COVID-19. In *How COVID-19 is Accelerating the Digital Revolution* (pp. 17–30). Springer. doi:10.1007/978-3-030-98167-9_2

Shah, I. A., Jhanjhi, N. Z., Humayun, M., & Ghosh, U. (2022). Impact of COVID-19 on Higher and Post-secondary Education Systems. In *How COVID-19 is Accelerating the Digital Revolution* (pp. 71–83). Springer. doi:10.1007/978-3-030-98167-9_5

Shah, I. A., Habeeb, R. A. A., Rajper, S., & Laraib, A. (2022). The Influence of Cybersecurity Attacks on E-Governance. In *Cybersecurity Measures for E-Government Frameworks* (pp. 77–95). IGI Global. doi:10.4018/978-1-7998-9624-1.ch005

Singh, M., Fuenmayor, E., Hinchy, E. P., Qiao, Y., Murray, N., & Devine, D. (2021). Digital Twin: Origin to Future. *Appl. Syst. Innov.*, *4*(2), 36. doi:10.3390/asi4020036

Singh, A. P., Pradhan, N. R., Luhach, A. K., Agnihotri, S., Jhanjhi, N. Z., Verma, S., Kavita, Ghosh, U., & Roy, D. S. (2020). A novel patient-centric architectural framework for blockchain-enabled healthcare applications. *IEEE Transactions on Industrial Informatics*, *17*(8), 5779–5789. https://ieeexplore.ieee.org/abstract/document/9259231. doi:10.1109/TII.2020.3037889

Russell, H. (2020). Sustainable Urban Governance Networks: Data-driven Planning Technologies and Smart City Software Systems. *Geopolit. Hist. Int. Relations*, *12*, 9–15.

Singh, M., Fuenmayor, E., Hinchy, E. P., Qiao, Y., Murray, N., & Devine, D. (2021). Digital Twin: Origin to Future. *Appl. Syst. Innov.*, *4*, 36.

Stojanovic, N., & Milenovic, D. (2018, December). Data-driven Digital Twin approach for process optimization: An industry use case. In *International Conference on Big Data (Big Data)* (pp. 4202-4211). IEEE.

Tao, F., Zhang, H., Liu, A., & Nee, A. Y. (2018). Digital twin in industry: State-of-the-art. *IEEE Transactions on Industrial Informatics*, *15*(4), 2405–2415. https://ieeexplore.ieee.org/abstract/document/8477101

Tagliabue, L., Cecconi, F., Maltese, S., Rinaldi, S., Ciribini, A., & Flammini, A. (2021). Leveraging Digital Twin for Sustainability Assessment of an Educational Building. *Sustainability*, *13*, 480.

Tao, F., Cheng, J., Qi, Q., Zhang, M., Zhang, H., & Sui, F. (2018). Digital twin-driven product design, manufacturing and service with big data. *International Journal of Advanced Manufacturing Technology*, *94*, 3563–3576. doi:10.100700170-017-0233-1

Tomin, N., Kurbatsky, V., Borisov, V., & Musalev, S. (2020). Development of Digital Twin for Load Center on the Example of Distribution Network of an Urban District. *Energy*, *209*, 02029.

Umrani, S., Rajper, S., Talpur, S. H., Shah, I. A., & Shujrah, A. (2020). Games based learning: A case of learning Physics using Angry Birds. *Indian Journal of Science and Technology*, *13*(36), 3778–3784.

Wright, L., & Davidson, S. (2020). How to tell the difference between a model and a digital twin. *Adv. Model. Simul. Eng. Sci.*, *7*, 13.

Yitmen, I., Alizadehsalehi, S., Akiner, I., & Akiner, M. (2021). An Adapted Model of Cognitive Digital Twins for Building Lifecycle Management.. *Appl. Sci.*, *11*, 4276.

Zhou, M., Yan, J., & Feng, D. (2019). Digital Twin Framework and Its Application to Power Grid Online Analysis. *CSSE J. Power Energy Syst.*, *5*, 391–398.

Chapter 3
A Comprehensive Study on Algorithms and Applications of Artificial Intelligence in Diagnosis and Prognosis:
AI for Healthcare

Sahana P Shankar
https://orcid.org/0000-0001-8977-9898
M. S. Ramiaiah University of Applied Sciences, India

Supriya M. S.
https://orcid.org/0000-0003-3465-6879
M. S. Ramiaiah University of Applied Sciences, India

Deepak Varadam
M. S. Ramiaiah University of Applied Sciences, India

Mushkan Kumar
M. S. Ramiaiah University of Applied Sciences, India

Harshita Gupta
M. S. Ramiaiah University of Applied Sciences, India

Rishika Saha
M. S. Ramiaiah University of Applied Sciences, India

ABSTRACT

Machine learning and deep learning are branches of artificial intelligence consisting of statistical, probabilistic, and optimisation techniques that allow machines to learn from previous observations recorded by humans. These machine learning algorithms, when combined with other technologies, can be used to perform very intuitive yet awkward human-like tasks. Using these algorithms, humans can enable computers to learn about certain things like recognising an object in an image. Prognosis is an important clinical skill, particularly for cancer patients' clinicians, neurooncologists. One of the biggest challenge for AI in prognosis is to verify and validate its models. Unlike diagnosis, the prognosis models are centered on predictive data that usually addresses the patient and not the disease. Prognosis models

DOI: 10.4018/978-1-6684-5925-6.ch003

were developed to aid in the decision-making of patients' treatment.AI can have bigger impact in the health care domain with more healthcare providers using AI to make the first diagnosis and prognosis more accurate and interpretable with the available patient data for better therapy.

INTRODUCTION

machine learning (and deep learning) are branches of artificial intelligence consisting of statistical, probabilistic, and optimisation techniques (often inspired by nature and its phenomenon) that allow machines (computers) to learn from previous observations recorded by humans. These machine learning algorithms, when combined with other technologies like especially Computer Vision, can be used to perform very intuitive yet awkward human-like tasks. Using these algorithms, humans can enable computers to learn about certain things like recognising an object in an image, classify text into different categories based on its feature(s), etc. Since machine learning can do these problematic tasks efficiently and without the requirement of human resources, the range of fields in which machine learning can be used, is extensive whether it be logistics, agriculture, information technology, healthcare, and many more. In the healthcare domain, machine learning isn't only providing ease of operations in many applications, but also creating new possibilities like the prediction of certain diseases without the need for professional medical personnel. The same can be extended to the fields of diagnosis and prognosis, as many machine learning models are coming up which are as useful as 96% or even more in diagnose of diseases like Alzheimer's, and perform some initial analysis even to suggest some primary treatment for the same. While the applications of machine learning in diagnosis and prognosis are still in an early phase and open to research, beneficial machine learning models are there for the diseases which can be diagnosed by some visual scans. These include Fractures (by analysing X-rays), Alzheimer (by analysing neuroimaging data), Cancer (by analysing CT Scans), COVID19 (a preliminary diagnosis can be made with the help of Chest X-Ray scans), and others. A variety of machine learning techniques, like Artificial Neural Networks (ANNs), Bayesian Networks (BNs), Support Vector Machines (SVMs) and Decision Trees (DTs). These have been generally applied in clinical exploration for the advancement of prediction models, bringing about viable and exact dynamic, for both diagnosis and prognosis. But the advantages of machine learning in diagnosis and prognosis isn't only limited to severe diseases requiring visual scans. The activity trackers which can monitor the heart rate, blood oxygen level, blood pressure, etc., health data is collected. This data can then be fed to a pre-trained machine learning model to analyse if the received information represents a healthy person, or are there few abnormal values. So, the activity tracker itself can notify the person about its health. And, many instances of such incidents have already been recorded where smartwatches or activity trackers sent distress signal when the patient's health data became very abnormal, and thus was able to save the patient. Not just diseases, but a healthy routine of an individual, a constant monitoring of a patient (also known as Remote Patient Monitoring), timely suggestions for calorie intake or to drink water, these are all done using machine learning models. AI in healthcare is creating new possibilities and making it available for an even more significant number of people at ease. In this chapter, detailed research is performed on the various applications of machine learning in healthcare (especially in diagnosis and prognosis), what are the current trends in it, and what future developments are possible.

Figure 1. Broad Spectrum of AI Applications in Healthcare

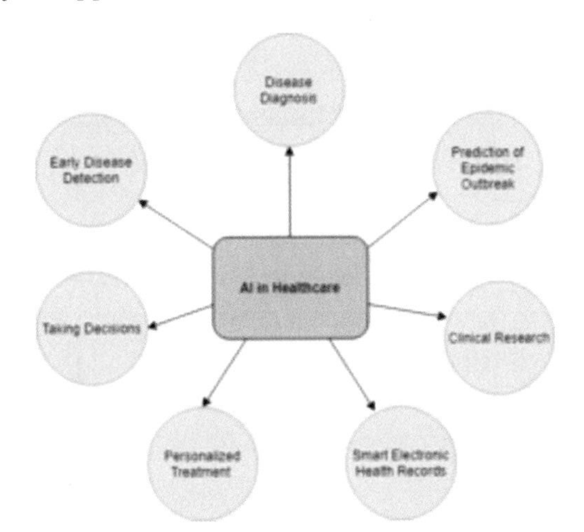

The key element of precision medicine to an explicit state of genetics is the identification of accurate biomarkers. To promote good and safe health for the communities, the screening and diagnosing of medical tests should be assessed and graded accurately. Recent years has seen an immense development in the prediction of the diagnostic and prognostic models, especially in the field of medicine.

Large scale clinical trials, data collection practices, cloud service providers and data storage capability are all accelerating the transformation of industry to the concept of a data-driven industry. Laterally with this transition, the growth of interest in biomarkers has led to the rise of deep learning methods. These methods allows the patient to mould diagnostic and prognostic choices for their treatment based on their specific features. The primary goal of the diagnostic and prognostic tools is to handle large amounts of data and their unique ability to distinguish between individuals with and without a well-defined condition. Deep learning models are able to produce good features in cases where there is a lack of understanding about the domain for feature engineering. In fact, the larger the data size, the better their performance. The training data plays a vital role in the selection of test data which results in the performance of the model. In machine learning terms, biomarker discovery depends on the collection of data sets for an enormous amount of individuals. This introduces the concept of feature selection based on the acquired data sets. The developed concept helps in the development of genome sequencing and other production of innovative technologies. The standard feature selection methods are commonly inadequate to process these data sets that encompasses more features than samples in order of magnitude. In the present day, failure of any component to the health monitoring system causes a major impact in the development of newer products. This threat is avoided by using robust diagnostic and prognostics technologies for accomplishing reliable and robust product availability for tomorrow's system environment. The newer products optimally lowers the operational cost and improvement of fault detection. Thereby the maintenance cost is reduced which results in greater efficiency of the products. The utmost perplexing issue to process the raw monitoring signal into information-rich features are solved through these developed products. These products helps our communities with safer and easier monitoring of good health. The major goal of these products helps to provide the accessibility at a reasonable cost and achieve in making precise health based decisions in real time environment avoiding catastrophic failures.

ARTIFICIAL INTELLIGENCE IN HEALTHCARE

Personalized healthcare is the next big step in the medical industry using technology. The rapid research and development in the field of AI, Machine Learning and data science has made the fusion of technology and medical science very smooth. The improvisation in the field of healthcare using the latest technologies and sensors also involves lowering the associated cost. It is now possible for individuals to track the human body's basic vitals such as blood pressure levels, heartrate, oxygen levels at the comfort of their home by making use of smart wearable devices that are available in the market. The integration of cloud computing technology with AI has made it possible to directly upload the patient's record onto the cloud servers which can be stored safely. This eliminates a lot of paper work and the hassle of safely maintaining the health records from the patient's side. Tracking every single detail of the patient's history is important for performing the correct diagnosis and prognosis of a disease.

Figure 2. AI in Digital Healthcare

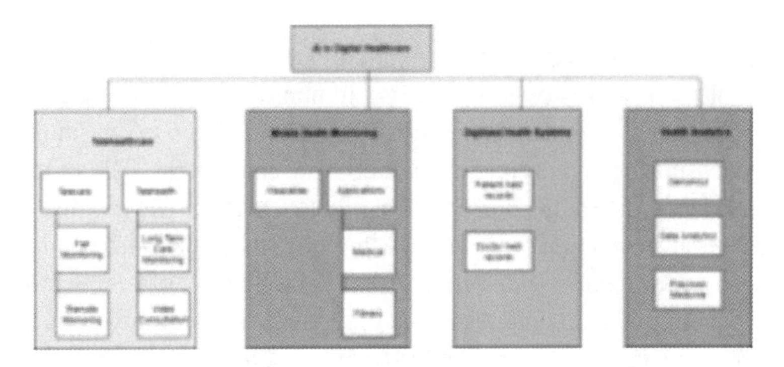

The Figure 2 discusses about the applications of AI in digital healthcare with respect to various divisons.With the advancement in the field of sensors, there is an increase in the use of robotic nurses that help to monitor the patient's health condition in a timely manner even in the absence of a physical practitioner. Accurate and automated diagnosis of the predicted disease, monitoring and treatment of remote patients, surgeries involving robots, online counselling for patients with psychiatry problems such as depression, anxiety and other mental health conditions are all covered under AI healthcare 5.0 i.e. implementing these using 5G mode of communication. Control, management and handling the various modules of a hospital management system on a unified platform remotely is the concept of the smart healthcare. This involves a chain of transactions right from the patient's OPD visit, to his admission and operation, pathological tests to discharge summary, where all the entities involved are treated as software units such as administrator, nurse, surgeon, front desk, accounts, and patient which are interconnected and in turn controlled by a main controller. The diagnosis of the patient's abnormalities by the pathologists and practitioners from the various sources such as images of scan reports, X-rays can be done quickly and accurately with the aid of AI algorithms. The AI algorithms have the capacity to analyse the huge data sets in shorter time that can further accelerate the patient's treatment. Other than these, the integration of AI with Internet of Things (IoT) can help in the implementation of smart blood banks and smart waste management.

APPLICATIONS AND ADVANTAGES

At the beginning of 1970s, conventional instruments like the flow became evident. Charts, trends and theorem of Bayes did not address most complex clinical problems. From the study, researchers could program and derive a cognitive phenomenon that has computational model which can be converted into Artificial Intelligence Programs. AI's applications are vast and its contribution in healthcare domain is tremendous. Artificial Intelligence (AI) can assist diagnosis and prognosis with higher degree of accuracy when compared to traditional models/ approaches. Such programs determine for every disease probable (diagnosis), whether it is to be expected the results given, recognize illness (diagnosis) a variety of findings that were required and rank the diseases in order with respect to their scores. To test the computational limits of AI, it proved to be diagnosing multiple disorders with multiple constraints. Therefore, such programs will reduce the number of diagnostic possibilities easily, using pathophysiological rationale effectively, and modelling of a particular patient's disease can be developed. The complexities generated by these models may interacting and overlapping by many diseases.

AI plays a vital role in fault detection and diagnosis. Perhaps, prognosis has also gained lesser attention in AI community because it's considered as a game-change technology to push machine safety boundaries administration. For healthcare equipment's, diagnosis are specified to include failure and fault isolation Identification, so that full diagnosis requires determination. The specific fault mode, not just the reporting mode, the sensor has an extraordinary value. The prognosis that the precursors of failure will be detected and that a lot of time will remain before a possible failure. The outlook for all these projects is the worst. Until you can treat them, you must be able to identify faults. In the same way, before performing prognosis, it should be able to diagnose the faults.

A method of AI that's very useful in prognosis is Fuzzy logic, when collaborated with machine learning method can lead to successful estimation in representing and managing the uncertainties. Prognosis is an important clinical skill, particularly for cancer patients' clinicians, neuro –oncology and many more. One of the biggest challenge for AI in prognosis is to verify and validate its models. Unlike diagnosis, the prognosis models are centered on predictive data that usually addresses the patient and not the disease or treatment. Prognosis models were developed to aid in the decision-making of patients' treatment. Thus, AI can have bigger impact in the health care domain with more healthcare providers using AI to make the first diagnosis and prognosis more accurate and interpretable with the available patient data for better therapy.

'Health is Wealth' as the saying goes, there is no denial on the importance of it in one's life. Considering its importance, much of the emphasis has been laid on research in the field of health sciences. With the advancements in the field of artificial intelligence and machine learning, most of the work is now carried out with the aid of tools or software developed using the same. The main reason why abundant research can be carried out in health sciences is because of abundance of data that is available. Earlier the doctors used to prescribe the same medicines to the patients who had similar symptoms and diagnosed with same ailments or diseases. However, it was observed that only a few patients recovered with those medicines. This baffled the physicians as they wondered why this happened. The AI based algorithms helped the physicians make a breakthrough in this area, where they aid the physicians to do diagnosis and provide the suitable treatments on an individual level. This is achieved as AI algorithms are able to identify specific patterns from wide variety of data sources that are available thereby providing insights that a human could not do (Paranjape et al., 2020). There are two broad applications of AI in healthcare. They can be classified as follows:-

i. Application of the AI algorithms to build healthcare products, devices and services.
ii. Use of AI algorithms to build cognitive systems that is able to understand a physician's abilities to do the tasks better than a physician.

The cognitive abilities include image recognition, face recognition, speech recognition, and natural language processing among other pattern recognition techniques. The main aim for the software developers who are developing the AI based projects is to develop algorithms that can behave and think rationally like a person (Shneiderman, 2020). There are variety of chronic disorders for which AI algorithms based personalized care is available today. Most popular ones include Parkinson's, Kidney Disorders, Oncology, Cardiovascular diseases and diabetes.

IMPORTANCE OF AI ALGORITHMS IN DISEASE DIAGNOSIS AND TREATMENT

The AI algorithms can help the health care industry do better than what it is doing right now in the following ways:-

i. Patient's DNA data, medical history along with his/her lifestyle and the current medical trends can be applied to provide personalized healthcare.
ii. Delay in disease progression and early detection and prevention of the chronic diseases.
iii. Individual patient needs understanding, medical treatments and treatment effectiveness on a day to day basis (Knickerbocker, Budd, Dang, Chen, Colgan, Hung, & Wen, 2018).

The AI and machine learning algorithms are widely used in the prediction of cancer given the current medical conditions. AI and machine learning algorithms are excellent at handling data whether labelled or unlabeled. Diagnosis of cancer is a challenging task in artificial intelligence domain. The classification of the available data whether he is a healthy person or not is completely based on the oncologist's expert advice and experience. Among all the cancers in women resulting in death, breast cancer is the second main reason. The exact cause of breast cancer isn't known. It mainly affects elderly women. Sufficient advancements have been made in the field of AI especially with regards to breast cancer prediction, that these algorithms are widely used in removing any human errors during screening process. Both supervised and unsupervised learning algorithms can be applied on the breast cancer datasets. Artificial Neural Network (ANN) can also be used in the task of breast cancer diagnosis. Many data repositories are available for the purpose of breast cancer research. One of the widely used repository is Wisconsin cancer database. Deep learning algorithms are used for classification of breast cancer in a good way. Prevention of the breast cancer by prediction is an efficient way of mitigating the disease. This can be achieved by using feature selection algorithms. A wrapper method is used where Bayesian classifier is merged with feature selection to provide a framework for prediction with good accuracy. Recursive feature selection algorithm can be used to further enhance the accuracy compared to the feature selection algorithm. For accurate detection of cancer cells in people, a hybrid model consisting of Recursive Feature Elimination and Support Vector Machine is employed. Another hybrid algorithm that is widely used for diagnosis of breast cancer is Extreme Learning Machine classification algorithm with Deep Belief Network. This algorithm is used in the extraction of the data from the breast cancer cells. Gradient boosting decision tree and multi-verse optimizer AI algorithms can be combined to classify the cancer into two groups namely malignant and benign. The other breast cancer datasets that are widely used for research are Surveillance, Epidemiology and End Results, Wisconsin Original Breast Cancer and Wisconsin Diagnostic Breast Cancer. AI algorithms such as cost sensitive support vector machine and genetic algorithm wrapper are also used in the detection of the false negatives during classification. These algorithms are used to reduce the error involved in classification of false negatives when compared with the false positives. Fast Correlation Based Feature is used in improving the quality of the classification by eliminating the repeating features (Rafi et al., 2021).

Figure 3. Application of AI Algorithms to Medical Datasets

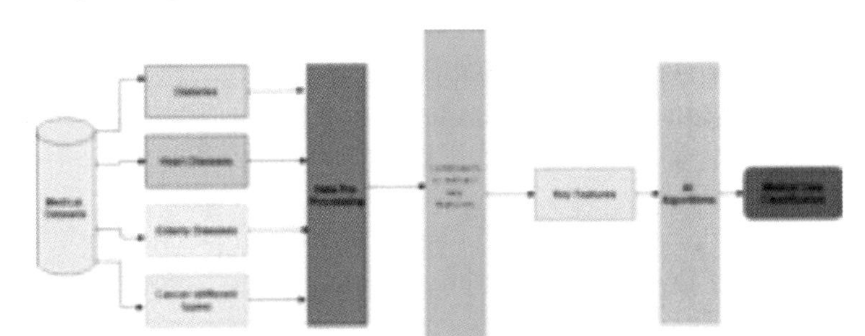

The Figure 3 discusses how the AI algorithms are applied to the various medical datasets for research. Cardiovascular diseases include wide range of diseases heart attack, Arrhythmia, Heart Valve Complications and Heart Failure. Using AI algorithms for prediction and training of heart patients is essential for the right diagnosis to be done by the doctors. Support Vector Machines, Random Forest, Random Under Sampling Boosting, Convolutional Neural Network are some of the AI algorithms that are applied on the patient's cardiovascular data (Alkhodari et al., 2021). Multiple applications are created for wearable devices using AI, ML and IoT technologies. These applications are used to monitor the cardiovascular activities such as heart rate among many others. AI algorithms is also used in robot assisted cardiac surgeries. Such surgeries are no more in theory and already in practice. Shorter duration of hospitalization is one of the main advantages of such operations performed by an AI empowered robot. AI algorithms can be combined with IoT and big data analytics thereby enabling in prediction of heart attacks in patients prior to the occurrence allowing the physicians to take appropriate measures on time. Some of the commonly used wearable IoT devices to assist in the mentioned tasks include earbuds, headband, glasses, camera clips, sensor patches, tablets, smart phones, wrist band, and smartwatch, embedded sensors in shoes, belts and clothes (Firouzi et al., 2020).

The robot nurses are widely used, to monitor and record the patient's health condition in the absence of an actual physician. Using such AI enabled nurses, real time data can be sent to the doctors to take appropriate actions in case of any need or emergency. IBM's Watson treatment recommendation made towards cancer patients had 99% accuracy and was in alignment of that of tumor board's recommendations. This study was conducted on a total of 1000 patients. The Watson had also made some recommendations based on which clinical actions had to be taken by the oncologists. The oncologists also say that such insights couldn't be obtained without the help of AI enabled Watson (Knickerbocker, Budd, Dang, Chen, Colgan, Hung, & Wen, 2018).

Given the fact that health is a very sensitive issue, integration of AI with healthcare should be done in such a way so that there will be accountability. This is possible with the aid of explainable AI. These are used to provide justifications for the results obtained using the AI models and the corresponding predictions made. The use of explainable AI has the following benefits when the applications of AI models in healthcare is explained to the stakeholders (Pawar et al., 2020):

i. Improvement in the models: Data is the powerhouse for the AI models, this data is used in the learning of the AI models to make predictions. The rules generated can be learnt using the XAI methods. This helps in identifying the errors in the predictions made so that it can be identified and eliminated thereby improvising the model.
ii. Tracing of the results generated: What factors resulted in obtaining an outcome by the AI system, can be traced back to the source using the XAI.
iii. Enhanced Transparency: Increased levels of trust from the stakeholders can be achieved as every decision taken can be explained using the XAI methods.

House call for the doctors or medical practitioners had been in practice for a very long time a few years ago. However, since the COVID-19 pandemic the medical field has revolutionized itself in order to adapt to the demanding changes. The requirement of maintaining social distancing has been the top most priority to avoid the spread of the infection. There are still a large number of extremely sick and elderly patients in our country who cannot make it to the hospital on their own and need house call assistance. On the other hand, among other patients who are not so sick, house calls can still be a good idea considering that many people hesitate to step out of the house to visit the hospital to avoid the risk of contracting COVID-19. The next major step that needs to be carried out by the hospitals is to decide whom to prioritize for the house call treatments among numerous calls they receive on a daily basis. This also implies growing data volumes of the patients along with combinatorics that needs to be considered. The AI models using optimization techniques can be used to solve the issue stated above by helping the hospitals in prioritizing the patients list for house calls. Various attributes are taking into consideration for making a decision such as the patient's ID, any major medications that the patient is already taking, the number of days that passed since the last hospitalization, type of medical incidence, any allergic conditions, any seasonal allergies to take proactive measures, patient's address, major drugs induced to the patients in the last week (Vuppalapati et al., 2020).

The AI models are also widely used in the prediction and modelling of the COVID-19 outbreak. It has been used to model and make predictions regarding the outbreak, treatment using the data available. The main challenge in the healthcare domain is the privacy concerns. Most of the organizations hesitate to share the patient's COVID related data for storage. Hence, there is a need to build a robust AI model that uses the real time patient data. Another challenge is building of a generalized prediction model that says one model fits all. The solution to the above problem can be obtained by combining blockchain technology with AI. The security concern can be handled using the blockchain technology. Abundance of promising results have been obtained since the COVID-19 pandemic due to lot of data of the X-rays and CT scans of the chest and use cases that are available. The blockchain protects the data identity by using formalized contracts for data access (Aich et al., 2021).

The AI technology is used in the optimization of ultrasound image quality. The reason is that the quality of the ultra sound images obtained depends on the skill of the radiologist. This AI model learns from the experts who do ultrasound scans and makes appropriate predictions in line with that of a radiologist (Annangi et al., 2020).

APPLICATIONS OF AI

Though artificial intelligence (AI) existed several years before, it has advanced dramatically in the last ten years for medical applications, and is currently employed for therapeutic, diagnostic and prognostic purposes in practically all sectors. Despite the fact that AI's application in different domains of medicine has yielded promising outcomes (Pérez & Grande, 2020). Some of its applications have been discussed here.

Hepatocellular Carcinoma (HCC)

HCC is a highly prevalent type of tumour and AI has been used extensively to diagnose, treat and prognosis of various illnesses in hepatology. HCC has unique radiological characteristics that allow it to be diagnosed without a histological examination. As a result, imaging test analysis is particularly important because their interpretation is not always straightforward, and they fluctuate outlook changes throughout the course of the disease and treatment reaction, both of that are influenced through a variety of circumstances. All of this results in a massive amount of data that AI can investigate due to its integration and quick processing.

Figure 4. Hepatocellular carcinoma with AI

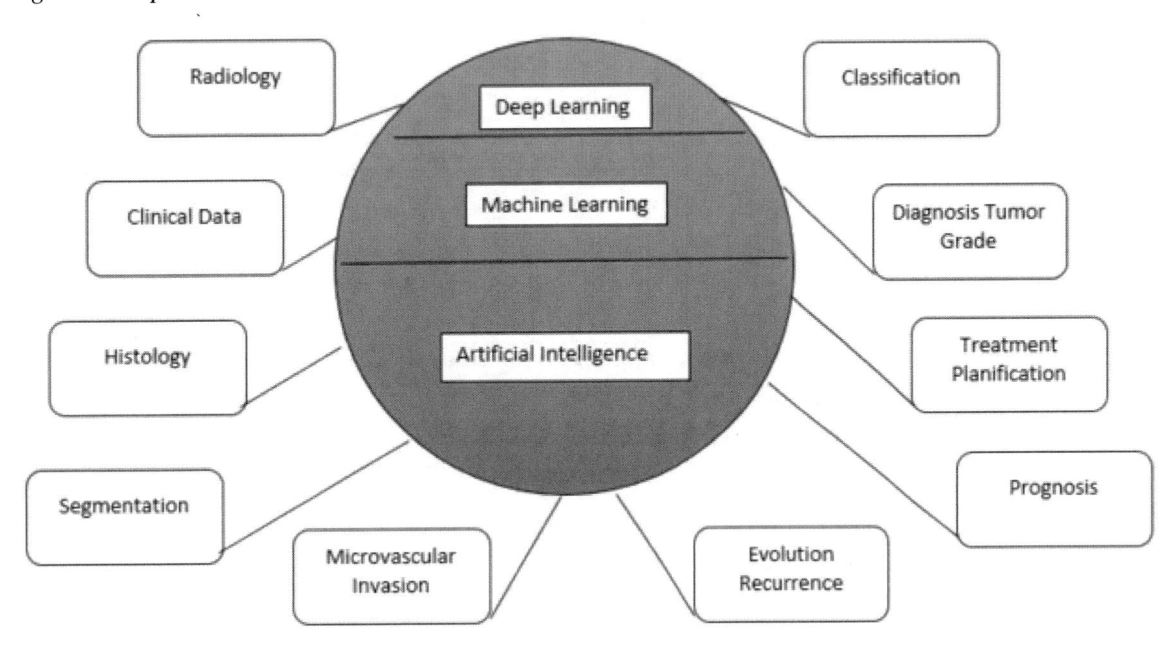

Figure 4 depicts how AI, in its various forms, can be used to look into a patient who has been diagnosed or suspected of having HCC. AI can incorporate clinical, radiological and histological data to generate data that can help with accurate diagnosis, tumour staging, and treatment planning utilizing segmentation approaches, and assessing the existence of microvascular invasion, as well as to provide estimate of prognosis (Pérez & Grande, 2020).

Breast Cancer

In recent years, AI, particularly machine learning and deep learning, has become increasingly prevalent in clinical research of cancer. Assumed its extraordinary precision level, that is even greater than the average for oncology statistical applications, AI is known to aid diagnosis and prognosis of cancer (Huang et al., 2020). Cancer is a disease that is aggressive the median survival rate is poor. Due of high recurrence and fatality rates, the treatment process is extensive and expensive. To improve the patient's survival percentage, accurate early cancer detection and prognostic prediction are critical (Huang et al., 2020). Breast cancer diagnosis and prognosis is common with the use of Artificial Neural Network (ANN). They've been utilized to forecast the prognosis of breast cancer patients. They can be used to analyse complex data in order to anticipate medical outcomes. Genetic Algorithms (GA), Evolutionary Algorithms such as Extreme Programming (EP), and Evolutionary Strategies (ES) have all been effectively employed in the selection of effective features for the classification of mammographic micro-calcifications for breast cancer diagnosis. Even fuzzy logics based on member functions are employed in the diagnosis and prognosis of breast cancer (Jain et al., 2000).

Sepsis

Sepsis is a dangerous illness that requires early detection and treatment are critical in lowering death rates. The majority of the papers included in the review focused on AI algorithms that can forecast whether or not a patient has sepsis or will progress this one in the future are being developed. Due to disease's complex pathogenesis and the variability of sepsis and the absence of reliable diagnostic tools, detecting sepsis in its early stages is challenging. AI can be used to extract data from a wide range of sources. To predict the intended outcome measures, algorithms practice clinical data, laboratory findings, patient's medical history, demographics, and clinical findings environment. Furthermore, real-time data streams are becoming more popular. The benefit of AI models is their immediate usefulness, especially when they are based solely on critical criteria. In circumstances where clinicians have yet to arrive considered to diagnose sepsis, an algorithm can raise alarms (Schinkel et al., 2019).

On prognosis, AI aids in the prediction of death in ICU and emergency department populations at various times in time. Models with AUROC values ranging from 0.79 to 0.90. These results are equivalent to commonly used APACHE-II score that has an AUROC of 0.8354. Some individuals who are not initially diagnosed with sepsis may experience a quick decline and a high risk of death. Antibiotics could provide a significant benefit to these people. Clinicians would benefit greatly from an AI strategy that might forecast these elevated death rates for specific patients (Schinkel et al., 2019).

Neuro-Oncology

Other CNS cancers, including CNS lymphoma and brain metastases, have seen the application of machine learning technologies, with the possibility to explain diagnostic difficult circumstances and increase workflow speed and precision. Image-processing techniques like three-dimensional template matching remained initially employed to identify and restrict brain metastases. Current research using three-dimensional CNNs shows collective potential, by the capability to aid in the planning of stereotactic radiation therapy. In several cases, available clinical and imaging paradigms make it impossible to distinguish between glioblastoma, brain metastases and primary CNS lymphoma (Rudie et al., 2019).

To solve this issue, decision tree and multivariate logistic regression model were used in dynamic susceptibility and diffusion tensor imaging to distinguish between these three entities, -weighted contrast-enhanced MRI measurements from the augmenting area were taken. Additional work used random forest analysis on collected radiomic texture and wavelet data to differentiate nonnarcotic glioblastoma from CNS cancer, outperforming three human readers. It is not uncommon for patients to be discovered to suffer from brain metastases with no recognized primary site. AIML methods can be useful to solve this scientific situation (Rudie et al., 2019).

Mental Disorders

Since it gives brain biomarkers, mental diseases prognosis and diagnosis is done by electroencephalography (EEG). Due to the intricacy of EEG signals, only highly qualified professionals can interpret them. The fundamental benefit of using DL to process EEG data is that, unlike standard machine learning algorithms, it can handle raw EEG data since it conducts Feature Engineering (FE) automatically. When creating a hand-crafted FE is not possible, an automatic FE can mine novel information from the raw data, improving the result in classification. Even if a large amount of data is not accessible, DL can still be used because pre-trained networks are used (Rivera et al., 2021).

Alzheimer's

Alzheimer's disease (AD) is the most common form of dementia, as well as one of the major causes of death in those over the age of 65. At present, no medication available to delay or stopover the development of AD. There is a growing consensus that disease-modifying therapy must prioritize the disease's initial phases, such as Moderate Cognitive Impairment (MCI) and pre-clinical stages. Creating an AD diagnosis and providing a prognosis in these primary stages are difficult jobs, but they are likely with the assistance of multi-modality imaging like MRI, FDG-PET, amyloid-PET, and the newly presented tau-PET, that provide dissimilar but opposite information. Statistical artificial intelligence approaches are widely used to do quantifiable analysis of multi-modality at the MCI or preclinical phases of Alzheimer's disease, picture data can be used to diagnose and predict prognosis. (Liu et al., 2018).

AD diagnosis in its initial stages necessitates pathological confirmation using renowned norms such as the NIA-AA criteria. Prognosis is equally crucial to diagnosis because it entails the quantification of illness development, such as estimating the time until dementia onset or predicting change within a specific period. A substantial quantity of present research emphases on forecasting MCI adaptation to AD (Liu et al., 2018).

Classic machine learning algorithms are still the most often employed methodology in current research. Despite its ubiquity in other fields of computer vision, DL-based algorithms take only been used to initial AD diagnosis and prognosis utilizing multi-modality imaging. Support vector machine, Multiple Kernel Learning, Random forest method are extensively used (Liu et al., 2018). New technologies these days have made it easier to work in every field especially in healthcare. Healthcare is one of the fields where technology is making new advancements every time. Recasting in healthcare such as using sensors and doing data analysis with healthcare. Due to these techniques we are able to detect all the chronic diseases at a very early stage.

Advancements in healthcare such as using sensors and analyzing situations is trending. Here, in this paper we have discussed about new technologies such as heterogeneous technology and tools that provide electronics for diagnosis and sensors. Data supports AI to give guidance in healthcare and gives solutions for patients and clients (Knickerbocker, 2018).

Examples of new technologies are as suppose:

i. Precision handling of components, sub components.
ii. Laser Micro component.

Figure 5. Artificial Intelligence in Healthcare

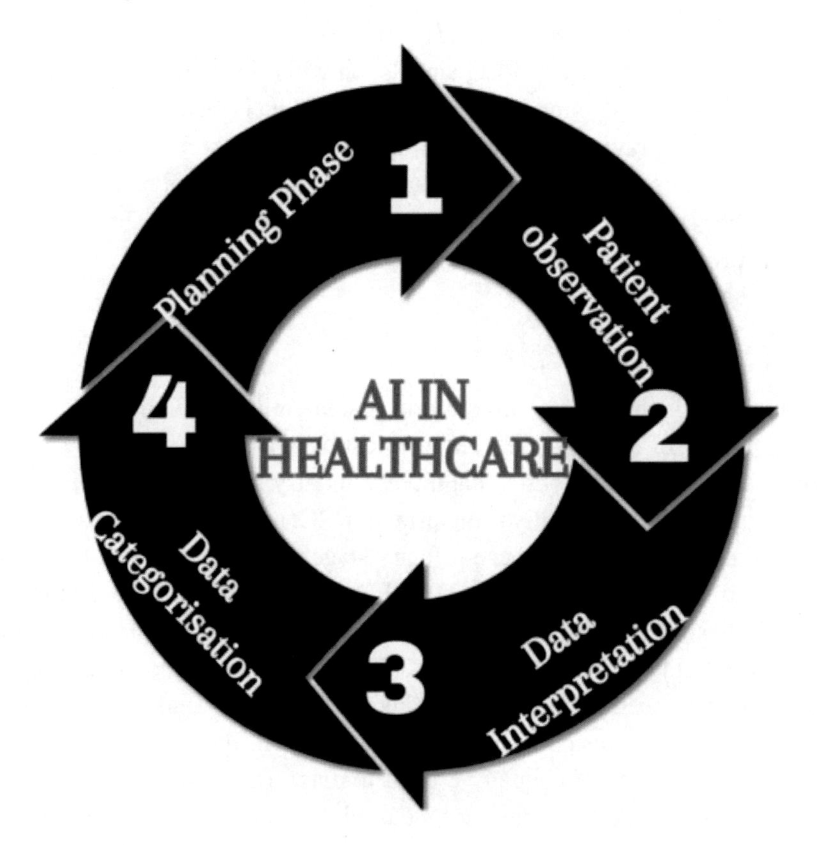

The figure 5 depicts the application of artificial intelligence in healthcare. A lot of research work is going on for the diagnostics, modeling and artificial intelligence. Healthcare technologies have also advanced to now be able to track population health and management tools (Tawalbeh & Habeeb, 2018). Using the AI-Blockchain EHR management system we can, use it for well-organized data integration (Wehbe et al., 2018). The changes in healthcare are constant. Defining the mechanisms is difficult but it gives positive responses for healthcare systems and medical research. Privacy is one of the prime concerns in medical research and there is also always a threat of data leaking. With all these problems, there are also a lot of challenges faced in large infrastructure disparities in field (Mohanta, 2019). Healthcare data is one of the primary sources of information for medical research. The main aim of this research is to study the requirements for AIBlockchain HER management framework. The blockchain in healthcare has been growing consistently. For a better analysis of human tumors, researchers are studying single cell composition such as mass cytometry along with computation which is known as CellCycleTRACER (Wehbe et al., 2018).

Figure 6. Applications of Blockchain in Healthcare

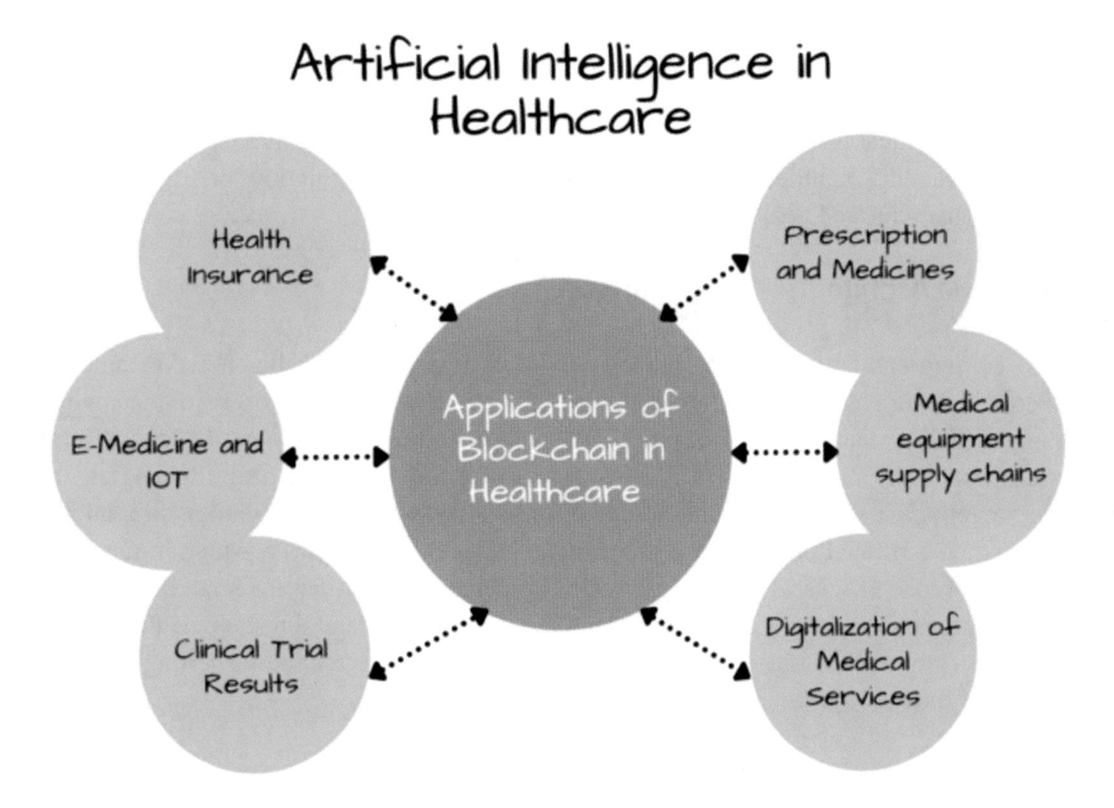

The figure 6 discusses how blockchain and different security aspects of blockchain is important for healthcare. At later times, mobile computing will become an essential part of our lives in healthcare systems as it will play a very important role as an interface between the patients and the doctors or organizations (Tyrväinen et al., 2018). Some disadvantages in this will be of very less battery lifetime and less storage space. Cloud computing framework mainly is dependent on network based sharing. There are new technologies coming up every day such as mobile computing, cloud computing and wireless communications. Some of the most popular examples of cloud computing are Google and Microsoft changing people's lives (Le Nguyen & Do, 2019). The healthcare field is undergoing a lot of changes due to growth in technology. The most beneficial advancement in healthcare is of the visibility of epidemiology in advance. We can say now that the near future approaching us can be more powerfully analysed. AI devices like smartphones, tablets, and laptops are helping the doctors and the health workers in a drastic manner (Lee et al., 2018). The main objective of introducing Ai in healthcare is due to certain reasons such as reduced costs in healthcare that makes it affordable and accessible for people in today's world. Using advanced machines and technologies to solve the complexities of diseases that occur and analyse the reason behind it (Soni et al., 2019).

Artificial Intelligence (AI) will make revolutionary changes in the utilization of medicine and alter the delivery of healthcare. The healthcare industry is developing drastically with the use of Artificial Intelligence and Machine Learning Algorithms. The technologies developed using Artificial Intelligence can forecast, detect, gain an understanding of the mechanism and function as required, whether it's employed to recognize association between genes or to control surgery-assisting robots. AI is used in early detection of various diseases, in drug discovery, in clinical trials, in maternal care, healthcare robotics and many more. Early diagnosis of numerous diseases by artificial intelligence helps in early commencement of the treatment for it, which reduces the spread of the disease, and hence, provides the patient with a better quality of life, which in turn brings down the economic burden involved in healthcare management (Manne & Kantheti, 2021). Here are some of the implementations of artificial intelligence in the field of medicine and healthcare.

Most used AI Architecture in Healthcare

Machine Learning and Deep Learning are the subgroup of Artificial Intelligence. Machine Learning refers to training a device to learn certain technologies. Deep learning refers to a set of machine learning algorithms, which are inspired by processing information and distributed communication in network of neurons (Amann et al., 2020). Neural network is one of the most used deep learning algorithm in healthcare automation. Neural networks basically imitate the way the way neurons in a human brain signal one other. Artificial Neural Networks are comprises of a node layer, which in turn comprises of an input layer, one or several hidden layers, and finally an output layer. Each node is also known as artificial neuron, attaches to one more neuron and has a linked load and threshold. If the output of any discrete node is greater than the set threshold value, that node is triggered, transporting data to the following layer of the network (Shaheen, 2021).

AI in Medicine

According to the newest research in AI, Machine Learning the subcategory of AI helps in generating personalized medicine by studying the reports of the patient and also by recognizing the trends in the medical history of the patient. AI and Machine Learning algorithms are also helpful in treating chronic diseases like cancer. Machine learning algorithms can be used to increase our interpretation of important genomic progression in lung cancer. One of the main reason in the triumph of AI for lung cancer is that many molecular irregularities have already been discovered, such as mutations in the skin epiderm tissue growth (Bartoletti, 2019).

AI for Clinical Trials

A clinical trial is a process in which freshly implemented treatments are given to the volunteers to test how effective they are. This process takes a significant amount of time, money and effort. The success rate, however, is quite low. The automation of clinical trials has proved to be a beneficial for AI and the healthcare business (Kaushik et al., 2020).

Challenges In AI

Absence of sufficient explanations of AI algorithms brings about some resistance by the medical fraternity. The algorithms which have a greater accuracy, such as neural networks and deep learning, require less explanations. Due to the "black box" phenomenon (algorithms whose inputs and operations are not visible to the user) healthcare professionals find it difficult to get used to working of the AI algorithms and trusting the accuracy of the algorithm. In the end, it becomes necessary for the medical staff to know verify the algorithm and trust its accuracy to use the automated healthcare technologies using AI on patients. Developers of these technologies will have to take this into account and prioritize both understandable and accurate.

As intellectuals predicted and researchers have already proved, we are entering an era of global artificial intelligence (AI) convergence. AI technology is getting more popular in a variety of fields, including health care. Artificial intelligence is also widely used and developed in the field of medical health, especially in areas such as health management, healthcare administrators, medical imaging, risk management, and so on. Rare diseases, which have a low incidence of occurrence, pose a serious threat to people's health such as haemophilia. They have a prevalence rate of less than 1/500000, as well as disorders with an incidence rate of less than 1/10000 in neonates. Therefore, gene sequencing is required to scientifically and successfully prevent and diagnose "rare diseases" (Fu, 2019). The concept of "precision medicine" has been developed. It's a type of medical treatment that relies on genes, genomes, and detection. It's also a method of disease detection and treatment, as well as a promising future medical direction. Gene detection is the process of extracting scientific and useful information from large amounts of data using a decoding approach (Fu, 2019) (Sasubilli & Kumar, 2020). It is currently very difficult to extract scientific and effective information from gene sequences since most of the decoding and recording of high-throughput sequencing technology is tough to complete gene interpretation. Simultaneously, artificial intelligence technologies can significantly improve the current scenario. The accuracy of the case data testing model is increased by using the initial mathematical model and introducing the full genome sequence and RNA sequence of healthy human beings into the model for training (Fu, 2019) (Augusto, 2020) (Cheng, 2019).

Furthermore, a smart dental gadget is created and built to do tooth image acquisition. According to various researches conducted, the prototype model collected 12, 600 clinical images from 10 private dental clinics and developed an automatic diagnosis model based on MASK R-CNN technique to determine and classify seven different dental diseases, including dental plaque, decayed teeth, fluorosis, and periodontal disease, with a diagnosis accuracy of up to 90% as shown in the Figure 7 (Liu et al., 2020).

Figure 7. Dental image analysis system flow using MASK R-CNN

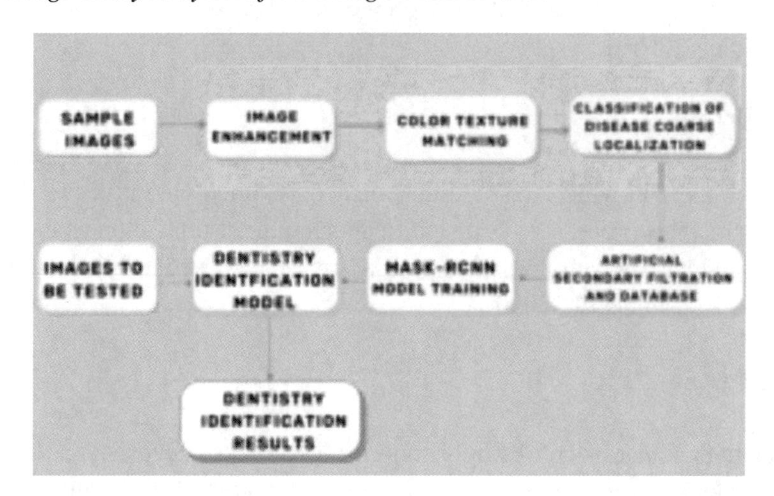

The most significant aspect of the intelligent dental Health-IoT platform is AI identification of dental disorders, and the major steps are shown in Figure 7. To achieve this purpose, the dental image improvement comparison chart includes the collecting of tooth cases photos, the creation of a sample set, and model training (Liu et al., 2020) (Cheng, 2019). The COVID-19 pandemic has caused havoc on the health of people all across the world. It has become a threat to mankind. COVID-19 has put the entire planet in a tough situation, suspending life and killing thousands of people all over the world. To solve COVID-19 pandemic problems that are affecting human health there are some of the AI- based approaches. The following describes those approaches:

The data must first be prepared for data mining, which is required for data interpretation, data preparation, and big data. Medical data, such as clinical reports, records, pictures, and other documents that can be converted into data that can be utilised to make choices, is the subject of this discussion. Understanding Data Objectives, data attributes, and identifying key data sources are just a few examples (Jamshidi et al., 2020) (Pham et al., 2020).

In addition, Deep Learning (DL) approaches could be employed in circumstances where huge or sophisticated data processing challenges machine learning (ML) or conventional data processing methods, such as data volume and total number of variables to summarize the data (Jamshidi et al., 2020). ANNs are employed in the diagnosis and tracing of symptoms at five levels as shown in Figure 8. Different AI-based solutions for assessing COVID-19-related infection concerns, such as high-risk patients, outbreak control, identifying, and imaging, were developed using RNN, LSTM, GAN, and ELM algorithms (Jamshidi et al., 2020) (Pham et al., 2020).

Using large-scale data from COVID-19 patients, advanced machine learning algorithms can assist researchers in better understanding the virus's spread pattern, increasing the speed and accuracy of diagnosis, discovering novel, successful therapy techniques, and even identifying individuals who are most susceptible to the disease based on their genetic and physiological traits are all goals (Jamshidi et al., 2020) (Sasubilli & Kumar, 2020).

Figure 8. Flowchart for applications of ANNs in diagnosis and tracing the symptoms in 5 layers

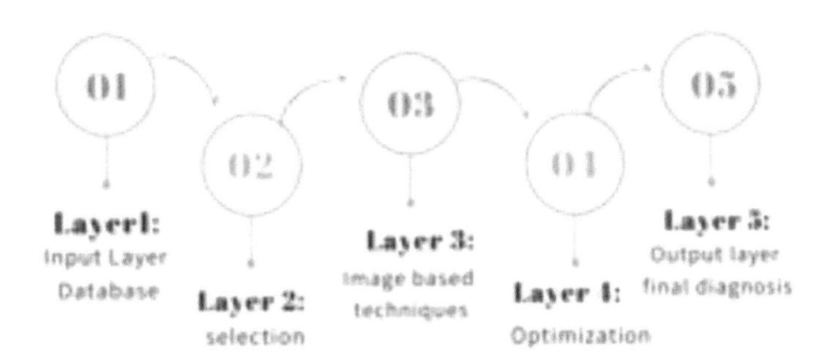

CONCLUSION

The AI along with the other machine learning algorithms has revolutionized the entire healthcare industry. From the small mobile applications that connects the patients to the doctors who is located globally, online consultations and even remote operations AI empowers both the patients and medical practitioners. The chapter here discusses all the different applications of AI in medical field including the latest COVID-19 pandemic. From this we can observe that the AI and related technologies are able to rapidly evolve to fit the current day medical needs. With so much advancement in the field of medicine and technology, there is much more scope for research in the years to come.

REFERENCES

Aich, S., Sinai, N. K., Kumar, S., Ali, M., Choi, Y. R., Joo, M. I., & Kim, H. C. (2021, February). Protecting Personal Healthcare Record Using Blockchain & Federated Learning Technologies. In 2021 23rd International Conference on Advanced Communication Technology (ICACT) (pp. 109-112). IEEE. 10.23919/ICACT51234.2021.9370566

Alkhodari, M., Rashid, M., Mukit, M. A., Ahmed, K. I., Mostafa, R., Parveen, S., & Khandoker, A. H. (2021). Screening cardiovascular autonomic neuropathy in diabetic patients with microvascular complications using machine learning: a 24-hour heart rate variability study. IEEE Access.

Amann, J., Blasimme, A., Vayena, E., Frey, D., & Madai, V. I. (2020). Explainability for artificial intelligence in healthcare: A multidisciplinary perspective. *BMC Medical Informatics and Decision Making*, *20*(1), 1–9. doi:10.118612911-020-01332-6 PMID:33256715

Annangi, P., Ravishankar, H., Patil, R., Tore, B., Aase, S. A., & Steen, E. (2020, September). AI assisted feedback system for transmit parameter optimization in Cardiac Ultrasound. In *2020 IEEE International Ultrasonics Symposium (IUS)* (pp. 1-4). IEEE. 10.1109/IUS46767.2020.9251501

Augusto, C., & … . "Test-Driven Anonymization in Health Data: A Case Study on Assistive Reproduction," *2020 IEEE International Conference On Artificial Intelligence Testing (AITest)*, 2020, pp. 81-82, 10.1109/AITEST49225.2020.00019

Bartoletti, I. "AI in healthcare: Ethical and privacy challenges." *Conference on Artificial Intelligence in Medicine in Europe*. Springer, Cham, 2019. 10.1007/978-3-030-21642-9_2

Cheng, Y. "A Development Architecture for the Intelligent Animal Care and Management System Based on the Internet of Things and Artificial Intelligence," 2019 International Conference on Artificial Intelligence in Information and Communication (ICAIIC), 2019, pp. 078-081, 10.1109/ICAIIC.2019.8669015

Firouzi, F., Farahani, B., Barzegari, M., & Daneshmand, M. (2020). Ai-driven data monetization: The other face of data in iot-based smart and connected health. *IEEE Internet of Things Journal*.

Fu, X. "Application of Artificial Intelligence Technology in Medical Cell Biology," *2019 International Conference on Robots & Intelligent System (ICRIS)*, 2019, pp. 401-404, 10.1109/ICRIS.2019.00106

Huang, S., Yang, J., Fong, S., & Zhao, Q. (2020). Artificial intelligence in cancer diagnosis and prognosis: Opportunities and challenges. *Cancer Letters*, *471*, 61–71. doi:10.1016/j.canlet.2019.12.007 PMID:31830558

Jain, A., Jain, A., & Jain, S. (2000). *Artificial intelligence techniques in breast cancer diagnosis and prognosis* (Vol. 39). World Scientific. doi:10.1142/4484

Jamshidi, M., Lalbakhsh, A., Talla, J., Peroutka, Z., Hadjilooei, F., Lalbakhsh, P., Jamshidi, M., Spada, L. L., Mirmozafari, M., Dehghani, M., Sabet, A., Roshani, S., Roshani, S., Bayat-Makou, N., Mohamadzade, B., Malek, Z., Jamshidi, A., Kiani, S., Hashemi-Dezaki, H., & Mohyuddin, W. (2020). Artificial Intelligence and COVID-19: Deep Learning Approaches for Diagnosis and Treatment. *IEEE Access: Practical Innovations, Open Solutions*, *8*, 109581–109595. doi:10.1109/ACCESS.2020.3001973 PMID:34192103

Kaushik, S., Choudhury, A., Sheron, P.K., Dasgupta, N., Natarajan, S., Pickett, L.A. and Dutt, V., 2020. AI in healthcare: time-series forecasting using statistical, neural, and ensemble architectures. Frontiers in big data, 3, p.4.

Knickerbocker, J. U., ... "Heterogeneous Integration Technology Demonstrations for Future Healthcare, IoT, and AI Computing Solutions," 2018 IEEE 68th Electronic Components and Technology Conference (ECTC), 2018, pp. 15191528, 10.1109/ECTC.2018.00231

Knickerbocker, J. U., Budd, R., Dang, B., Chen, Q., Colgan, E., Hung, L. W., & Wen, B. (2018, May). Heterogeneous integration technology demonstrations for future healthcare, IoT, and AI computing solutions. In 2018 IEEE 68th electronic components and technology conference (ECTC) (pp. 1519-1528). IEEE.

Knickerbocker, J. U., Budd, R., Dang, B., Chen, Q., Colgan, E., Hung, L. W., . . . Wen, B. (2018, May). Heterogeneous integration technology demonstrations for future healthcare, IoT, and AI computing solutions. In 2018 IEEE 68th electronic components and technology conference (ECTC) (pp. 1519-1528). IEEE.

Lee, Y., Tsung, P., & Wu, M. "Techology trend of edge AI," 2018 International Symposium on VLSI Design, Automation and Test (VLSI-DAT), 2018, pp. 1-2, 10.1109/VLSI-DAT.2018.8373244

Le Nguyen, T., & Do, T. T. H. "Artificial Intelligence in Healthcare: A New Technology Benefit for Both Patients and Doctors," *2019 Portland International Conference on Management of Engineering and Technology (PICMET)*, 2019, pp. 1-15, 10.23919/PICMET.2019.8893884

Liu, L., Xu, J., Huan, Y., Zou, Z., Yeh, S.-C., & Zheng, L.-R. (2020, March). A Smart Dental Health-IoT Platform Based on Intelligent Hardware, Deep Learning, and Mobile Terminal. *IEEE Journal of Biomedical and Health Informatics*, *24*(3), 898–906. doi:10.1109/JBHI.2019.2919916 PMID:31180873

Liu, X., Chen, K., Wu, T., Weidman, D., Lure, F., & Li, J. (2018). Use of multimodality imaging and artificial intelligence for diagnosis and prognosis of early stages of Alzheimer's disease. *Translational Research; the Journal of Laboratory and Clinical Medicine*, *194*, 56–67. doi:10.1016/j.trsl.2018.01.001 PMID:29352978

Manne, R., & Kantheti, S. C. (2021). Application of artificial intelligence in healthcare: Chances and challenges. *Current Journal of Applied Science and Technology*, *40*(6), 78–89. doi:10.9734/cjast/2021/v40i631320

Mohanta, B., P. Das and S. Patnaik, "Healthcare 5.0: A Paradigm Shift in Digital Healthcare System Using Artificial Intelligence, IOT and 5G Communication," 2019 International Conference on Applied Machine Learning (ICAML), 2019, pp. 191-196, 10.1109/ICAML48257.2019.00044

Paranjape, K., Schinkel, M., & Nanayakkara, P. (2020). Short Keynote Paper: Mainstreaming Personalized Healthcare–Transforming Healthcare Through New Era of Artificial Intelligence. *IEEE Journal of Biomedical and Health Informatics*, *24*(7), 1860–1863. doi:10.1109/JBHI.2020.2970807 PMID:32054591

Pawar, U., O'Shea, D., Rea, S., & O'Reilly, R. (2020, June). Explainable ai in healthcare. In *2020 International Conference on Cyber Situational Awareness, Data Analytics and Assessment (CyberSA)* (pp. 1-2). IEEE.

Pham, Q.-V., Nguyen, D. C., Huynh-The, T., Hwang, W.-J., & Pathirana, P. N. (2020). Artificial Intelligence (AI) and Big Data for Coronavirus (COVID-19) Pandemic: A Survey on the State-of-the-Arts. *IEEE Access: Practical Innovations, Open Solutions*, *8*, 130820–130839. doi:10.1109/ACCESS.2020.3009328 PMID:34812339

Pérez, M. J., & Grande, R. G. (2020). Application of artificial intelligence in the diagnosis and treatment of hepatocellular carcinoma: A review. *World Journal of Gastroenterology*, *26*(37), 5617–5628. doi:10.3748/wjg.v26.i37.5617 PMID:33088156

Rafi, T. H., Shubair, R. M., Farhan, F., Hoque, M. Z., & Quayyum, F. M. (2021). Recent Advances in Computer-Aided Medical Diagnosis Using Machine Learning Algorithms with Optimization Techniques. *IEEE Access: Practical Innovations, Open Solutions*, *9*, 137847–137868. doi:10.1109/ACCESS.2021.3108892

Rivera, M. J., Teruel, M. A., Maté, A., & Trujillo, J. (2021). Diagnosis and prognosis of mental disorders by means of EEG and deep learning: A systematic mapping study. *Artificial Intelligence Review*, 1–43.

Rudie, J. D., Rauschecker, A. M., Bryan, R. N., Davatzikos, C., & Mohan, S. (2019). Emerging applications of artificial intelligence in neuro-oncology. *Radiology*, *290*(3), 607–618. doi:10.1148/radiol.2018181928 PMID:30667332

Sasubilli, G., & Kumar, A. "Machine Learning and Big Data Implementation on Health Care data," 2020 4th International Conference on Intelligent Computing and Control Systems (ICICCS), 2020, pp. 859-864, 10.1109/ICICCS48265.2020.9120906

Schinkel, M., Paranjape, K., Panday, R. N., Skyttberg, N., & Nanayakkara, P. W. (2019). Clinical applications of artificial intelligence in sepsis: A narrative review. *Computers in Biology and Medicine*, *115*, 103488. doi:10.1016/j.compbiomed.2019.103488 PMID:31634699

Shaheen, M. Y. (2021). *Applications of Artificial Intelligence (AI) in healthcare: A review*. ScienceOpen Preprints.

Shneiderman, B. (2020). Design lessons from AI's two grand goals: Human emulation and useful applications. *IEEE Transactions on Technology and Society*, *1*(2), 73–82. doi:10.1109/TTS.2020.2992669

Soni, R., Guan, J., Avinash, G., & Saripalli, V. R. "HMC: A Hybrid Reinforcement Learning Based Model Compression for Healthcare Applications," 2019 IEEE 15th International Conference on Automation Science and Engineering (CASE), 2019, pp. 146-151, 10.1109/COASE.2019.8843047

Tawalbeh, L. A., & Habeeb, S. "An Integrated Cloud Based Healthcare System," *2018 Fifth International Conference on Internet of Things: Systems, Management and Security*, 2018, pp. 268-273, 10.1109/IoTSMS.2018.8554648

Tyrväinen, P., Silvennoinen, M., Talvitie-Lamberg, K., Ala-Kitula, A., & Kuoremäki, R. "Identifying opportunities for AI applications in healthcare — Renewing the national healthcare and social services," 2018 IEEE 6th International Conference on Serious Games and Applications for Health (SeGAH), 2018, pp. 1-7, 10.1109/SeGAH.2018.8401381

Vuppalapati, C., Ilapakurti, A., Kedari, S., Vuppalapati, R., Vuppalapati, J., & Kedari, S. (2020, December). Stratification of, albeit Mathematical Optimization and Artificial Intelligent (AI) Driven, High-Risk Elderly Outpatients for priority house call visits-a framework to transform healthcare services from reactive to preventive. In 2020 IEEE International Conference on Big Data (Big Data) (pp. 4955-4960). IEEE.

Wehbe, Y., Zaabi, M. A., & Svetinovic, D. "Blockchain AI Framework for Healthcare Records Management: Constrained Goal Model," 2018 26th Telecommunications Forum (TELFOR), 2018, pp. 420-425, 10.1109/TELFOR.2018.8611900

Chapter 4
Appositeness of Digital Twins in Healthcare

Arjun Arora
UPES, India

Aditya Raj
UPES, India

Sarthak Srivastava
UPES, India

Sahil Bansal
UPES, India

ABSTRACT

Machine learning is a branch of artificial intelligence (AI) and computer science which focuses on the use of data and algorithms to imitate the way that humans learn, gradually improving its accuracy. Machine learning is a significant part of the developing field of information science. Using factual strategies, calculations are prepared to make characterizations or forecasts, revealing key experiences inside information mining projects. These bits of knowledge thusly drive decision making inside applications and organizations, preferably affecting key development measurements. As large information proceeds to extend and develop, the market interest for information researchers will increment, expecting them to aid the recognizable proof of the most significant business questions and accordingly the information to respond to them.

INTRODUCTION

Why is Machine Learning Important?

Machine learning is significant on the grounds that it provides ventures with a perspective on patterns in client conduct and business functional examples, as well as supports the improvement of new items. A considerable lot of the present driving organizations, for example, Facebook, Google and Uber, make AI a focal piece of their tasks. AI has turned into a critical cutthroat differentiator for some organizations (Zhang et al., 2020; An & Chen, 2021).

DOI: 10.4018/978-1-6684-5925-6.ch004

Some Machine Learning Methods

Machine learning algorithms are often categorized as supervised or unsupervised.

- **Supervised machine learning algorithms** calculations can apply what has been realized in the past to new information utilizing named guides to foresee future occasions. Beginning from the examination of a known preparation dataset, the learning calculation delivers an induced capacity to make forecasts regarding the result values. The framework can give focuses to any new contribution after adequate preparation. The learning calculation can likewise contrast its result and the right, expected result and track down mistakes to adjust the model appropriately.
- In contrast, **unsupervised machine learning algorithms** are utilized when the data used to prepare is neither grouped nor named. Solo learning concentrates on how frameworks can derive a capacity to depict a concealed design from unlabeled information. The situation doesn't sort out the right result, however it investigates the information and can attract deductions from datasets to portray concealed structures from unlabeled information.
- **Semi-supervised machine learning algorithms** fall some place in the middle of managed and solo learning, since they utilize both named and unlabeled information for preparing - normally a modest quantity of named information and a lot of unlabeled information. The frameworks that utilization this technique can significantly further develop learning exactness (Wang et al., 2021; Zhang et al., 2021). As a rule, semi-administered learning is picked when the obtained marked information requires gifted and important assets to prepare it/gain from it. Any other way, securing unlabeled information for the most part doesn't need extra assets.
- **Reinforcement machine learning algorithms** is a learning strategy that interfaces with its current circumstance by creating activities and finds mistakes or rewards. Experimentation search and postponed reward are the most significant qualities of support learning. This strategy permits machines and programming specialists to naturally decide the best conduct inside a particular setting to expand its presentation. Straightforward award input is expected for the specialist to realize which activity is ideal; this is known as the support signal.

How Machine Learning Works

UC Berkeley breaks out the learning system of a machine learning algorithm into three main parts.

1. **A Decision Process:** as a rule, AI calculations are utilized to make an expectation or arrangement. In view of a few information, which can be named or unlabeled, your calculation will deliver a gauge regarding an example in the information.
2. **An Error Function:** A mistake work effectively assesses the forecast of the model. On the off chance that there are known models, a mistake capacity can make a correlation with survey the precision of the model (Von Rueden et al., 2021; Ross et al., 2013; Ahamed & Farid, 2018).
3. **An Model Optimization Process:** If the model can fit better to the relevant elements in the preparation set, then, at that point, loads are changed in accordance with diminish the inconsistency between the known model and the model gauge. The calculation will rehash this assess and enhance process, refreshing loads independently until a limit of exactness has been met.

APPLICATIONS OF MACHINE LEARNING

Machine Learning is the current popular expression for nowadays' time innovation clearing across the worldwide business scene. It's far an umbrella time span for a bunch of strategies and apparatuses that help PCs learn and adjust all alone. It addresses an essential advance forward in how PCs can break down and learn (Ahmad et al., 2018; Kushwaha & Kumaresan, 2021).

Machine Learning (Shailaja et al., 2018) has caught the famous creative mind, conjuring up dreams of advanced self-picking up/breaking down AI and robots. AI is ordinarily thought about to be a subfield of man-made consciousness, and, surprisingly, a subfield of software engineering in certain viewpoints. AI contains considerations and thoughts that have been acquired throughout some stretch of time outline and adjusted from various disciplines, delivering it a genuine multidisciplinary and interdisciplinary region.

Machine Learning is significant in light of the fact that it provides association with a perspective on patterns in client conduct and undertaking functional examples, as well as helps the improvement of most recent product. AI has ended up being a huge contender for some associations (Rohan et al., 2020; Vyas et al., 2019).

An essential component to remember is that this is definitely not a far-reaching posting of fields or area names however a substitute an impression of the key contraption acquiring information on subject areas. We are utilizing AI in our ordinary day to day routine even without realizing it for instance Maps, menial helpers' advertisement Alexa, and so forth The significant fields or spaces connected with AI incorporate the accompanying:

Figure 1. Different areas of application of machine learning

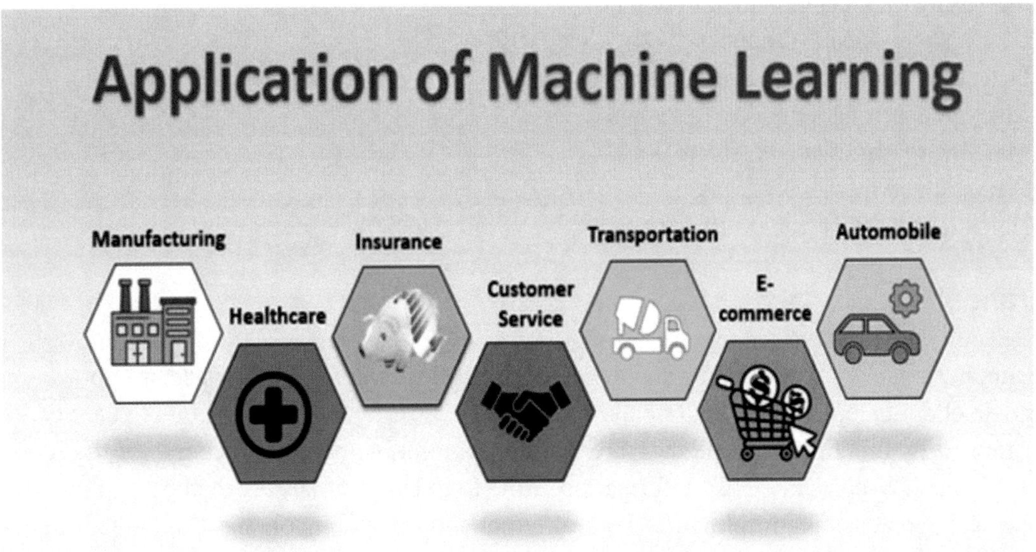

Manufacturing

Fabricating items can be pricey and a muddled interaction for the ones that don't have the legitimate instruments and assets to deliver quality items. AI assumes basic part in assembling area:

- Locate new efficiencies and cut waste to save money
- Recognize market trends and modifications
- Meet regulations and industry standards, enhance safety, and decrease their impact on environment.
- Enhance product quality
- Find and remove bottlenecks in production system
- Enhance visibility into supply chain and distribution networks
- Detect the earliest signs and symptoms of failure or anomalies to reduce downtime and perform maintenance extra quick
- Perform more accurate root cause analysis to improve system
- Optimize equipment lifecycle

Healthcare

Machine Learning for medical services advances gives calculations self-learning brain networks which can upgrade the nature of therapy by breaking down outer information on a patient's condition, their X-beams, CT checks, different tests, and screenings. Following are the uses of ML in Healthcare area (Dol & Geetha, 2021; Ramesh & Shashikanth, 2020):

- Managing medical information or data
- Facilitates in medical diagnosis
- Detecting diseases at an early stage
- Machine learning in medical assistance
- Machine learning in decision making
- Personalized medicinal drugs
- Helps finding the errors in Prescriptions

Insurance

The Insurance business is developing suddenly and the utilization of AI/man-made brainpower methods to upgrade client care, fabricate better endorsing models, cost forecast, claims taking care of, etc. It is doing as such by utilizing the huge measure of information obtained in the course of the most recent couple of years (Wojtusiak, 2012). Information is the foundation of any AI method and the protection business had been catching information from different sources and involving it for fixing fundamental business issues and speed up business. A portion of the purposes cases for the Insurance business are as per the following:

- Insurance advice/offers to the clients
- Fraud Detection and prevention
- Easy Claims processing and prediction

- Client retention
- Recommendation System

Customer Service

To contend successfully in the present cutthroat business display, it's more vital than any other time to give uncommon and awesome client assistance experience. Probably the best way to deal with work with those endeavors is through innovation that is improved with man-made consciousness and AI (Alcaraz et al., 2018). Recorded beneath are not many ways by which AI upgrades client assistance experience for organizations of all sizes and degrees:

- Offer superior personalization
- Provide faster, more efficient assistance
- Recognize your customer needs
- Reach the right customer at the right place
- Enhance customer analytics
- Match people with products
- Perceive fraud more without difficulty
- Constantly improve customer experiences
- Understand customer intent
- Enjoy efficient data tagging

Transportation

Lately, ML methods have become a piece of savvy transportation. Through profound learning, ML investigated the mind-boggling connections of streets, expressways, traffic, natural elements, crashes, etc. ML has additionally striking limit in everyday rush hour gridlock the executives and the assortment of traffic information. Referenced beneath are a few highlights of ML in transportation:

- Expediting Resolution of Delays
- Ensuring Highly Secure Routes
- Generating Accurate ETAs (Estimated time of arrival)
- Predicting Vehicle Breakdowns
- Driving Prescriptive Analytics

E-Commerce

AI is helping online business improvement partnerships take the shopper experience to a whole new level. It is likewise making them more light-footed. AI is helping web based business organizations produce income in manners that they would never done beforehand. There are a couple of ways by which the force of AI can release the maximum capacity of an internet business.

- Customer segmentation, personalization of services, and targeted campaigning.
- Optimized pricing

- Fraud safety
- Optimized search outcomes
- Product recommendations
- Customer support
- Managing supply and demand
- Predictions about customers
- Curating relevant marketing campaigns
- Advertising boosted by machine learning
- Web search

Automobile

From parts suppliers to vehicle makers, specialist co-ops to rental vehicle partnerships, the auto and related portability ventures stand to acquire essentially from executing AI at scale. We see the immense automakers making an interest in evidence of-idea projects at different stages, while disruptors in the field of independent driving are attempting to fabricate absolutely new organizations on an underpinning of man-made brainpower and machine learning (Arora et al., 2018; Arora et al., 2017; Kaur & Arora, 2020).

Figure 2. Common Applications of AI

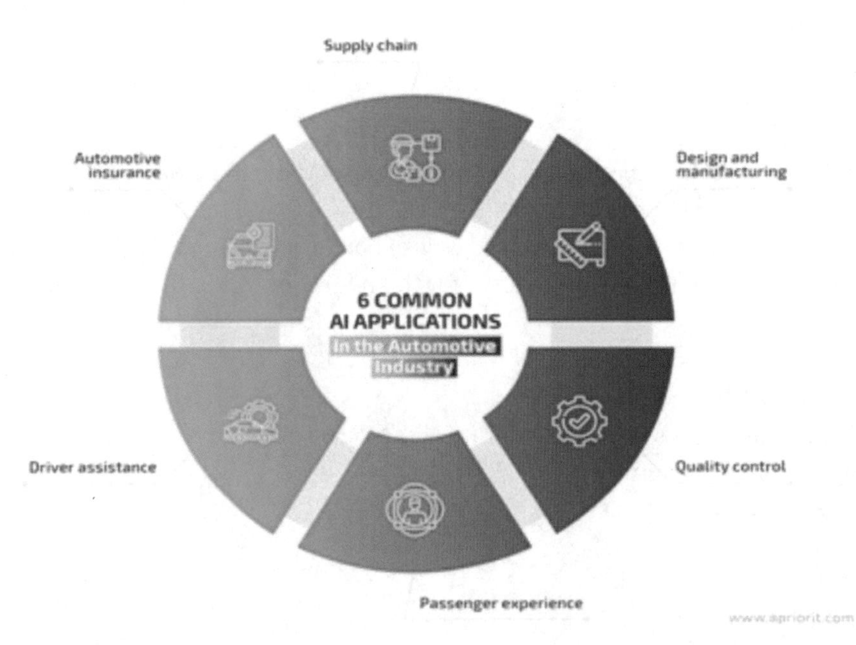

- EFFECTIVE INCORPORATION OF ANALYSIS
- ENABLING PREVENTIVE/PREDICTIVE MAINTENANCE
- ENHANCING OVERALL IN-VEHICLE USER EXPERIENCE

APPLICATION OF MACHINE LEARNING IN OUR EVERYDAY USE

1. Image Recognition
2. Product Recommendations
3. Sentiment Analysis
4. Speech Recognition
5. Auto Pilot Cars
6. Email Spam / Malware Filtering
7. Virtual Assistants / Chatbots
8. Language Translation
9. Medical Diagnosis
10. Online Fraud Detection
11. Weather Forecast

DIGITAL TWIN TECHNOLOGY

Digital Twin technology is an arising idea that has turned into the focal point of consideration for industry and, in later years, the scholarly community.

A computerized twin is basically an advanced portrayal of a true article, interaction or administration. A computerized twin can go about as an advanced clone of an article in the actual world, for example, guard frameworks or wind cultivates, or considerably bigger things like structures, and so forth.

- The computerized twin innovation can be utilized to imitate processes to gather information to foresee how they will perform.

An advanced twin is a PC program that utilizes true information to make reenactments that can foresee how an item will perform. These projects can incorporate the IoT (Internet of Things), computerized reasoning and programming investigation to upgrade the result.

With the headway of AI and factors, for example, enormous information, these computerized twins have turned into a staple in current designing to drive development and further develop execution (Arora et al., 2016).

So, making one can permit the improvement of key innovation patterns, forestall expensive disappointments and furthermore, by utilizing progressed logical, observing and prescient abilities, test cycles and administrations.

- Consider an advanced twin a scaffold between the physical and computerized world.

First savvy parts which use sensors are utilized to recognize and gather constant information.

The parts are associated with a cloud specialist co-op that gets and processes the information which is then broke down against business of other relevant information.

- Enhancements to the item can be made conceivable by gaining from the reproductions and carrying out them.

There are various sorts of computerized twins in view of the item amplification.
There can be more than one computerized twin in an item.

- **Component Twins/Part Twins**: Component twins are essentially the example of the simplest working component.
- **Asset Twins**: At the point when at least two than two parts cooperate it is known as a resource. These resource twins permit us to get the cooperation between these parts
- **System/Unit Twins**: Framework or Unit twins empowers us to perceive how these resources co-operate and shape a whole working framework.
- **Process Twins**: Process twins on a wide level uncover how frameworks cooperate to make a whole working office. Process twins can assist with deciding the exact planning plans that at last impact generally speaking viability.

ADVANTAGES OF USING DIGITAL TWINS

Better Research and Development

The utilization of computerized twins empowers more successful examination and plan of items, with an enormous measure of significant information in regard to the item. That data can prompt experiences that assist organizations with making required item enhancements.

Greater Efficiency

Indeed, even after another item has gone into creation, computerized twins can assist with watching out for the working of the item, helps in accomplishing and keeping up with top productivity all through the whole assembling process.

Product End-of-life

Advanced twins might assist makers with choosing how to manage items that arrive at the finish of their lifecycle. By utilizing advanced twins, they can figure out which item materials can be gathered.

Industry and Market Use of Digital Twins

While computerized twins are valued for what they offer, they aren't excessively normal and isn't good for each producer. Only one out of every odd venture is perplexing to the point of requiring that extreme and ordinary information checking.

Then again, a few enterprises flourish with the utilization of the computerized twin innovation.

- Actually, enormous ventures like structure, spans and other huge designs that are limited by severe standards of designing.
- Precisely intricate ventures like autos, airplanes and stream turbines. These twins can assist with further developing proficiency inside confounded hardware.

- Power gear that can be utilized to create and communicate power.
- Fabricating projects: Digital twins can be utilized to make the assembling system productive and smoothed out.

APPLICATIONS OF DIGITAL TWINS

Some of the current used applications of digital twins include

Structures and Their Systems

During the design phase big physical structures like buildings, bridges can be improved through the use of digital twins. Digital twins give multi-dimensional views into how an asset is designed and how it's performing, including occupant behavior, use patterns, space utilization, and traffic patterns. A digital twin offers a means to test "what-if" scenarios, including the impact of design changes, weather disruptions, and security events. It collects substantial data under one environment.

Figure 3. Physical Structure Design

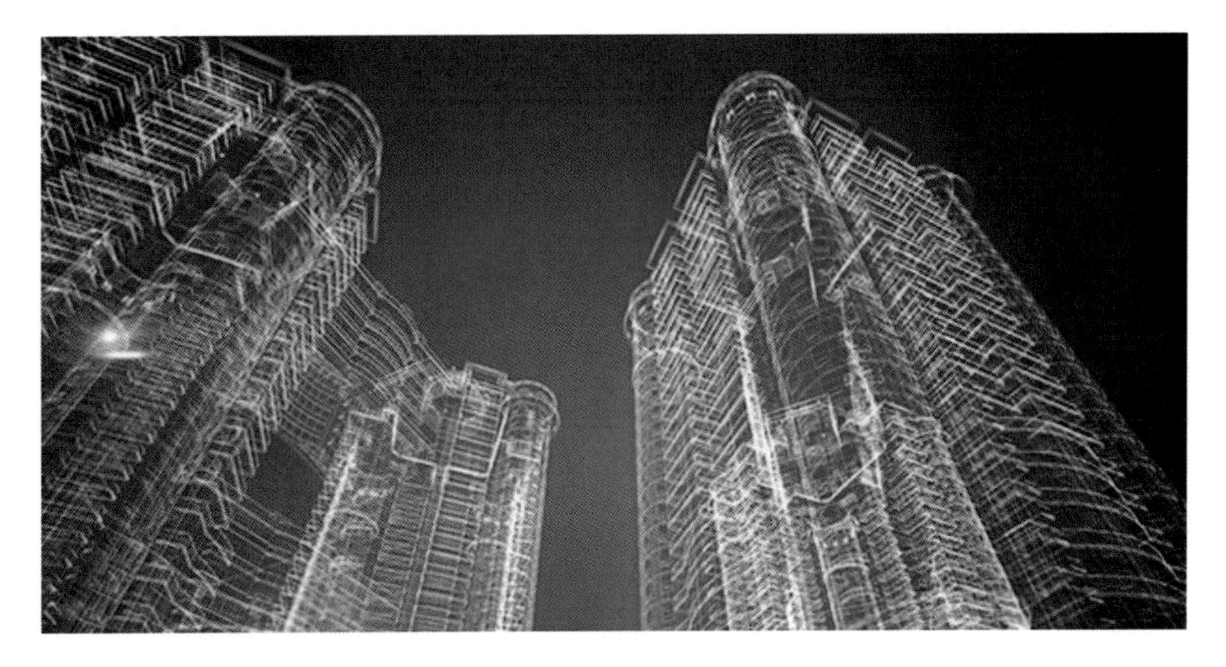

Healthcare Systems

Various types of digital twin sensors can be used to track, monitor and analyze various healthcare related data. Digital Twins allow the creation of handy virtual models and medical simulations based on the data gathered from wearable devices, patient records, drugs and pharmaceutical companies, device manufacturers and other healthcare departments. This helps streamline the overall clinical and care-giving processes. Promising areas of digital twins technology under healthcare are development of customized treatments and drug administration, advanced surgical procedure planning, enhanced care-giver efficiency and experience, testing of new age medical devices and drugs and lastly improvement in flexibility of supply chain.

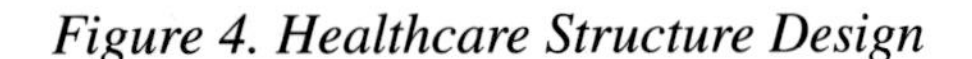

Figure 4. Healthcare Structure Design

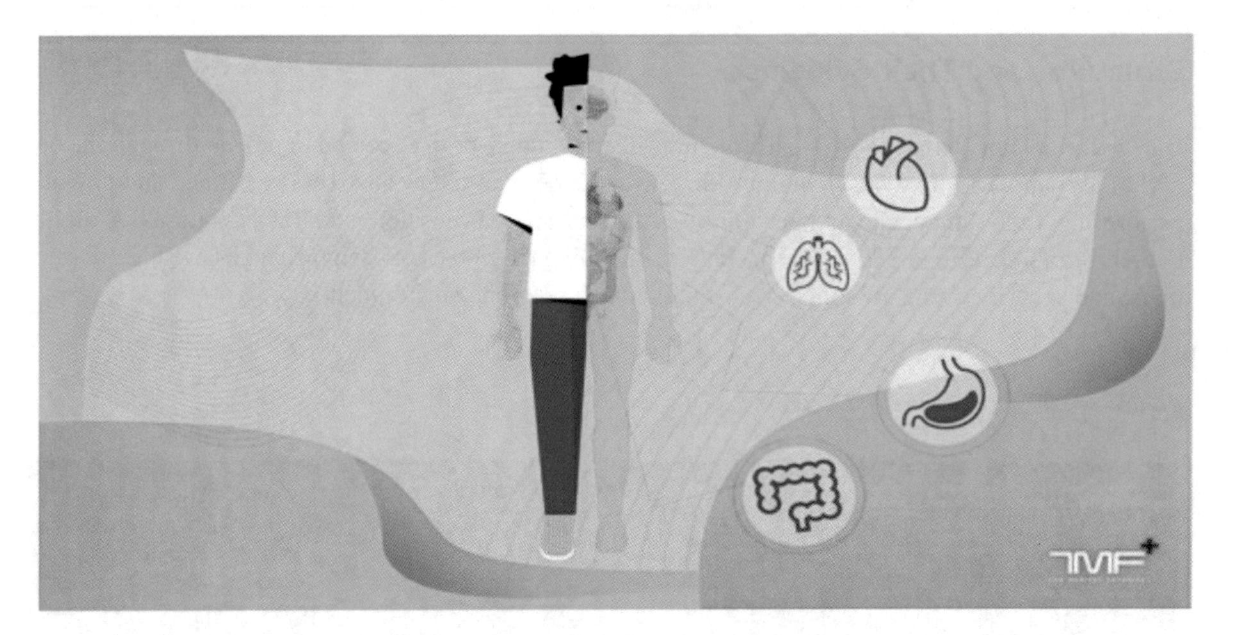

Urban Planning

Digital twins can be use essentially to make a 3D/4D blueprint that can provide spatial data in real-time. The digital twin encompasses the current landscape of buildings, transit, trees, daylight and shadows, and points of interest. It also contains proposed and under construction buildings and serves as an archive. Digital twins 3D virtual replicas of a given system, place or thing, allow cities and property owners to test out changes before they enact them in the real world. It offers an opportunity for modification to the cityscape with potential forecast how changes to a structure can impact its surrounding. The concept of the digital twin is beneficial in every sense, for use in both large and small scale building projects. The interesting aspect is the sheer advantages in regards to the implementation of a digital twin in urban planning.

Automotive Industry

Digital twins can be extensively used in auto-design as cars use various co-functioning components. Digital twins can be used to improve performance as well as make the production efficient. Digital twin in automotive industry is a virtual replica of an entire car, software, mechanics, electrics, and physical behavior of a vehicle. The digital twin holds all real-time performance; sensor and inspection data, as well as service history, configuration changes, parts replacement and warranty data. Digital twins benefit overall automotive industry by unifying data, easing verifications, avoiding failures and predicting customer demands.

Figure 5. Urban Planning Design

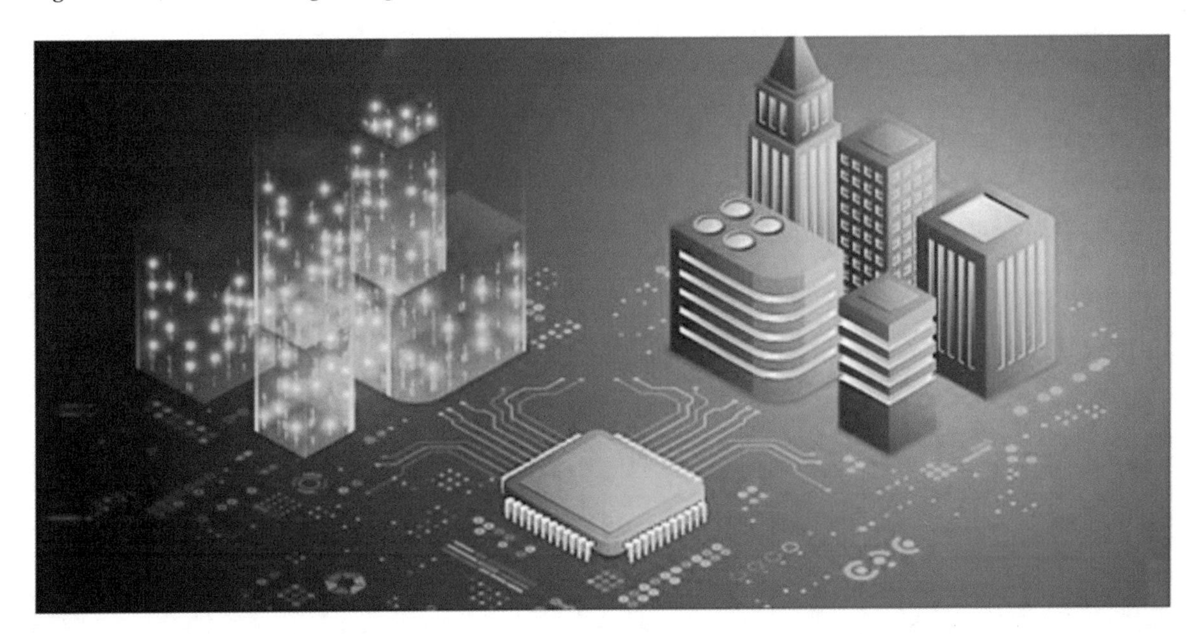

Figure 6. Automotive Industry Design

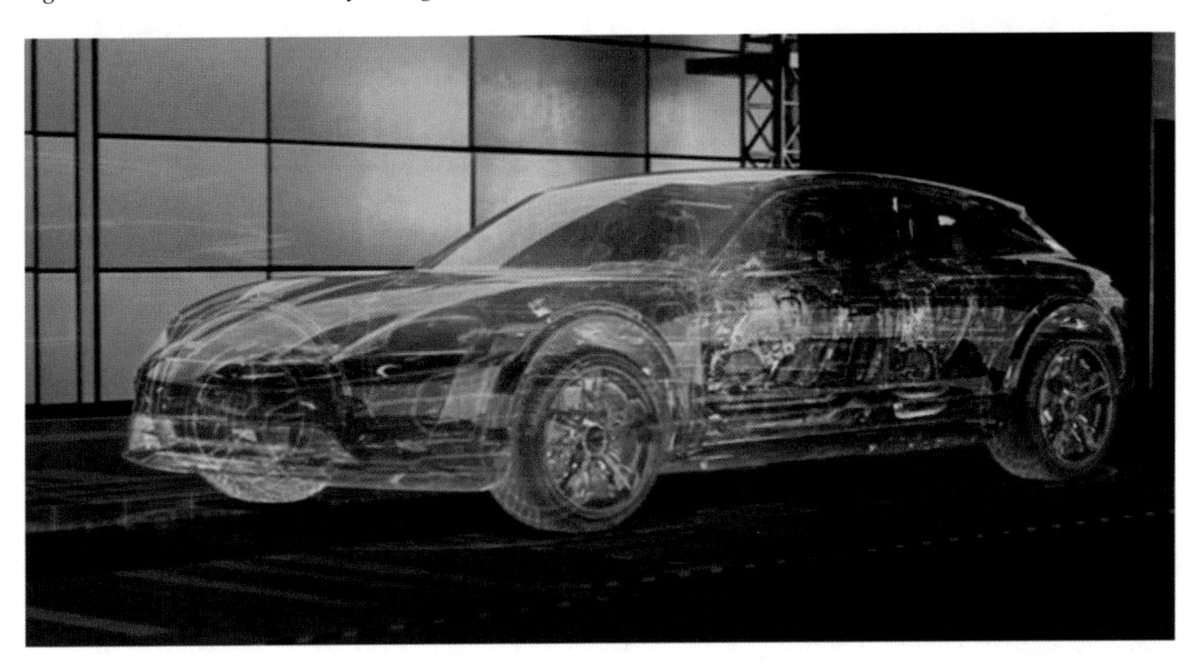

Power Generation Equipment

Be it jet engines, locomotive engines or turbines in power generation digital twin refers to the mapping of physical asset models in a digital platform, where a virtual digital replica model is created. This is created using asset-related data obtained from various sources; combined with deep domain knowledge about the asset. This virtual model is built using information from massive amounts of design, manufacturing, inspection, repair, sensor and operational data. Lot of high-fidelity computational physics based analytics models are housed in the virtual model to analyze and forecast health and performance of operating assets over their lifetime. The digital twin technology informs about the asset behavior and allows the user to take necessary actions. Resulting in the asset being kept in the optimal level of operation, rather than performing random, uncertain and reactive maintenance.

Figure 7. Power Generation Equipment Design

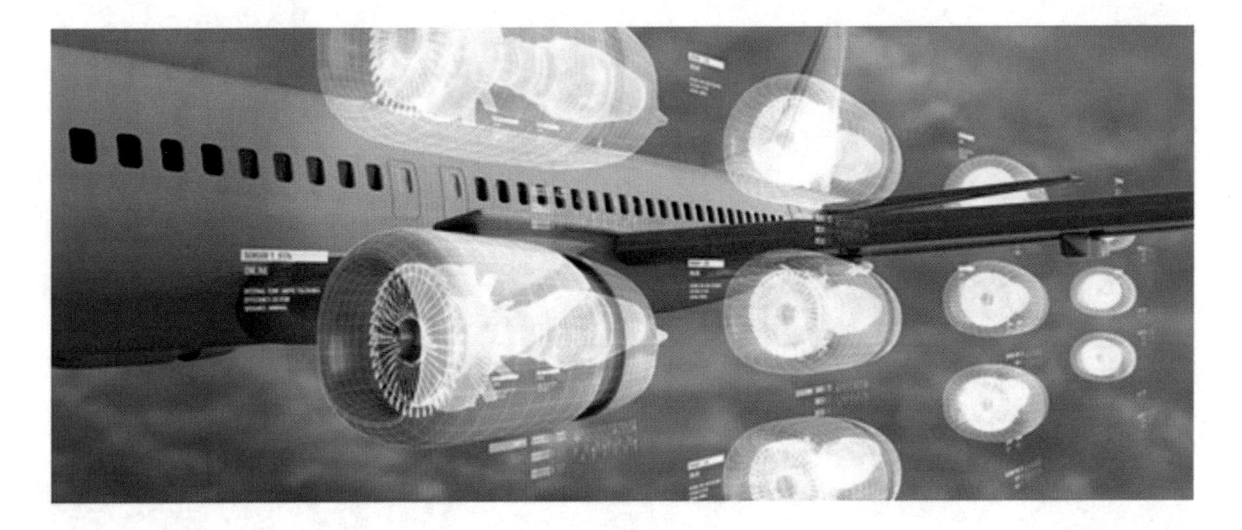

CONCLUSION

In the near future it is expected that the digital twins would be a widely used for digitalization in multitude of fields such as smart cities, healthcare, manufacturing etc. Industries such Automotive, Transportation and also the Defense Sector will greatly be taking benefits from the concept of digital twins. Digital Twins have shown strength as well as potential in varied types of interconnected physical assets and their corresponding communication with each other. Security is a major concern in such technologies as they are susceptible to misuse which could cause delay in the decision making resulting in enormous negative outcomes.

Secure deployment of digital twins on a varied set of underlying infrastructure is a key area of concern. Such underlying infrastructures generally consists of multiple possible vectors which are susceptible to attacks. A large number of threats tent to pose a huge risk towards the privacy, safety and security. A much newer concept coming in is the meta-verse which tends to amalgamate the VR technology and associated technologies with digital twins. The security again becomes a major concern in case of meta-verse. Future works are likely to include findings into possible countermeasures for threats as well as developing a compact framework for security for the digital twin technology based on block-chain, smart contracts etc.

REFERENCES

Ahamed, F., & Farid, F. (2018, December). Applying internet of things and machine-learning for personalized healthcare: Issues and challenges. In *2018 International Conference on Machine Learning and Data Engineering (iCMLDE)* (pp. 19-21). IEEE. 10.1109/iCMLDE.2018.00014

Ahmad, M. A., Eckert, C., & Teredesai, A. (2018, August). Interpretable machine learning in healthcare. In *Proceedings of the 2018 ACM international conference on bioinformatics, computational biology, and health informatics* (pp. 559-560).

Alcaraz, J. C., Moghaddamnia, S., Poschadel, N., & Peissig, J. (2018, September). Machine learning as digital therapy assessment for mobile gait rehabilitation. In *2018 IEEE 28th International Workshop on Machine Learning for Signal Processing (MLSP)* (pp. 1-6). IEEE. 10.1109/MLSP.2018.8517005

An, D., & Chen, Y. (2021, July). Digital Twin enabled methane emission abatement using networked mobile sensing and mobile actuation. In *2021 IEEE 1st International Conference on Digital Twins and Parallel Intelligence (DTPI)* (pp. 354-357). IEEE. 10.1109/DTPI52967.2021.9540133

Arora, A., Mishra, K. K., & Rakesh, N. (2016, December). Reconsidering the cloud approach towards VANET communication. In *2016 Fourth International Conference on Parallel, Distributed and Grid Computing (PDGC)* (pp. 22-27). IEEE. 10.1109/PDGC.2016.7913157

Arora, A., Rakesh, N., & Mishra, K. K. (2017). Scrutiny of VANET Protocols on the Basis of Communication Scenario and Implementation of WAVE 802.11 p/1609.4 with NS3 Using SUMO. In Advances in Computer and Computational Sciences (pp. 355-371). Springer, Singapore.

Arora, A., Rakesh, N., & Mishra, K. K. (2018). Reliable Packet Delivery in Vehicular Networks Using WAVE for Communication Among High Speed Vehicles. In *Networking Communication and Data Knowledge Engineering* (pp. 65–77). Springer. doi:10.1007/978-981-10-4585-1_6

Dol, M., & Geetha, A. (2021, August). A Learning Transition from Machine Learning to Deep Learning: A Survey. In *2021 International Conference on Emerging Techniques in Computational Intelligence (ICETCI)* (pp. 89-94). IEEE. 10.1109/ICETCI51973.2021.9574066

Kaur, B., & Arora, A. (2020, September). Emotional Intelligence: Rendering Association amongst the Technology Approach and Non-Fiscal Efficiency Aspects. In *2020 IEEE 1st International Conference for Convergence in Engineering (ICCE)* (pp. 11-15). IEEE.

Kushwaha, P. K., & Kumaresan, M. (2021, November). Machine learning algorithm in healthcare system: A Review. In *2021 International Conference on Technological Advancements and Innovations (ICTAI)* (pp. 478-481). IEEE. 10.1109/ICTAI53825.2021.9673220

Ramesh, T. K., & Shashikanth, A. (2020, November). A Machine Learning based Ensemble Approach for Predictive Analysis of Healthcare Data. In *2020 2nd PhD Colloquium on Ethically Driven Innovation and Technology for Society (PhD EDITS)* (pp. 1-2). IEEE.

Rohan, T. I., Yusuf, M. S. U., Islam, M., & Roy, S. (2020, June). Efficient approach to detect epileptic seizure using machine learning models for modern healthcare system. In *2020 IEEE Region 10 Symposium (TENSYMP)* (pp. 1783-1786). IEEE. 10.1109/TENSYMP50017.2020.9230731

Ross, M., Graves, C. A., Campbell, J. W., & Kim, J. H. (2013, December). Using support vector machines to classify student attentiveness for the development of personalized learning systems. In *2013 12th international conference on machine learning and applications* (Vol. 1, pp. 325-328). IEEE. 10.1109/ICMLA.2013.66

Shailaja, K., Seetharamulu, B., & Jabbar, M. A. (2018, March). Machine learning in healthcare: A review. In *2018 Second international conference on electronics, communication and aerospace technology (ICECA)* (pp. 910-914). IEEE. 10.1109/ICECA.2018.8474918

Von Rueden, L., Mayer, S., Beckh, K., Georgiev, B., Giesselbach, S., Heese, R., Kirsch, B., Walczak, M., Pfrommer, J., Pick, A., Ramamurthy, R., Garcke, J., Bauckhage, C., & Schuecker, J. (2021). Informed machine learning-a taxonomy and survey of integrating prior knowledge into learning systems. *IEEE Transactions on Knowledge and Data Engineering*, 1. doi:10.1109/TKDE.2021.3079836

Vyas, S., Gupta, M., & Yadav, R. (2019, February). Converging blockchain and machine learning for healthcare. In *2019 Amity International Conference on Artificial Intelligence (AICAI)* (pp. 709-711). IEEE. 10.1109/AICAI.2019.8701230

Wang, Y., Cao, Y., & Wang, F. Y. (2021, July). Anomaly Detection in Digital Twin Model. In *2021 IEEE 1st International Conference on Digital Twins and Parallel Intelligence (DTPI)* (pp. 208-211). IEEE. 10.1109/DTPI52967.2021.9540116

Wojtusiak, J. (2012, December). Semantic data types in machine learning from healthcare data. In *2012 11th International Conference on Machine Learning and Applications* (Vol. 1, pp. 197-202). IEEE. 10.1109/ICMLA.2012.41

Zhang, S., Dong, H., Maschek, U., & Song, H. (2021, July). A digital-twin-assisted fault diagnosis of railway point machine. In *2021 IEEE 1st International Conference on Digital Twins and Parallel Intelligence (DTPI)* (pp. 430-433). IEEE. 10.1109/DTPI52967.2021.9540118

Zhang, Z., Lu, J., Xia, L., Wang, S., Zhang, H., & Zhao, R. (2020, June). Digital twin system design for dual-manipulator cooperation unit. In *2020 IEEE 4th Information Technology, Networking, Electronic and Automation Control Conference (ITNEC)* (Vol. 1, pp. 1431-1434). IEEE. 10.1109/ITNEC48623.2020.9084652

Chapter 5
Digital Twin in Healthcare Present and Future Scope:
Digital Twin in Healthcare

Kavita Thapliyal
https://orcid.org/0000-0003-2099-3241
Amity International Business School, Amity University, India

ABSTRACT

With the massive digital innovation and adaptions, healthcare is also changing quickly to digital health care. The term 'digital twin' refers to a wide-reaching concept that comprises the structure via amalgamating many technologies and functionalities for digital transformation in the healthcare sector. The digital twin (DT) will enable the healthcare industry to reform, enhance, and optimize comprehensive and complicated clinical trials. This chapter will feature digital twin broadly, using the 4P Medicine framework for a sustainable medical solution. DT will enable personalized, predictive, participative, and preventive medical solutions for patients of today to an improved state of patient of tomorrow by incorporating pre-specified covariate modifications.

INTRODUCTION

The Objective of The Chapter

1. Unprecedented times have taught us the need of medical doctors, consultancy, and the importance of digital medical healthcare. So, the prime objective is to explore how digital twins are transforming the future of healthcare.
2. Digital Twin applications in hospital and healthcare industry for enhancing operational productive efficiency.
3. To know how medical simulations and trainings on digital twin will enable pre- and post-surgical interpretations in mitigating damage to human anatomy.

DOI: 10.4018/978-1-6684-5925-6.ch005

BACKGROUND

We all have witnessed how COVID19 pandemic has revolutionized the healthcare industry. Today healthcare sector is moving with a fast pace and at all three levels – Design, Development & Delivery- Digital innovations are the future. Artificial Intelligence (AI), Blockchain, Virtual Reality (VR), Augmented Reality (AR), Internet of Things (IOT) and Quantum Computing are all modernizing and transforming the future of healthcare. Among the most advance technical interface Digital Twin is the most symbolic term that is creating a new paradigm. This technique is evoking speed, accuracy and is saving time, energy, and stress of patients and medical practitioners. The Chapter will highlight the importance of smart healthcare adaption's using digital twin.

Digital twin is the future of sustainable healthcare. We all know how COVID19 reveals the launch of biological wars and has created a havoc to human lives. Medical aids and support systems collapsed during the pandemic tides worldwide. Hence, we require a robust system where there is a process of automation supporting man with the help of advance machine. With the emerging new age technological innovation, new types of medical concerns are emerging and to handle the high medical demands of huge population it is becoming utmost important to be equipped with higher- quality medical services. Digital Twins are vitally helping in Virtual Organs, Genomic Medicine, Personalized Health Information, Customized Drug Treatment, Complete Body Scanning, Planning of Surgery, Improvement in Healthcare Organization, Driving Efficiency, Supply Chain Resilience, Improving Caregiver Experience, Shrinking Critical Window Treatment, Value Based Healthcare, Faster Construction of Hospitals, Call Centre Interaction Streamlining, Medical Device and Drug Manufacturing & Development, Medical Device Software's, Drug Risk Classification, New Product Line Stimulations, Improvement in Device Uptime, Drug Delivery Improvement, Post Market Surveillance, Human Variability Stimulation and Digital Twin Labs etc.

The innovative healthcare models and ideas help in addressing critical and sensitive healthcare problems with much more precision and accuracy. This chapter we will broadly highlight the modern technologies in medicine industry that are going to shape better sustainable solutions to human in future. Digital twins (DT) are one of the modern virtual techniques which can help medical practitioners to innovate, design, develop a human clone where all testing and monitoring of imposed medicine and results can be evaluated. This helps the researchers to thoughtfully investigate the imposed drug and treatment on the patient and find the characteristics for effective delivery. The Digital Twins can create models of high use from information gained through wearable devices, patient's records, and processes and then connect vital links in the medical healthcare ecosystem of doctors, span patients, drugs and device manufacturers. They are showing remarkable promises in customizing medical treatments to patients based on their exclusive genetics, behaviour, anatomy and many other traits. Researchers are already encouraging medical fraternity to collaborate further in scaling Digital Twin research and operations across mass personalization platforms and sync it with most modern customer data platforms of today.

The evolution of technology innovation has remarkably modernised each sector today. Things which were an imagination earlier are real today. One of such innovation in healthcare industry is Digital twin which works in heath precision management solutions. DT has its wide-reaching impact and lays a foundation in understanding human body, its biological, social, and psychological aspects and is an asset to both patients and health providers. Today digital twin is not only supporting health researchers and diagnostic management systems in acquiring the right blend of data collection for communicating meaningful clinical outcomes in understanding patient history, simulations, mutations, for better predictions for disease management and beyond. At present health care sector requires effective and efficient diagnostic and treatment, valuable consultancy management for a healthy and protected citizen. (Erol, 2020) With this innovative industry 4.0 technology and best solutions for diagnosis and further treatment can be provided in real time. Nowadays we witness digital technological practices successfully running in various manufacturing firms and are providing fruitful results by industrial and engineering enterprises. The same has now been innovated in the healthcare sector with a promise to maximise and enhance better healthcare solutions for all. To further understand this it is important to know that with the help of digital twin medical professionals can advance human modelling using smart digital practices and modern technologies, like smart sensor technology, artificial intelligence, data analytics using algorithms, IoT, Big Data in order to sense, perceive and prevent medical trails and failures by systematic personalised care and advance system performance, to and discover innovative opportunities for surgeons and medical practitioners to explore better and more patient-centric health solutions to cure and prevent fatal and pandemic health disasters by advance diagnosis, surgical pre and post care management. It is a complete solution to patient and hospital operations and to medical research fraternity (Peng, 2020). Traditional Building Information Modelling (BIM) in hospital management is being overhauled by innovative constant lifecycle integration model under digital twins which facilitates early movement contracts and contactors. There is instant artificial intelligent diagnosis and real time visual management, hereby saving time, cost and energy. (Volkov, 2021) Smart health cares in smart cities are well supported by Internet of Things, Mobile medicines and Digital Twins. The idea of smart healthcare as element of smart planet was initiated in 2009 by IBM. Similarly, many leading technologies and vivid approaches are aligning to better handle complex environments.

Conceptually, a digital twin is a digital replica or representation of a physical object, process, or service, but also much more than that. It is a virtual model (data plus algorithms) with special features not found in traditional models and simulations, one that dynamically pairs the physical and digital worlds, and leverages modern technologies, such as smart sensor technology, data analytics, and artificial intelligence (AI) to detect and prevent system failures, improve system performance, and explore innovative opportunities.

As digitalization is defining and reshaping the future, digital twins are designed to create better and healthy simulations that can help to predict the multiple output of product and services to perform with more accuracy and intelligence.

Broadly Digital Twins Have Two Major Functions and Purposes

1. Digital twin assist and support us in understanding the physical functionality of a world and with the most advance technological interface we can deduce accurate insights about the status of the individual object that it symbolises as a twin.
2. Digital twins are advanced digital applications that advocate futuristic decision making for adapting more advanced techniques combining people, processes, and new age adaptive techniques for a sustainable tomorrow.

A digital twin is virtually designed to predict and understand the physical functionality on the virtual twin to predict the physical counterpart's implementing characteristics. It helps in simulating and predicting optimum output of the product systems and build the possibility of accurate operating outcomes investigating the real physical prototypes.

Figure 1. Digital Thread

Product
Design & Product Efficiency
Production
Manufacturing & Product Planning
Performance
Analysis & Decision Making on operational data

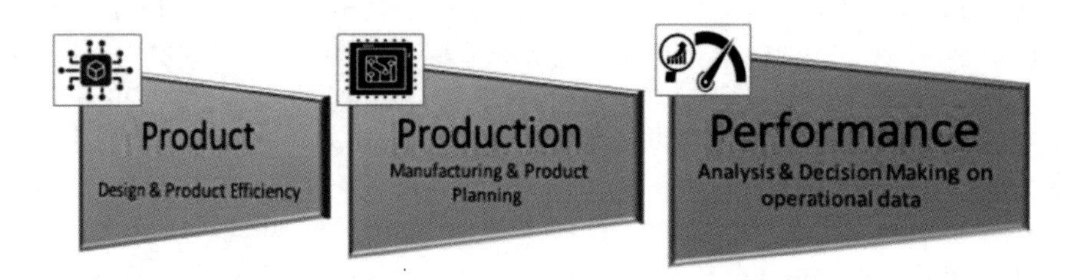

With rigorous research and incorporating multi-physical scenarios, data interpretation using data analytics using machine learning techniques digital twins are capable to reveal the impact of design changes. They are high designed virtual programmed models that help in usage scenarios keeping all environmental parametric variables in mind and help in eradicating the need of physical prototypes which help in mitigating development and process time and helps in refining quality of concluded products or process.

Digital Twin, use data from sensors installed on physical objects to ensure accurate modelling over the entire lifetime of a product to efficiently determine the objects real-time performance with the existing operating systems and incorporate changes over the period. While using the data the digital twin continuously keeps updating and progressing to reflect any change occurred to the physical counterpart during the product lifecycle via generating a closed loop of reactions occurred in the virtual environment that enables digital innovators, companies, researchers, and companies to constantly optimize their products to more reliable and high oriented performance at the most affordable cost.

Based on the lifecycle stage of the product digital twin depend on broad three stages- Product, Production and Performance. Here it is very important to understand the deep connection between the three stages of product, production, and performance- as these three stages develop and process together, they are just connected like a thread, a digital thread involved in brining collective data from all the stages of lifecycles.

Technology is transforming ecology including human lives in a big way. Education, learning processes, work, transportation, communication, and foremost healthcare have all benefitted enormously by the digital fusion which is constantly evolving. Life has become a lot simpler using technology and its very user friendly. Standard of living has gone up due to the digital transformation and it has added multiple progressive dimensions to the global economy.

Digital Twin is the new mantra that is transforming the health care systems worldwide. Here innovative and adaptive computer models are used to create replicas of people, process, systems, and tools integrating technology for creating a multiple digital database to be processed for varied business processes including healthcare, labs, and hospital environments. It's vital for human physiology and psychology to be in sync with the futuristic medical amalgamations. Data covering environment, population traits and individual are merged to create virtual twins. Digital twin technology is vital to generate diversified models, review strategies for operations, and regroup staffing & care replicas for best suitability as per the prevailing environment. This enables the path to right resource optimization and risk mitigation & novel management strategies. It is believed that around 70% investments in healthcare are digital twin centric today. This is because digital twin is enhancing the performance and viability of health care systems by planning present and futuristic needs through personalization and customization of patients' needs including their medicines, diagnosis, devises, and surrounding infrastructure facilities. (van der Valk, 2021) Digital twins are vastly dependent on their cases subject to individual usages. The digital twin concept, cases and usage in healthcare is totally different from different set of specialized characters used in engineering domain. Yet real time updates are the common binding factors derived from similar and shared underlying characteristics and technology used.

Digital tools like AI and Data Science are used leveraging real time and historical data of healthcare operations and surrounding environments to create replicas or digital twins to enable management to foresee and correctly forecast equipment shortages, infrastructure loopholes and simultaneously optimize staff scheduling including patient room operations. This improves resource efficiency, reduces redundancy, augments performances, and foremost brings down operational costs. It's a strong deterrent against risk through checks and measures to test system performance changes like device maintenance, new installations and staff count including operation room availabilities. Though there are some serious challenges like data privacy, data quality and limited adoption yet.

History, Conceptualization, Research, Innovation and Adaption of the Digital Twin

Dr. Michael Grieves, research professor at Florida Institute of Technology is considered as the creator and man behind the conceptualization of Digital Twin. Digital Twin got recognition after his presentation on Technology at the University of Michigan in 2002. Dr. Grieves stressed on the intricate management of a product lifecycle centre and its enhanced development. Taking technology and digital platforms as a spearheading tool, it integrated real space, virtual space, elements of digital twin and information flow with data from real to virtual space. Though, newer technologies and terminology for the same evolved over the years, the conceptualization entity of creating a digital and physical twin as one has remained same since its inception. Although NASA, has been using this technology concept for space programming since 1960s by replicating systems at space to physical systems at grounds for research. During the Apollo 13 Launch this technology was used for a health safety survival scare in the 1970 to assess and stimulate varied conditions on board and further tested on ground with success on physical systems. With age and technological advancements physical systems have made way for digital or virtual systems which save time, cost, and manpower. Digital Twin or DT was configured as a virtual model or copy of the physical entity or physical twin which were interconnected in real time by data swapping. (David Jones, May 2020) The digital twin has a complete product lifecycle starting with a digital twin prototype, then digital twin instance, followed by digital twin aggregate and ending with a digital twin environment

After its global recognition in 2002, it became an area of prominence for research and innovation. Till 2017 it had become one of the top technological trends worldwide and became implemented in varied businesses. Digital Twins enabled by IOT, and Big Data revolutionized the business processes making them cost effective innovations and real time saviours. Seeing its popularity and continuous top trending spree, the future belongs to digital twin technology including physical systems and aligning software models. It is widely estimated that soon more than half of the large businesses will utilize this technology, thus connecting digitally with more than 22 billion sensors globally. This will immensely cut down operation and maintenance & repair costs and around 65% of the quality and product performance will be mapped will be done using digital twins from the offices. With the outcome, growth and usage of digital twin being of high relevance, its continuous usage in turning around systems have been predicted for numerous centuries in future.

DIGITAL TWIN NEED OF THE HOUR

Digital Twins are evolving industry 4.0 and have embraced data exchange, AI, automation, and other digital technologies for the better. They have become the new buzzword of the industry and medical fraternity is truly benefitting from it immensely as they are a boon to them as cost effective life savers. The digital twins due to their revolutionary technologies are transforming businesses with unlimited new possibilities. The digital twin industry is most likely to grow in abundance due to its big USP in saving time, planning and cost of product development.

Digital twins are creating complex virtual models which are of high proficiency as their original physical counterpart. This twin replica could be anything, be it a human, animal, bridge, building, car or even an aero plane. Collected data is mapped from physical entities to virtual replicated models through sensors.

Today cutting edge medical technologies like Digital Twin and Remote Sensing integrations are being envisioned, aspired and created for healthcare systems in the field of Remote Patient Monitoring, Artificial Intelligence Tools, 5G Enabled Devices, Machine Learning, Mental Health, Internet of Medical Things, Tricorders, Nano Medicine, Telemedicine, Personalized Healthcare, eHealth, mHealth, PGHD, Pharmaceutical, Data Platforms, Diagnostics, Next-Gen Imaging, Lab Chip, Bio Ventures, Digital Assistants, Smarter Pacemakers, Cancer Immunotherapy, 3D Printing, Augmented Reality, Virtual Reality, Robotic Surgeries, Quantum Computing, Internet Medicine, Blockchain, MedTech, Purpose Wearables, Genomics, Tele Health, Brain Tech, Data Science Digital Therapeutics, Biotech, Data Security and Medical Devices etc. The AI enabled healthcare market is expected to grow enormously surpassing $34 billion by 2025. Reduction in the treatment of non-communicable diseases through digital health can be to the tune of $45 trillion. We have seen that the pandemic has accelerated the digital technology & telemedicine arena.

DIGITAL TWIN MODEL FRAMEWORK FOR HEALTHCARE

Digital twin will enable Personalized, Predictive, Participative and Preventive medical solutions for patients of today to an improved state of patient of tomorrow by incorporating pre-specified covariate modifications. By the help of advanced digitalized automation DT will foster to create smart medical facilities connecting human with smart intelligent futuristic machine by synchronization of physical and digital twin in near time for an equilibrium from tradition medical care to personalised medical care for a productive outcome.

Digital twin is an innovation which is designed based on the virtual representation of a physical object by collating all physical needs, genetic data, biomedical signals, behavioral, social, and psychological determinants keeping all current updates of its real physical counterparts. By the help of all imposed data DT enables preemptive decision making and help in optimizing most fruitful predictions for a sustainable healthcare system. A digital twin is a digital cloned computer designed program that reflects the physical entities of a particular person, processes, devices, and systems that uses real world data

Figure 2. Digital health platforms supporting digital twin

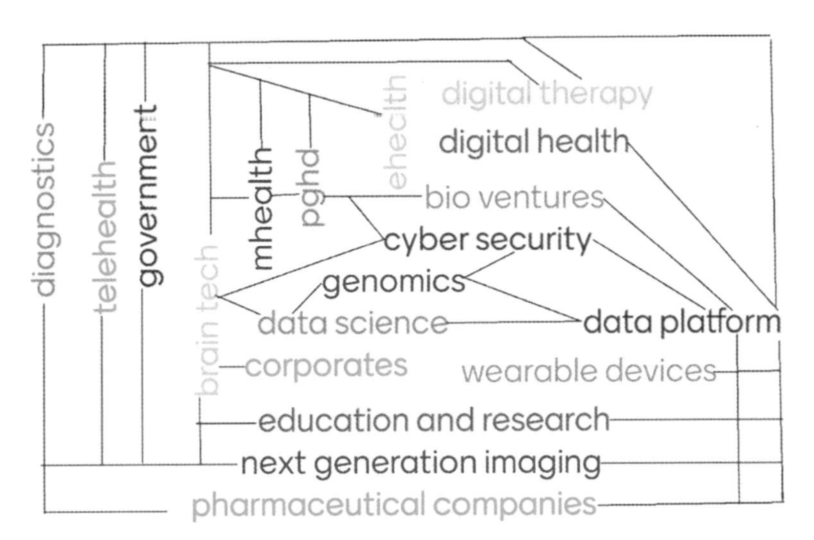

to construct and produce simulations via IoT, artificial intelligence, machine learning using technical algorithms, 3D simulations, virtual reality, and augmented reality. All these modern technologies like cloud computing, data science, smart sensors and prototypes are used for testing and interpreting more effective research for high performance outcomes. (Qia, 2018) Cyber physical integration is seamlessly

Figure 3. Digital Twin 4P's Healthcare framework for a sustainable medical solution

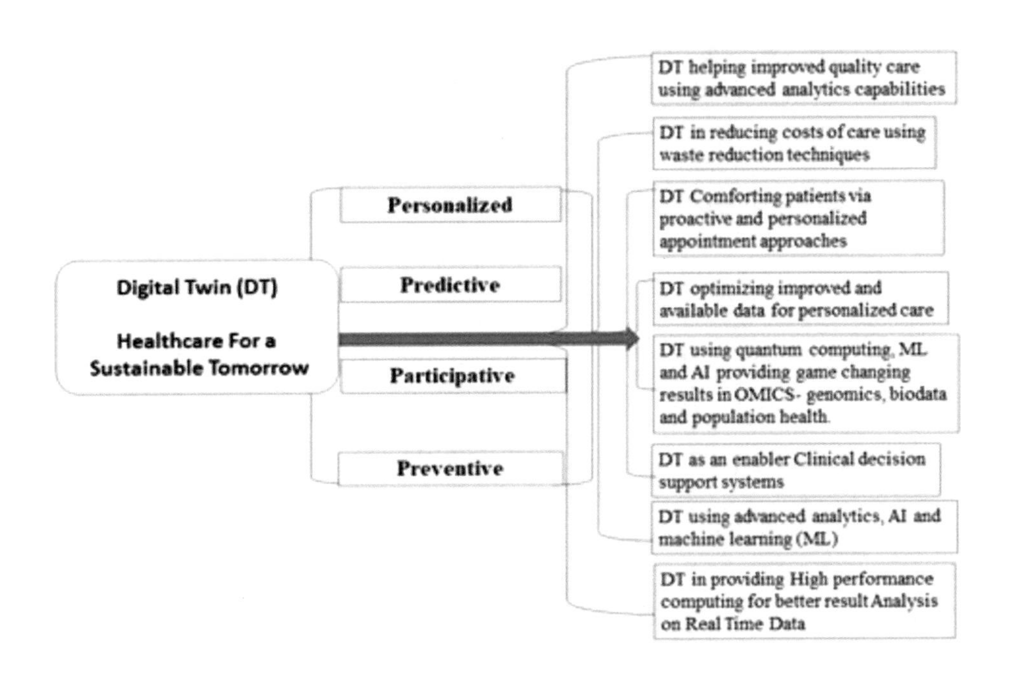

embedded in manufacturing by digital twin and can fundamentally change the product design & manufacturing and other services towards smart production houses.

The objective of DT modelling is to effectively run environmentally friendly and cost-effective simulations. With the help of data models medical practitioners and life sciences experts can effectively capture all required information to perform operations and diagnostics based on the captured data. The prime concern of digital twin technology is developed for creating effective predictions for patients, hospital management and pharmaceutical industry for an outcome-oriented analysis. Frugal innovations and adaptations to technologies like artificial intelligence, virtual reality (VR), blockchain, IoT, quantum computing all have changed the orientation towards future and the healthcare industry is witnessing a big boom and reflecting noteworthy benefits within abundant developments.

DIGITAL TWIN AND MEDICINE

Various literature in the recent past describes the importance of digital twin. In the smart city people are getting sensitive about their fitness (Barricelli; Casiraghi; Gliozzo; Petrini; Valtolina), various infections due to viral, remote surgery and innovative healthcare concerns and management are the prime field of discussions.

By the advancement of technologies like artificial intelligence, blockchain, big data, iot, data science healthcare industry can immensely be benefited from the digital technology and digital twins will be able to provide more personalized and customised evaluation and analysis for faster and reliable healthcare solutions.

The use of digital twins in healthcare is transforming clinical trials and is improving hospital management by developing robust systems to enhance medical care with digital tracking and expanding progressive digital modelling of the human body. Thus, by the help of digital twin human can avoid trials and experiments to happen in their real body and can use all the experiments in the clone that is their digital twin for a better medical solution. It is going to be a great help to researchers in exploring and researching diseases, mutations, exploring new drugs, technology, developing medical devices and systems. Soon digital twins may support and assist physicians enhance and boost the functionality and executing and implementing customised performance of patient-specific medication and concern plans. The advancement in digital innovations is going to foster life-saving innovations and best practices by integrating and implementing vast amount of data and predictions which will be more pocket friendly with high safety and privacy to the patience and will be comfortable to understand and cope with. (Saddik, 2022) Smart cities can use this virtualization of industrial processes to improve the healthcare, wellbeing, and quality of their resident's life with this state of art DT technology.

DIGITAL TWIN TOWARDS SMART MEDICAL FACILITY

The expertise of digital twin will help hospitals to create a digital replica of the system and critically and intelligently examine the hospital management functionalities like capacity, resources, footfall, lab and treatment care and concerns and will help in mitigating the risk and image building. It will further by correct predictive analysis help hospital management systems to generate a good balance between various stakeholders, doctors, patients, and staff.

Figure 4. Digital twin in personalized medicine

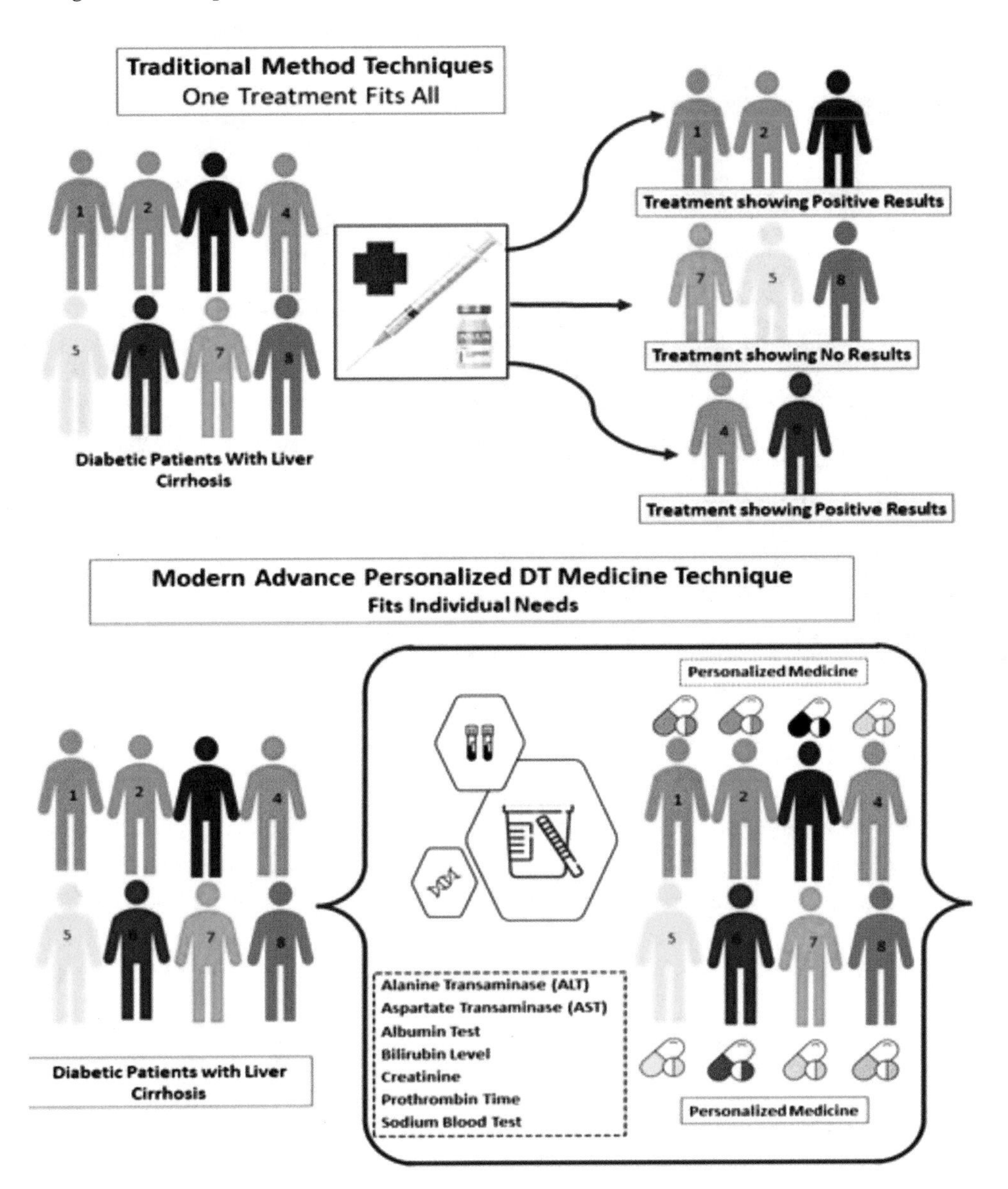

Resource Optimization: Digital twin can maximise real-time data of hospitals in mapping the resource flow and shortages. It can help the hospital management in streamlining the systems better by obtaining real time insights into patient's health and workflows. This system will be helpful in reducing stress and effective planning, organizing, staffing, controlling, and executing things in an amicable manner. (Boulos, 2021) Digital twin has evolved personalized medicine to public health precision. Erstwhile names in the sixties from mirror space model to information mirror model have transformed to digital twin concept as of today.

Figure 5. Digital Twin Linking Client Operations and Hospital Management Support Systems

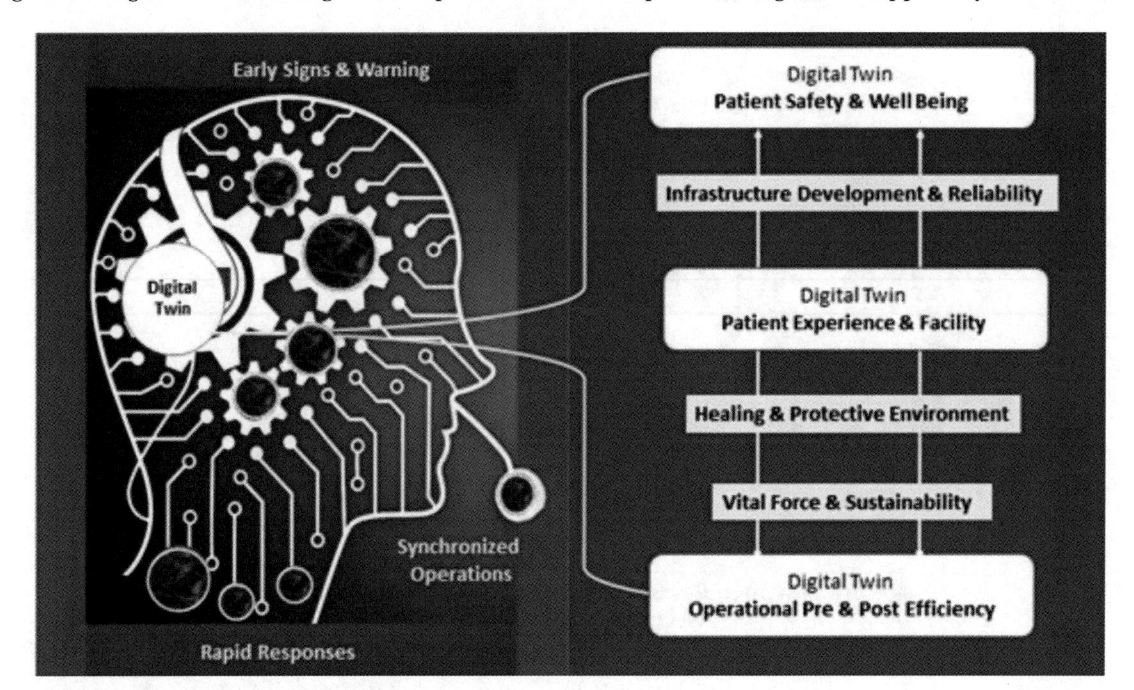

Technology Shaping Healthcare

When we cannot eat the same kind of food all the time or would not like to dress the same cloth 24*7, we must take this call also in same manner with the medical treatment and healthcare concerns of an individual. Why most of us get the same kind of medication? This question is very important from personal care point of view and that's why it is becoming utmost important to have a personalized health care solutions and towards the steppingstone for personalized care- Digital twin are the first seed of thought.

Human Body Digital Twin

This is the most vital and interesting conception of digital twin as it explores the complexities of human body and its functions. Applications for individual genetic makeup, lifestyle, habits, characteristics, genes, physiology, psychology, cells, and organs are minutely researched and studied for creating individual medicine, treatment, and rehabilitation. These human body internal assessment replicas through personalized diagnosis and treatment planning, help in the overall rejuvenation of the patient and is a must for a complete 360-degree recovery. Vital data is collected from respective patients and their doctors to analyse body metabolism including body parts functionality, blood pressure, and oxygen levels and helps to track persistent conditions and patients' priorities during prior and post treatments. This forms as a solid base for research data development and clinical trials at Labs.

Here focus is client based and treatment is not based on mass driven samples. There is customized simulation to track the suitability of patient to different treatment, thus enhancing the chances of accurate treatment plan for the respective patient. So, there is a great demand, interest and work being done on personalized medicine but digital twin application for actual patients has a long way to go. Through

Figure 6. Human digital twin & advance technology amalgamations

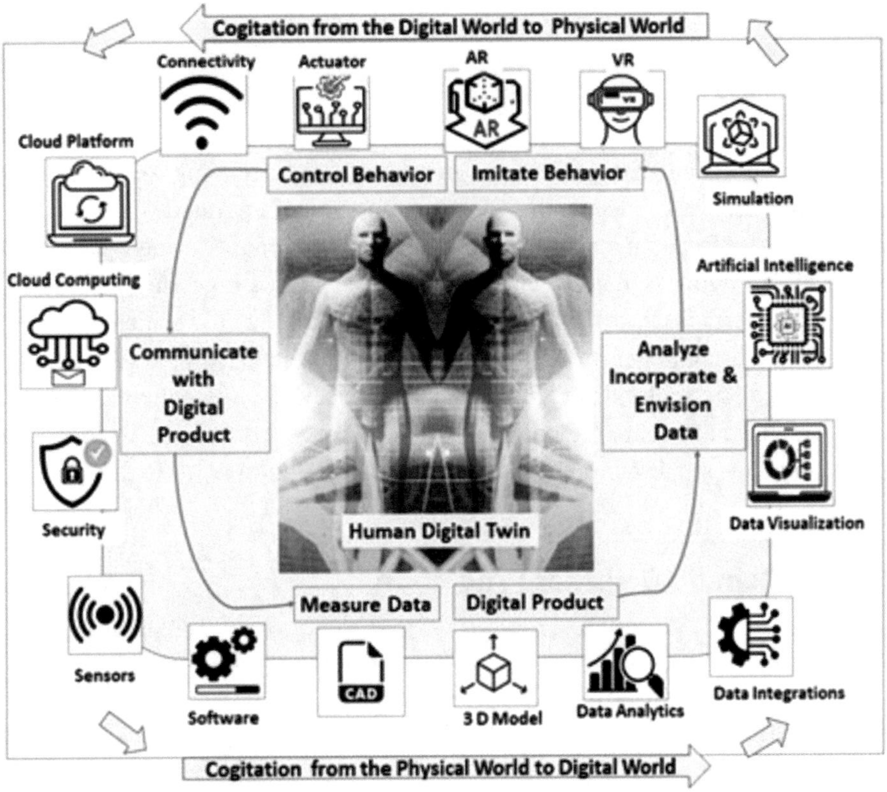

advance and intrinsic modelling of human body the doctors can determine the pathology before the complexities are evident. This helps them to change the treatments and have a wider scope of surgery research.

Among the most famous specialized centres of personalized medicine is the **Linkoping University of Sweden** where animals' RNA (**mice**) has been mapped through digital twin to research and predict futuristic effects of medications.

LEADING GLOBAL MEDICAL TWIN HEALTHCARE IMPACTING SOLUTION PROVIDERS

PrediSurge- France (Patient Anatomy Simulations)

Digital twins of patient's anatomies are created by this start-up using simulation technology. 3D models of anatomy are generated for specific patients for personalized research. Preferred medical implants of the digital models are selected from the database to run pre-set numerical simulations of the intervention. So, tailor made optimized care is made available to patients through precise decisions and treatment made by surgeons. Cardiovascular surgeries often use implants like stent grafts, however at times altered parameters or material properties of the grafted stent can adversely change the course of critical treatment. Proceeding interventions and predicted outcomes are made by creating 3D simulations of patient's anatomies.

NUREA Designs- France (Medical Imaging Software)

This start-up helps cardiovascular surgeons through its digital twin imaging software. The design, development and marketing are well conceptualized and supported by integrated Artificial Intelligence (AI). This software generates 3D automated reconstruction from patients CT angiograms enabling patient specific vascular digital twins. Surgeons with the software's help use geometrical data to perceive the growth of bulge in the aorta and work on early treatment to minimize the critical impact of the disease. The aorta bulge or aorta aneurysm often ruptures and causes internal bleeding among artery walls, leading to complex cardiovascular disorder. To measure its severity the patients, undergo multiple CT and MRI scans, which is harmful to the body due to radiation exposure risk. To reduce the complexity of this treatment, start-ups are developing virtual model based digital twins to prejudge and drive better treatments.

Predictiv- USA (Genetic Disorder Prediction)

This US based start-ups uses DNA to create digital twins and forecast frequency of severe individual genetic disorders. DNA is extracted from patient's fingernails, to be collected and make their digital twins. A preventive personalized healthcare plan is prepared because of the genetic based risk assessment test report. DNA is a complex building block of cells loaded with infinite information about each organism. Through their DNA digital twins' scientists can plan and predict personal treatments, making futuristic concerns more transparent and avoidable. Today it's an evolving process but their advanced digital trails on surgical and medical applications are already becoming a boon for patient's safety.

Virtonomy.io-Germany (Virtual Medical Device Testing)

Clinical trials are conducted on medical devices through virtual patients for humans and animals by this innovative medical twin. This data driven platform accelerates medical device development with digital twin amalgamations. V-patients are introduced to medical device developers to carry out testing and research & development in a digitally enabled environment. This speeds growth reduces risks, expenses, and regulatory blocks. Here end to end simulation solution through digital twin based on anever-expanding database, analytical analysis of actual clinical data showcases variations in the anatomies, pathological states, and demographic diversities. Anatomies of people are mimicked through simulations to be used by medical equipment producers for ready references. Clinical evidences substituted with digital evidence throughout the product development lifecycle making it more affordable and resource proficient. The demand for innovative and efficient medical equipment and medicines are growing, so are the development costs, profitability and reaching markets and clients are on the high. These technology start-ups are providing options to test addresses of medical devices instead of human trails in initial stages to cut costs, safety, and time. Thus, providing with scores of patient's lifesaving and affordable treatments, this is a real time boon for them.

Q Bio -USA (Whole Body)

A clinical platform is built by this digital twin start-ups Q Bio Gemini. It is powered by the Mark 1 Q Bio whole body scanner software. The patient's body is scanned in 15 minutes flat and there is no risk of claustrophobia and radiation. Securely shared dashboards present detailed real time inputs to medical professionals including concerned doctors. Such features make the whole-body scanning procedure much safer and reliable. Whole body scans recommended by doctors, provide more precise diagnosis and treatment procedures, but can need to radiation problems like cancer in the body. This makes it a costly and risky affair. So, AI enabled novel screening, digital twin technologies are providing more accessible comprehensive diagnostic safety and relief to patients.

INDIA ALSO CONTRIBUTING GLOBALLY TO TWIN TECHNOLOGY IN DIVERSE SECTORS INCLUDING MEDICAL INTEGRATIONS

Twin Health (Medical): This medical start-up has invented the whole-body digital twin. It helps the medical fraternity and patients to avert and repeal the metabolic chronic diseases. By improving physical health and energy it is extending the lifespan of the patients considerably. Merging medical science with advanced new age technology, this medical twin is healing the most dynamic and complex human metabolism system. Here more than 3000 health signals are replicated daily through a digital twin body. The non-invasive sensors used are perfectly safe and time saving. By constantly analysing these health signals, this medical health twin becomes a complete health guide, which reflects on the exact need to heal the damaged metabolism to reverse diabetes and other diseases. It also advises on personalized nutrition, sleep, activities and breathing procedures through a user-friendly app.

SwitchOn (Manufacturing): This start-up uses deep technology through digital twins to predict the performances on the shop floors. The conception is automating quality inspection procedures using AI and digital twins to forecast performance. By adding innovation, it further enables intelligence and smart systems in the manufacturing sector. Though AI is highly innovative and has been very adaptive in the enterprise and consumer eco system, but it is still emerging in the manufacturing sector. The solutions provided by this digital twin is predicting present and future shop floor performances enabling real time intelligence and cost saving measures from shop to top floor.

Pratiti Technologies (Solar Energy): This digital twin analytics systems start-ups is based on product development for solar energy assets sector. Integrating remote monitoring systems and SCADA (Supervisory Control and Data Acquisition), it is today one of the top energies impacting organization in India. Focusing on IoT and SMAC (Social Mobility Analytics and Cloud) it amalgamates Big Data and Cloud Computing driven by digital transformation. It improves the solar Photo Voltaic (PV) and adds to the renewable energy sector plants performance and procedures. This novel digital twin enables renewed energy with astute analytics, which adds to its USP.

Intangles (Transport): Fleet operators get precise projections for day-to-day operations and logistics. This real time predictive diagnostic twin is enabled by Start-ups Programme of Intel. It is responsible for providing the much-needed accurate insight to managers and owners to correctly map the performance of vehicles and save huge costs by better planning management. This helps the decision makers to take informed decisions by simulating real world environment virtually and thus analysing data physics based on analytics and deep learning. This has revolutionized the transport industry as any feedback of the vehicle which was till now made available only after physical inspection or service can now be accessed through its digital twin sitting anywhere or from your office.

Genesys International Corp (Geospatial): This geospatial solution start-ups integrates all the processes and actions that are having spatial details and are embedded inherently in the workflow of businesses. Through innovative advanced products like Geo AI, Geo Twin, Wonobo, Geo Loc & Geo Census very precise and high-quality geospatial content is delivered to its end users. They provide unique tailor-made end to end solutions for diverse sectors like Agriculture, Mining, Forestry, Utilities, Water Resources, Urban, Retail, Infrastructure, Insurance, Real Estate and Banking etc.

DIGITAL TWIN ADVANTAGES

Due to its plethora of advantages, data twin is seen as a milestone in industry 4.0 including downsizing excesses of uncertainties, inefficiencies, errors, costs, time, processes, and systems. It further helps in removing the hiccups in the integrations of compartments and divisions within a complex traditional organization structure which tend to work solo and in isolation. (Aidan Fuller, 28 May 2020) Not to mention that data twin is a boon for healthcare, manufacturing, and smart city concepts. Its rich IOT enabled environment is essential for product & service fault detection and maintenance predictions, enabling safe manufacturing and smart systems processes.

Cost Saving: Since most of the resources used in the creation of digital twins are virtual in nature, the overall cost of prototyping gets reduced a lot with time. There are lots of expenses incurred in traditional prototyping and the time taken is much more. Use of extensive labour, physical materials and catastrophic tests can bring an abrupt end to the costly prototype. Here using the digital twin, products can be created, recreated, and potently tested any number of times without any materialistic additional costs. So even if those initial costs are at par, the eventual costs reduce. Inflation can cause the physical costs to increase at the inception as time progresses, the virtual costs gradually decrease to a great extent. Digital twin allows product to be tested without additional costs under diverse operating circumstances, including disastrous ones which carry highest risks. This extends the life span of assets and equipment's and reduces the operating costs once put into practice.

Product Redesigning and Speed Prototyping: The analysis and design cycles are reduced heavily due to the simulations and investigations being based on varied scenarios. This makes the complete process of redesigning and prototyping much faster and easier. Digital Twin can be used in diverse stages of product design procedures from idea conceptualization of a product to its actual testing. Above all it creates and prospective opening for personal product customization based on patients need and usage of possible data. Since there is lifetime connectivity between the physical twin and its digital twin, regular comparative analysis on actual and forecasted performance is possible. This allows product design and engineering team to rework and rethink on their hypothesis of the earlier designed product.

Planning Systems and Predicting Problems: Systems can be planned accordingly as problems and inaccuracies of physical twin can be forecasted using their digital twin. Predicting problems in advance becomes easy due to free flow of real time data between the digital twin and the physical twin. Products having intricate compositions, numerous parts and having been constituted of multiple parts are the most beneficial with this technology like factory equipment, vehicles, and aircraft etc. It is so because it's always harder to forecast component breakdowns using conservative techniques in higher complex productivity scenarios.

Optimizing Solutions and Improving Maintenance: Conventional maintenance methods are based on plans derived from prior experience with similar problems and worse conditions scenarios, instead of material specification, structural constitution, and usability of the product. This makes them reactive instead of being proactive. With digital twin you can foresee the deficiencies and irregularities in the system, material, or plant & machinery. This helps to plan and schedule advance maintenance of the defaulting arena much easily, saving cost, time, and further damage. The digital twin after accessing the multiple scenarios stimulates the most suitable option or servicing strategy, making the whole system flexible and easier to use. We can get better validation and optimization of the system process constantly through constant feedback loop between the physical twin and its digital twin.

Easy Viability and Accessibility: The digital twin is highly accessible as its physical device can be remotely monitored and controlled. Virtual systems or the digital twins can be shared widely and can be used distantly. We have seen the vitality of distant working in the pandemic where remote monitoring and controlling of systems and equipment's became a necessity when physical access became limited due to health and government restrictions.

Safety and Reliability: In extreme and hazardous conditions like mining, oil & gas where safety is of high concern, digital twin scores through its ability to remotely access and predict things accurately. This not only reduces accident risks and fatal failures but abstains from unwanted human contact and on-site monitoring, leading to safety measures as well. During the pandemic, almost one third companies have used digital twin technology to remotely monitor men, material, systems as counter safety and risk mitigation tools & measures.

Reducing Wastage: Waste is reduced to a great extent when digital twins are used to test product and system prototypes in a virtual setup. The researched, tested, and simulated designs can be explored and examined virtually under diverse scenarios before zeroing in on the final product before production stage. All this cuts down development costs, material wastage and time taken for product to reach market.

Documenting and Communicating Seamlessly: Digital twin are created by synchronizing data spread across different hard copies, databases, and software applications to minimize the process of maintenance and accessibility of data at one place. Due to its enhanced understanding of system responses, it can be utilized to effectively communicate and document the mechanism and behavioural patterns of its physical twin.

Training and Development: Enhanced, instructive, and more efficient safety training and development programmes can be developed using the digital twins. These are more impactful and practical than the traditional ones. Digital twin helps the operational team to practice and train beforehand on the diverse procedures and scenarios before exposing them in high-risk zones or in the usage of hazardous plant and machinery. This educates them and exposes them to handle any such miss happenings in advance. This makes the team confident and better equipped to handle tricky situations like Mining, Oil Riggs, Explorations, and Tunnels. Here the use of digital twin, helps to train new employees how to use such plant and machinery in volatile situations easily and handle emergencies in accordance, so it's a great learning and risk mitigation tool to fill the knowledge gap which can arise in unpredictable and isolated environments.

PRESENT ARENA

Till now digital twin was more leveraged in manufacturing and aerospace sectors and still infancy in other sectors like healthcare, construction, agriculture, and automobiles etc. During the pandemic there were many driving factors that pushed for the digital twin demand in pharmaceutical, healthcare and the manufacturing industries. The Covid -19 gave digital twin the platform to grow and be life saviors. 'Cardio Twin' developers consider that their product can prevent heart stroke in future. So digital twin, has all the capability to give personalized and cost-effective medical care to every person, which he so very much deserves. Globally more and more governments are generating interest and adapting digital twins in their states and cities to be better planned and managed in mitigating present and future risks. In high-risk prone incidents like tsunamis, cyclones and earthquakes, digital twins can serve the stakeholders faster as they are prone to resolve critical issues quickly as seen in the pandemic where they were able share local strategies at a much faster rate in multiple cities. In future more and more technologies can be aligned with the digital twins for enhanced results. Better visualization can be achieved for remote supervisory inspections using it with mixed reality. Education is benefitting when DT is combined with Virtual and Augmented Reality (VR/AR) in engineering, construction, and architecture streams. This developed digital pedagogy is immensely valuable for teachers in remote lecture deliverances in emergencies or regular online learning platforms.

DIGITAL TWIN GROWTH & CHALLENGES IN PRESENT AND FUTURE

Technology namely Artificial Intelligence (AI), Internet of Things (IOT), Big Data, Industrial Internet of Things (IIOT), Cloud Computing, Simulation is integrated in a loop for composing Digital Twin. These technologies keep evolving constantly, so in accordance DT must evolve itself to be relevant. Therefore, the true potential of digital twins is yet to be mapped as it still must evolve from the dense fog that surrounds the business complexities. As per global market expectations DT is expected to grow by more than 50% and reach 50 billion $ in next five years. The pandemic has been one of the main growth factors as digital twin has gained prominence in times of uncertainties, it is expected to grow at a faster rate post pandemic as the industry will now push for further full steam digitalization. Of course, human will play pivotal role in the development of digital twin as it will be vital for symbiotic relationship between machine and humans soon. This will be an indispensable part of machine development and researchers are already predicting the 'digital triplet' as the next generation evolution. Here "intelligent activity world" will sync with cyber and physical worlds. Digital Triplets will have the human interaction with processes and system accounted for where data will create value from human knowledge and intelligence, unlike in digital twin where systems and process. The plan of digital triplet will be to garner support and make the engineering plans of a product life cycle more fool proof. This means the digital triplet will be more involved in the design, manufacturing, usage, circulation of recourses, maintenance, remanufacturing, and scaling of the process by integrating the three worlds as the digital twin is already doing.

IMPLEMENTATION CHALLENGES

Novel Evolving Technologies: Though there are several challenges as digital twin is a mammoth arena. Its implementation is one of the challenges as are its development and complexities of technology while scaling. Digital twin is in its infancy stage with great potential and its implementation is complicated due to technical, engineering, and commercial hiccups. Other complications like uncertainties in understanding the concept of digital twin, usage of appropriate tools, expensive research and development, data compatibility issues and deficient rules and regulations. So as an emerging technology, it is vital for individuals, businesses, and industries to imbibe practical and technical knowledge of digital twin professionally so that seamless adaptations can be implemented across organizations. Being a novel concept there is limited research, case studies of business models, or accurate cost factors to be implemented on a very mass scale. Since aligning technologies that make digital twin a highly emerging potent are themselves at developing stages, it hampers the pace of evolution of the digital twin technology. To augment the efficacy of the digital twin, infrastructure must be upgraded in accordance. Further futuristic research is needed in the aligning DT with areas of result enhancing technologies such as real time technology, high performance computing, machine learning, real-virtual interactive machines, connection technology and intelligent perception units etc. A plethora of aligning supporting software must be created to be integrated with DT for smooth solutions like the present ones from Azure from Microsoft, Predix by GE, ABB Watson by IBM, Digital Enterprise Suite by Siemens, PTC, 3D by Dassault. The best suitable platform must be carefully identified for catering to separate product lines for maximum output and most appropriate service to respective industries.

Cost and Time Factors: Digital Twin is still an early-stage start-ups and of high cost at the research and development stage but sharply streamlines as itis implemented on ground. So, it is vitally important to judiciously manage this high potential digital twin cost in the early bird stage. Since ultra-high fidelity computer software, hardware and digital models are involved in the simulation process, it's a costly and time taking affair. To add to it, factors like computational power consuming, high labour intensity and time-consuming research makes it of high-cost proposition. The digital twin system needs to be embedded with data collection sensors, best software, and hardware to process and store huge data banks. So, cost and time naturally increases to be well supported by latest IT infrastructure of highest performance. The outcome though is of the high-test order and matches the best cutting age technology globally.

Data Security and Synchronization: Digital Twin works on huge data banks, which is a critical aspect to storage, transparency, confidentiality, privacy, risk, and ownership rights etc. Here company and client policies and agreements come into foreplay, which is beyond the intricacies of engineering and technology. Digital Twin must strike a careful and judicious balance with a well drafted policy while sharing this confidential data to its internal and external stakeholders. This mismatch can lead to data blocks within departments or businesses, hampering flow of information. Also sharing data among different digital twins at different hierarchical levels or interoperability is complex and needs high precision. Cyber security and risk mitigation of vital importance while handling data as it can lead to disruptive performance and cybercrimes. Data governance and convergence is also a major challenge as big data loads can make or break a project.

Mismatching Life Cycles: Products having long life cycles like cities, ships, aircrafts, buildings, plant & machinery are challenging for digital twins because of time bound validations by the integrated software used in simulations, design, and data storage compatibility. There is high risk of software becoming obsolete with time or being locked in new version update by concerned vendors or tool authorization entities.

Lacking in Regulations and Standards: Even as there is surplus of literature on the architecture and models of the digital twin, there is still no concrete framework for their standardization and regulations. Across the industry, these interfaces and standardization rules must be mutually understood and abided so that there is a firm consensus for setting parameters and compliances. Since it is a high proposition product carrying sensitive data, its security and policy becomes even more strategic. Here standardized models, interfaces, protocols are essential for human and product safety, integrity, and data security across diverse industries. ISO 23247, or the Digital Twin Manufacturing Framework is being developed for setting guidelines and roadmap for manufacturing, developing, and adapting the DT. The framework intends to cover the general principles and its overview, architecture references, sharing of information and digitally representing of the physical manufacturing elements.

CONCLUSION

Though digital twin as a concept was used years ago by NASA, its real conception, impact, and adaption is a recent phenomenon. It is already making a high impact in the globe as a technological marvel due to its unique proposition to diverse industries. Though Digital Twin is a intricate technology, however if it's implemented judiciously, it can be a solution to the most complex problems and be a real lifesaver in medical and other industries. It can be used to replicate workflows, staffing systems, care delivery models, capacity planning to improve overall medical mindfulness. Digital Twin is leading to clinical advancement by proposing novel ways of research while exploring illness. There are numerous medical use cases; digital twin s being closest to reality form medical device development to personalized medicine. The USP of digital twin is that it evolves seamlessly with diverse technologies and end use industries, thus reducing time and operational costs. Simultaneously it adds to the production by enhancing systems, improving maintenance, and upgrading security. This eases accessibility and creates a safe working environment. As a potent industry 4.0 tool, it simulates and predicts outcomes, stores, and shares vital data and is crucial for trouble shooting measures. It can reduce costs, increase outputs, be accessed remotely, and streamlines operations and services. (BergthorBjornsson, 2019) The Digital Twin clinical will require implementation that will entail solving of a wider range of medical, ethical, theoretical and technical challenges. You can compare the complexities and cost to a Human Genome Project (HGP), but the after affects and results of improved health care and disease understanding mechanisms, technical development, research potential apart from novel research integration surpasses everything with vast magnitude comprehensively. Thus, we can convincingly say Digital Twin or DT is the technological future of different industries, promising exponential growth and viability globally and needs to be pursued and supported relentlessly.

REFERENCES

Aidan Fuller, Z. F. (28 May 2020). Digital Twin: Enabling Technologies, Challenges and Open Research. *IEEE.*

Barricelli, B.; Casiraghi, E.; Gliozzo, J.; Petrini, A.; Valtolina, S. (n.d.). Human Digital Twin for Fitness Management. *IEEE* doi:. doi:10.1109/ACCESS.2020.2971576

BergthorBjornsson, C. B. (2019). Digital twins to personalize medicine. *Biomedical Central-. Genome Medicine.*

Boulos, M. N. (2021). *Digital Twins: From Personalised Medicine to Precision Public Health.* Researchgate.

David Jones, C. S. (May 2020). Characterising the Digital Twin: A systematic literature review. *Science Direct*, 36-52.

Yang Peng, M. Z. (2020). Digital Twin Hospital Buildings: An Exemplary Case Study through Continuous Lifecycle Integration. *Resaerch Gate.*

Qia. Q. F. Y. (2018). Digital Twin Service towards Smart Manufacturing. Elsevier, 237-242.

Saddik, A. E. (2022). *Digital Twin for Healthcare: Design, Challenges and Solutions.* Elsevier.

Tolga Erol, A. F. (2020). *The Digital Twin Revolution in Healthcare.* Research Gate.

van derValk, H. H. (03 Dec 2021). *Archetypes of Digital Twins.* Springer.

Volkov, I. G. A. (2021). Digital Twins, Internet of Things and Mobile Medicine: A Review of Current Platforms to Support Smart Healhcare. Springer.

Chapter 6
Digital Twins Enabling Technologies, Including Artificial Intelligence, Sensors, Cloud, and Edge Computing

Subramaniam Meenakshi Sundaram
https://orcid.org/0000-0003-2352-0714
GSSS Institute of Engineering and Technology for Women, Mysuru, India

Tejaswini R Murgod
Nitte Meenakshi Institute of Technology, Bengaluru, India

Sowmya M.
GSSS Institute of Engineering and Technology for Women, Mysuru, India

ABSTRACT

With the fast growth of big data, IoT, industrial internet, and intelligent control technology, digital twins are extensively employed as a novel form of technology in many aspects of life. Digital twins have emerged as the ideal connection between the real world of manufacturing and the digital virtual world, as well as an effective technological way of realizing the interaction and cooperation of the real and information worlds. Digital twins rely on knowledge mechanisms, digitization, and other technologies to build digital models. They use IoT and other technologies to convert data and information in the physical world into general data. Its necessity is mainly reflected in the massive data processing and system self-optimization in the digital twin ecosystem, so that the digital twin ecosystem is orderly and intelligent cloud travel, and it is the central brain of the digital twin ecosystem. The rapidly expanding digital twin market indicates that this technology is already in use across many industries and is demanded to rise at an estimated USD 48.2 billion in 2026.

DOI: 10.4018/978-1-6684-5925-6.ch006

INTRODUCTION

The idea of digital twin technology was first voiced in 1991, with the publication of Mirror Worlds, by David Gelernter. However, Dr. Michael Grieves (then on faculty at the University of Michigan) is credited with first applying the concept of digital twins to manufacturing in 2002 and formally announcing the digital twin software concept. Eventually, NASA's John Vickers introduced a new term "digital twin" in 2010. However, the core idea of using a digital twin as a means of studying a physical object can actually be witnessed much earlier. In fact, it can be rightfully said that NASA pioneered the use of digital twin technology during its space exploration missions of the 1960s, when each voyaging spacecraft was exactly replicated in an earthbound version that was used for study and simulation purposes by NASA personnel serving on flight crews.

Advanced computer technologies such as Artificial Intelligence (AI), cloud computing, digital twins, and edge computing and big data have been applied in various fields as digitalization has progressed. A digital twin is a virtual representation of an object or system that spans its lifecycle, is updated from real-time data, and uses simulation, machine learning and reasoning to help decision-making. The purpose of a digital twin is to run cost-effective simulations. The digital twin uses IoT sensors, log files and other relevant information to collect real-time data for accurate modeling of assets. These models are then combined with AI-powered analytics tools in a virtual setting. Digital twins can significantly improve enterprises' data-driven decision-making processes. They are linked to their real-world equivalents at the edge and businesses use digital twins to understand the state of the physical asset, respond to changes, improve operations, and add value to the systems. These digital assets can be created even before an asset is built physically. Research the physical object or system that will be mimicked and integrate sensors into physical assets or monitor log files and other sources to collect data. This is further integrated into the virtual model with AI algorithms. Later by applying analytics into these models, data scientists and engineers get relevant insights regarding the physical asset. The digital twins are commonly used in manufacturing which provide lower maintenance costs via predictive maintenance, improved productivity, faster production times, testing prior to manufacturing and improved customer satisfaction.

Although simulations and digital twins both utilize digital models to replicate a system's various processes, a digital twin is actually a virtual environment, which makes it considerably richer for study. The difference between digital twin and simulation is largely a matter of scale: While a simulation typically studies one particular process, a digital twin can itself run any number of useful simulations in order to study multiple processes.

For example, simulations usually do not benefit from having real-time data. But digital twins are designed around a two-way flow of information that first occurs when object sensors provide relevant data to the system processor and then happens again when insights created by the processor are shared back with the original source object. By having better and constantly updated data related to a wide range of areas, combined with the added computing power that accompanies a virtual environment, digital twins are able to study more issues from far more vantage points than standard simulations can with greater ultimate potential to improve products and processes.

Alexopoulo et al. (2020) pointed out that the digital twin's model can be used to accelerate the ML training phase by generating an appropriate training data set and automatically labeling it through a simulation tool chain, thereby reducing user participation in the training process. These synthetic datasets may be expanded and cross-validated using extensive real-world data that does not require considerable use. Fan et al. (2021) investigates and proposes a vision of a disaster city digital twins concept, which can realize the interdisciplinary integration of information and communication technology (ICT) in crisis informatics and disaster response. This involves incorporating AI algorithms and methods to enhance situation assessment, decision-making, and coordination among different stakeholders, thereby increasing visibility into the dynamics of intricate disaster response and humanitarian assistance.

According to Rasheed et al.'s (2019) study, digital twins are adaptive models of complex systems. Digital twins are currently a significant rising trend in a wide range of applications. Also known as computing giant models, device shadows, mirroring systems, avatars, or synchronized virtual prototypes. As a result, digital twins play a transformational role not only in how we build and manage cyber-physical intelligent systems, but also in how we promote the modularization of multidisciplinary systems to solve fundamental obstacles.

A fundamental change to existing operating models is clearly happening. A digital reinvention is occurring in asset-intensive industries that are changing operating models in a disruptive way, requiring an integrated physical plus digital view of assets, equipment, facilities, and processes. Digital twins are a vital part of that realignment. The future of digital twins is nearly limitless, due to the fact that increasing amounts of cognitive power are constantly being devoted to their use. So digital twins are constantly learning new skills and capabilities, which means they can continue to generate the insights needed to make products better and processes more efficient. According to Gaur et. al. (2021) machine learning (ML) based AI applications are commonly regarded as a promising technology in the manufacturing industry. Nevertheless, the ML method needs a huge number of high-quality training datasets. In the case of supervised ML, manual input is frequently necessary to label these datasets. This method is costly, error-prone, and time-consuming, particularly in a complicated and dynamic manufacturing setting. Santosh et. al. (2022) evaluates AI and machine learning (ML) algorithms in dealing with challenges that are primarily related to public health. It also helps find ways in which we can measure possible consequences and societal impacts by taking into account open public health issues and common AI solutions. Rana et. al. (2021) has proposed a theoretical framework to adopt artificial intelligence (AI) and machine learning (ML) as a protective measure for interaction between the customers. Gaur et. al. (2021) gives a study of both theoretical and practical to the multidisciplinary domains of computer science, information systems and uses data using visual analytics techniques for digital twins.

TYPES OF DIGITAL TWINS

There are various types of digital twins depending on the level of product magnification. The biggest difference between these twins is the area of application. It is common to have different types of digital twins co-exist within a system or process. Let's go through the types of digital twins to learn the differences and how they are applied.

i) Component Twins/Parts Twins

Component twins are the basic unit of digital twin, the smallest example of a functioning component. Parts twins are roughly the same thing, but pertain to components of slightly less importance.

ii) Asset Twins

When two or more components work together, they form what is known as an asset. Asset twins let you study the interaction of those components, creating a wealth of performance data that can be processed and then turned into actionable insights.

iii) System Or Unit Twins

The next level of magnification involves system or unit twins, which enable you to see how different assets come together to form an entire functioning system. System twins provide visibility regarding the interaction of assets, and may suggest performance enhancements.

iv) Process Twins

Process twins, the macro level of magnification, reveal how systems work together to create an entire production facility. Are those systems all synchronized to operate at peak efficiency, or will delays in one system affect others? Process twins can help determine the precise timing schemes that ultimately influence overall effectiveness.

BENEFITS OF DIGITAL TWINS

Some of the benefits of digital twins include:

i) Better R&D

The use of digital twins enables more effective research and design of products, with an abundance of data created about likely performance outcomes. That information can lead to insights that help companies make needed product refinements before starting production.

ii) Greater Efficiency

Even after a new product has gone into production, digital twins can help mirror and monitor production systems, with an eye to achieving and maintaining peak efficiency throughout the entire manufacturing process.

iii) Product End-Of-Life

Digital twins can even help manufacturers decide what to do with products that reach the end of their product lifecycle and need to receive final processing, through recycling or other measures. By using digital twins, they can determine which product materials can be harvested.

APPLICATIONS OF DIGITAL TWINS

Digital twins are already extensively used in the following applications like:

i) Power-Generation Equipment

Large engines — including jet engines, locomotive engines and power-generation turbines — benefit tremendously from the use of digital twins, especially for helping to establish timeframes for regularly needed maintenance.

ii) Structures And Their Systems

Big physical structures, such as large buildings or offshore drilling platforms, can be improved through digital twins, particularly during their design. Also useful in designing the systems operating within those structures, such as HVAC systems.

iii) Manufacturing Operations

Since digital twins are meant to mirror a product's entire lifecycle, it's not surprising that digital twins have become ubiquitous in all stages of manufacturing, guiding products from design to finished product, and all steps in between.

iv) Healthcare Services

Just as products can be profiled through the use of digital twins, so can patients receiving healthcare services. The same type of system of sensor-generated data can be used to track a variety of health indicators and generate key insights.

v) Automotive Industry

Cars represent many types of complex, co-functioning systems, and digital twins are used extensively in auto design, both to improve vehicle performance and increase the efficiency surrounding their production.

vi) Urban Planning

Civil engineers and others involved in urban planning activities are aided significantly by the use of digital twins, which can show 3D and 4D spatial data in real time and also incorporate augmented reality systems into built environments

DIGITAL TWINS AND SIMULATIONS

A digital twin is a virtual model designed to accurately reflect a physical object. The object being studied for example, a wind turbine is outfitted with various sensors related to vital areas of functionality. These sensors produce data about different aspects of the physical object's performance, such as energy output, temperature, weather conditions and more. This data is then relayed to a processing system and applied to the digital copy. Once informed with such data, the virtual model can be used to run simulations, study performance issues and generate possible improvements, all with the goal of generating valuable insights which can then be applied back to the original physical object.

Although simulations and digital twins both utilize digital models to replicate a system's various processes, a digital twin is actually a virtual environment, which makes it considerably richer for study. The difference between digital twin and simulation is largely a matter of scale: While a simulation typically studies one particular process, a digital twin can itself run any number of useful simulations in order to study multiple processes. For example, simulations usually don't benefit from having real-time data. But digital twins are designed around a two-way flow of information that first occurs when object sensors provide relevant data to the system processor and then happens again when insights created by the processor are shared back with the original source object. By having better and constantly updated data related to a wide range of areas, combined with the added computing power that accompanies a virtual environment, digital twins are able to study more issues from far more vantage points than standard simulations can with greater ultimate potential to improve products and processes

DIGITAL TWINS AND INTERNET OF THINGS

Many organizations want to create models that demonstrate how the various elements of the internet of things (IoT) will be brought into their operating reality and merged with existing ISO, Six Sigma and total quality management (TQM) aligned methods for ensuring reliability. To achieve this, they have to apply rigor to specific areas where they define the *what*, *when*, *how* and *why* of their IoT deployment. These decision points align with the Internet of Things knowledge domain:

1. **Source**: The ready availability of digital twins will revolutionize the process of on boarding complex equipment. On boarding is often a siloed process, rife with paperwork and prone to human error. When industrial equipment is purchased, maintenance plans must be built based on multiple conversations with original equipment manufacturers (OEMs). Materials lists must be created and entered into systems manually, and stocking occurs based on assumed part criticality and allocated budgets. With each stage managed by a different team, the process is plagued with inefficiencies and can take months to complete. For example, digitizing something as large and complicated as an entire oil refinery could take as long as five or six months. This assumes it would be based on physical blueprints and paper documents from its structure to its equipment inventory, processes and failure modes. An initiative like this would completely dominate the time of plant engineers. Digital twins can streamline this process to get the system up and running immediately. Rather than rely on slow, manual processes, the digital twin leverages existing digital replicas of the individual components that reside within the larger system. (These digital assets would have been created by the owners of the components during the development process.)

2. **Connect**: Many in the industry say that IoT sensors continue to drop in price every year. This is to encourage organizations to enable their enterprises with the IoT now. But, people often underestimate the various requirements that come with connecting their equipment, their enterprise and their industry. Additionally, there are many application programming interfaces (APIs) and other development approaches. And, many questions on issues, such as access, information flow and storage, must be answered before an organization can build a truly secure and purposeful digital nervous system. Every connection point creates a possible vector for a cyber attack. Therefore, each connection needs to be designed, developed

and deployed to be secure; every single one. This is a lot of work without a platform that helps drive uniformity.

Digital twins that are used in operations with live data, as well as in collaborative development situations with manufacturers, operators and other third parties, require secure workspaces and communications. Otherwise, the integrity of the digital twins and the data they house cannot be maintained. Connectivity with asset sensors allows organizations to get closer to a full operating twin that mimics the experiences of the physical assets. But, it demands that the system is protected and facilitated as it's shared and updated by multiple parties.

3. Collect: Digital twins create a logical taxonomy of the data from the IoT, as well as the categorization and use of that data. The ability to shape the data set based on physical, digital and electromechanical attributes allows enterprises to manage their data requirements. Digital twins manage by exception and operating processes, such as anomaly detection, asset modifications and customizations. They *filter* the massive volumes of operating data that flows through the enterprise, limiting what needs to be captured, cleansed, stored, reused and actioned. By definition, the digital twin encompasses this collection phase, pulling in everything it knows to be true about the physical asset.

The vision of the Digital Twins is to enable good decisions that deliver value to physical and digital operations and support ongoing industry transformation

4. Analyze: As mentioned in data collection, data analysis is more effective based on volume of data. But it's less efficient based on the need to manage, merge and cleanse the volumes of data to create data sets that analysts and data scientists can use. By employing digital twins to categorize data and visualize and contextualize it, teams can compartmentalize their activities, create hypotheses and communicate results to non-technical or non-analytical peers. The addition of statistical analysis tools and models that execute a plethora of calculations on a rich model with multiple attributes makes it easier to predict failure, flow and feasibility. Modeling tools that enable the simulation of an issue or enhancement in a future state are already common in the virtual reality space, whereas digital twins allow physics to guide the analysis in a pseudo real-world sense. As such, whole production lines, factories, vehicles and systems can be tested before major investments or reductions in investments are made. This leads to the benefit artificial intelligence (AI) can bring to improving operations for physical assets. The digital twin holds the data that is collected and fed into the AI models to uncover key insights.

5. Do: If done correctly, a digital twin allows owners and operators to perform simulation and what-if analysis on their physical assets. If the physical asset is IoT enabled and accepts commands to actuate on the asset, remote and autonomous operation becomes possible. By combining the IoT with AI for anomaly detection and prediction, you create the asset of the future.

The vision of the digital twin is to enable good decisions that deliver value to your physical and digital operations and support your ongoing industry transformation. While the digital twin will solve many issues, the achievement of its vision isn't possible unless you digitize your physical assets and their subassemblies. We must also work together to develop standards for how digital twin resources should be structured to achieve consistency across consumption technologies.

Regardless of the challenges, there is no question that even in the very physical, asset intensive industries (e.g., energy and utilities, oil and petroleum, manufacturing and industrial products), digital assets are becoming just as essential as physical ones. Digital twins are a revolutionary solution to help ensure that companies achieve efficiency and efficacy in their operations, and that they continue to bring value to their customers.

DIGITAL TWINS AND ARTIFICIAL INTELLIGENCE

Software applications have also evolved over the decades in many ways, one of the most notable being the dramatic acceleration of the application adoption cycle. In the past two decades alone, users have shifted at alarmingly fast rates from treating applications as interesting novelties, to turning to them as a convenience, to expecting them to work flawlessly all the time. At each adoption stage, a user's expectation rises, meaning the product must also evolve and mature at very fast, scalable rates. The combination of the hardware and software trends formed an interesting convergence of product development requirements. New 'critical need' applications suddenly must include higher capacity of real-time processing, time-sensitive decision-making, high to very high availability, and expectations that platform-generated decisions be correct, every time. This combination formed the initial need for both ML and AI, to allow for the expectation of explosive adoption and growth.

While most people think of AI primarily as an end-user resource, AI has become necessary to enable faster product design and development. From the earliest stage of a chipset design or layout of a circuit all the way through end-product validation, emulators have become necessary to emulate complex interfaces and environments. These emulators, known as digital twins, are a virtual manifestation of a process, environmental condition, or protocol capable of serving as a 'known good signal.' In test terms, a digital twin can be a simple signal generator, a full protocol generator, or a complete environment emulator. Using a digital twin allows developers to rapidly create a significantly wider range of test conditions to validate their product before shipping. High performance digital twins typically contain their own AI engines allowing them to automatically troubleshoot and regression test new product designs.

The shift to AI-driven development using automating test functions and digital twins has become necessary due to the large amount of functionality and autonomous decision-making expected in new products. Basic design principles specify features and functionality of a product, then set up individual tests to validate them. The sheer number and complexity of interface standards makes that virtually impossible to construct by hand. By using digital twins, a much wider set of functional tests can be programmed in much less time than a developer could even imagine on their own. AI functionality then automates test processes based on what it discovers and predicts actions that might be needed based on a current state. To understand this better, it's useful to understand the core of what makes any AI possible.

In its simplest form, software decision-making starts with algorithms. Basic algorithms run a set of calculations, and if you know what constitutes acceptable vs. unacceptable results, you can create a finite state machine using decision tree outcomes. This would hardly be considered intelligent. By adding a notation of state, however, and inserting a feedback loop, your basic algorithm can now make outcome decisions a function of both the current conditions compared to the current state. Combine this while evolving the decision tree into a behavior tree and you have formed the genesis of AI.

We are all at the early stage of AI and digital twins, which means lots of products will be making lots of claims. Whether the AI you are examining is in your development lab, a cloud software application you are using, or in the autonomous driving car you own, it is there for a reason. Understanding what it's supposed to deliver will allow you to assess its criticality. Same is true for the digital twin. Once we isolate the intended signal(s), condition(s) or decision outcome(s) either is designed to replicate, evaluating its efficacy becomes the easy part.

FUTURE ASPECTS OF DIGITAL TWINS AND ARTIFICIAL INTELLIGENCE

Digital twin technology promises to transform design and give product developers, manufacturers and businesses a 360-degree view of products and systems throughout the entire lifecycle. Armed with an enriched pool of data provided by the Internet of Things (IoT), the design technology stands poised to deliver previously impossible opportunities. Unfortunately, meeting these goals lies beyond the reach of traditional design technologies. To address the new demands, designers are turning to artificial intelligence (AI), the missing element in the engineer's toolbox. But even with the current crop of AI technologies, developers and analysts have to perform a number of balancing acts. For instance, they have to find algorithms that can achieve the right balance of speed and accuracy. They must also acknowledge that the size of the data pool sometimes matters less than the quality of the data in it.

Furthermore, and this may make or break the technology's success, digital twin software providers will have to find a way to reduce implementation demands so that more users can enjoy the benefits of the technology. How can AI help to fulfill the promise of the digital twin? Developers of the virtual design tool see AI as providing the catalyst for a major shift in product development.

Technology developers see AI as a way to accelerate design processes, allowing engineers to quickly evaluate many possible design alternatives. By changing design parameters and running AI algorithms, digital twin design software providers contend that engineers could quickly evaluate possible best fits based on the results of the algorithms. The use of AI in this context is still in the early stages. Most successful digital twin technologies use AI systems to make predictions of situations where data is abundant and where the processes being evaluated are relatively simple. But this is changing. "We are in the midst of a second wave of digital twin technologies, which has truly game-changing attributes," says Juan Betts, managing director of Front End Analytics. "In this new framework, the digital twin is not just predicting overall product performance based on user preferences, but it is also adapting and predicting the performance and state of key individual components of the system to achieve user-specific individualized performance enhancements." A good way to see how these benefits are delivered is by viewing the various stages of a digital twin implementation. This examination begins with conventional computer design tools and migrates to more cutting-edge AI-based processes.

The typical starting point for implementing one of these virtual designs is with an existing 3D simulation model, created using a product lifecycle management (PLM) platform or CAD tool. These models typically describe what the physical entity will look like and provide dimensions and possibly descriptions of materials to be used in construction.

The engineer or sometimes the analyst begins to create a digital twin of the physical product by overlaying the existing 3D simulation model with real-time data from associated sensors, deployment details and operational conditions. At this point, the engineer encounters a major challenge. Conventional design software often takes hours or even days to complete simulations using the operational and sensory inputs required to create the digital twin. As a result, tasks such as design optimization, design space exploration and what-if analyses become impractical because they simply require too many simulations.

To bypass this obstacle, digital twin developers implement an AI-driven process called surrogate modeling also known as reduced order modeling which mimics the behavior of complex simulation models as closely as possible in a less computationally intensive way. The analyst constructs surrogate models using a data-driven, bottom-up approach, taking the critical aspects of a detailed model and reducing them to simpler algorithms that are executed in real time or faster. Multiple techniques can come into play here, with the engineer combining computations from online and offline phases and using decomposition methods. The surrogate model can use truncation, subspace and response surface methodologies, neural networks and ensemble-based heuristics

INDUSTRIAL APPLICATIONS OF DIGITAL TWINS

Artificial intelligence in digital twins is a universally applicable theoretical and technical system, with many applications, such as product design, equipment manufacturing, medical analysis, aerospace and other fields. At present, the most in-depth application in China is in the field of engineering construction, and intelligent manufacturing has gained the most attraction in the research field.

***a)* The Use of Digital Twins in The Aerospace Field.** The notion of digital twins was originally presented for use in the aerospace field. For example, digital twins are used in the maintenance and quality assurance process of flight simulation and aerospace flight machines27. The real aircraft model is established in the digital space, and then the sensors are used to integrate the digital space. The status of the aircraft is synchronized with the status of the flying aircraft in reality. In this way, the process of each aircraft taking off and landing is simulated and stored in the digital space. Through the data analysis of the digital space, it is possible to clearly understand whether the aircraft needs maintenance and whether it can proceed to the next flight.

The purpose of the research by Yurkevich et al. (2021) is to develop a neural model for digital air traffic control. This method adopts the concept of a physical self-organizing social network of a distributed organization and technical system, and its components are connected to wireless 4G and 5G networks. The advantage of this method is that the principle of analysis and management is very promising, and it has complex integration with hybrid artificial intelligence.

Dai et al. (2021) showed that the autopilot Unmanned Aerial Vehicle (UAV) system, as a safety-critical system, requires continuous improvement in its reliability and safety. Testing a complicated automatic pilot control system, on the other hand, is a time and money-intensive project that necessitates several outside flight tests during the project growth period. Therefore, an internal automated testing system for automatic driving platform is presented as a way to increase the efficiency and safety of UAV development. With the development of unmanned aircraft technology, unmanned aircraft are being employed in an increasing number of applications and are regarded as an essential component of the future smart city infrastructure. Simultaneously, the security and privacy threats connected with drone-based applications require proper testing and surveillance techniques. For a platform that facilitates the administration and performance of drone-based applications on common drone architecture, Grigoropoulos et al. (2020) supplied an analog environment and digital twins support. First, the simulation environment can perform in-depth testing of the platform itself and the functions of the applications running on the platform, and it can then be deployed to the actual world. After deployment, the digital twin is used to discover gaps and expected behaviors between applications, which in turn can be used as an error indicator when the simulation test is executed or malfunctions have not been found. Maintenance has evolved from "post-incident maintenance" and "preventive maintenance" to "predictive maintenance," making it one of the most critical components of aviation.

Precision maintenance is the future development path, with the purpose of ensuring operational safety and lowering the collaborative optimization goal and operating cost. To improve the effect of engine predictive maintenance, Xiong et al. (2020) studied a digital twin-driven aircraft engine predictive maintenance framework, and discovered an implicit digital twin IDT (Implicit Digital Twins) model.

The model's validity is determined by evaluating the concordance of virtual and actual data assets. The usefulness of the approach is demonstrated by integrating the data-driven deep learning (DL) method40 with the LSTM (Long Short-Term Memory) model41 and using an aviation engine as an example.

***b)* The Use of Digital Twins in The Intelligent Automated Driving.** AI applications are quickly developing as deep learning and big data analysis technologies advance. Among them, it is imperative to use artificial intelligence algorithms to develop autonomous driving systems. In real life, autonomous driving technology can reduce traffic accidents, realize the efficiency of time and space and other resource utilization, and even provide great convenience for the driving process of the disabled. However, due to the high technical requirements of autonomous driving, the need for digital twins to simulate driving in a virtual simulation environment has become an indispensable step.

***c)* The Use of Digital Twins In Intelligent Manufacturing**. With the continuous development of intelligent manufacturing technology in various countries around the world, the informatization level of the manufacturing industry is gradually improving. In order to enhance product production rates and deal with emergencies in the production process in a timely manner, enterprises must strengthen the management and control measures of each module in the production workshop to improve the company's ability to control the production process. Moreover, consumers' higher individual requirements for products have caused companies to face a large amount of data, data requirements and data structures in the production process, which has made it difficult for companies to manage and analyze data. Therefore, in the manufacturing process, how to effectively and timely feedback the use status of the equipment in the production workshop and early warning of failures has become a major problem in the current intelligent manufacturing industry.

***d)* The Use of Digital Twins In Smart Cities.** The concept of digital twins is simply to map people, objects, relationships, and processes in real-world to virtual-world, and realize the research and control of real objects by observing and analyzing the digital twin in virtual space. Applying this concept to the field of urban transportation is undoubtedly a boon to the construction of smart cities. The major functional region management of an urban area is a spatial organization and strategy that promotes urban and regional development with space control as the main goal. The research of Gao et al. (2017) shows that: the construction program of urban functional areas is optimized and analyzed according to big data and GIS (Geographic Information System). The primary goal of urban functional area management is to limit or regulate reasonable use of land and to establish a foundation for the efficient use of city area.

CHALLENGES FOR ARTIFICIAL INTELLIGENCE IN DIGITAL TWINS

Due to the rapid development of the global intelligent internet automotive industry, research on automotive internet related technologies is of great significance to promote the development of automotive Internet. The parameterization and generalization technology of traffic scene simulation shows that the test process and working conditions of autonomous driving simulation can be said to have no boundaries. Whether the car is running normally or not, it can be tested repeatedly to facilitate the discovery and location of problems. However, in the process of vehicle dynamic simulation test, the simulation sensor and sensing system enter the automatic driving control and decide to form a closed-loop test and system verification test equipment by pure software, which is also an important challenge for the current automatic driving hardware equipment.

The main function of automatic driving is to control the simulation car corresponding to the real car in the simulation system by receiving the real-time position, speed, acceleration, heading angle and other information of the real car sent by the data collection visualization system. Realize the real vehicle control and the simulation vehicle runs in the virtual scene, so that the motion states of the two are synchronized, and realize the basic function of the real vehicle in the loop. Although the current stage of research has formed a highly open digital twin autonomous driving test capability, a friendly and open test and verification environment has also been established to support a variety of autonomous driving algorithm experiments and provide open testing services for research companies related to autonomous driving. However, there are still challenges to solve the test solution:

i) **Testing Cost Issues**. The current test system for autonomous driving is not complete yet, but it has already produced high test costs. This is a very big challenge for automobile manufacturers. The most important issue for automobile manufacturers is how to maximize benefits and minimize costs. Therefore, the establishment of an efficient and low-cost test environment, a structured test process, and a strong test standard are all key issues in reducing test costs;
ii) **Testing Flexibility Issues**. The auto-driving system of automobiles covers various sensors, processors and controllers such as cameras, lidars, millimeter-wave radars, etc. The virtual test environment is no longer a single scene, and needs to meet the requirements of multiple cars driving test schemes. Therefore, this requires the test environment not only to support a single car test, but also to support multiple cars driving at the same time, and to ensure that no traffic accidents occur. The accident puts forward higher requirements on the test environment.
iii) **Smooth Advancement of The Test System**. Autonomous driving technology solutions for automobiles will definitely face tremendous changes and reforms in the future. First of all, the test system needs to smoothly adapt to technological advancement. During the test, the vehicles, pedestrians, road conditions, traffic signs, etc. in the system must be kept stable and orderly. Of course, it also needs to be tested according to the test. The number of objects grows and the types of cars undergo system upgrades from time to time.

CONCLUSION

Advanced computer technologies such as Artificial Intelligence (AI), cloud computing, digital twins, and edge computing and big data have been applied in various fields as digitalization has progressed. A digital twin is a virtual representation of an object or system that spans its lifecycle, is updated from real-time data, and uses simulation, machine learning and reasoning to help decision-making. The purpose of a digital twin is to run cost-effective simulations. The digital twin uses IoT sensors, log files and other relevant information to collect real-time data for accurate modeling of assets. These models are then combined with AI-powered analytics tools in a virtual setting.

Although simulations and digital twins both utilize digital models to replicate a system's various processes, a digital twin is actually a virtual environment, which makes it considerably richer for study. The difference between digital twin and simulation is largely a matter of scale: While a simulation typically studies one particular process, a digital twin can itself run any number of useful simulations in order to study multiple processes

Machine Learning (ML) based AI applications are commonly regarded as a promising technology in the manufacturing industry. Nevertheless, the ML method needs a huge number of high-quality training datasets. In the case of supervised ML, manual input is frequently necessary to label these datasets. This method is costly, error-prone, and time-consuming, particularly in a complicated and dynamic manufacturing setting.

There are various types of digital twins depending on the level of product magnification. The biggest difference between these twins is the area of application. It is common to have different types of digital twins co-exist within a system or process. The vision of the digital twin is to enable good decisions that deliver value to your physical and digital operations and support your ongoing industry transformation. While the digital twin will solve many issues, the achievement of its vision isn't possible unless you digitize your physical assets and their subassemblies. We must also work together to develop standards for how digital twin resources should be structured to achieve consistency across consumption technologies.

Regardless of the challenges, there is no question that even in the very physical, asset intensive industries (e.g., energy and utilities, oil and petroleum, manufacturing and industrial products), digital assets are becoming just as essential as physical ones. Digital twins are a revolutionary solution to help ensure that companies achieve efficiency and efficacy in their operations, and that they continue to bring value to their customers.

Digital twin technology promises to transform design and give product developers, manufacturers and businesses a 360-degree view of products and systems throughout the entire lifecycle. Armed with an enriched pool of data provided by the Internet of Things (IoT), the design technology stands poised to deliver previously impossible opportunities.

Technology developers see AI as a way to accelerate design processes, allowing engineers to quickly evaluate many possible design alternatives. By changing design parameters and running AI algorithms, digital twin design software providers contend that engineers could quickly evaluate possible best fits based on the results of the algorithms. The use of AI in this context is still in the early stages. Most successful digital twin technologies use AI systems to make predictions of situations where data is abundant and where the processes being evaluated are relatively simple.

Artificial intelligence in digital twins is a universally applicable theoretical and technical system, with many applications, such as product design, equipment manufacturing, medical analysis, aerospace and other fields. At present, the most in-depth application in China is in the field of engineering construction, and intelligent manufacturing has gained the most attraction in the research field.

Due to the rapid development of the global intelligent internet automotive industry, research on automotive internet related technologies is of great significance to promote the development of automotive Internet. The parameterization and generalization technology of traffic scene simulation shows that the test process and working conditions of autonomous driving simulation can be said to have no boundaries. With the continuous development of intelligent manufacturing technology in various countries around the world, the informatization level of the manufacturing industry is gradually improving. The concept of digital twins is simply to map people, objects, relationships, and processes in real-world to virtual-world, and realize the research and control of real objects by observing and analyzing the digital twin in virtual space. Applying this concept to the field of urban transportation is undoubtedly a boon to the construction of smart cities. In 2020, the digital twin market was valued at USD 3.1 billion. Some industry analysts speculate it could continue to rise sharply until at least 2026, climbing to an estimated USD 48.2 billion.

REFERENCES

Alexopoulo, K., Nikolakis, N., & Chryssolouris, G. (2020). Digital twin-driven supervised machine learning for the development of artificial intelligence applications in manufacturing. *Int J Comp Integ M.*, *33*(5), 429–439. doi:10.1080/0951192X.2020.1747642

Dai, X., Ke, C., Quan, Q., & Cai, K.-Y. (2021). RFlySim: Automatic test platform for UAV autopilot systems with FPGA-based hardware-in-the-loop simulations. *Aerospace Science and Technology*, *114*, 106727. doi:10.1016/j.ast.2021.106727

Fan, C., Zhang, C., Yahja, A., & Mostafavi, A. (2021). Disaster City Digital Twin: A vision for integrating artificial and human intelligence for disaster management. *International Journal of Information Management*, *56*, 102049. doi:10.1016/j.ijinfomgt.2019.102049

Gao, X., & Cai, J. (2017). Optimization analysis of urban function regional planning based on big data and GIS technology. *Technical Bulletin.*, *55*(11), 344–351.

Gaur, L., Afaq, A., Solanki, A., Singh, G., Sharma, S., Jhanjhi, N. Z., & Le, D. N. (2021). Capitalizing on big data and revolutionary 5G technology: Extracting and visualizing ratings and reviews of global chain hotels. *Computers & Electrical Engineering*, *95*, 107374. doi:10.1016/j.compeleceng.2021.107374

Gaur, L., Solanki, A., Wamba, S. F., & Jhanjhi, N. Z. (Eds.). (2021). *Advanced AI techniques and applications in bioinformatics*. CRC Press. doi:10.1201/9781003126164

Grigoropoulos, N., & Lalis, S. (2020). Simulation and digital twin support for managed drone applications. *IEEE/ACM 24th International Symposium on Distributed Simulation and Real Time Applications (DS-RT)*. (pp. 1–8). IEEE.

Rana, J., Gaur, L., Singh, G., Awan, U., & Rasheed, M. I. (2021). Reinforcing customer journey through artificial intelligence: a review and research agenda. *International Journal of Emerging Markets.*

Rasheed A, San O, & Kvamsdal T. (2019). Digital twin: Values, challenges and enablers.

Santosh, K. C., & Gaur, L. (2022). *Artificial Intelligence and Machine Learning in Public Healthcare: Opportunities and Societal Impact*. Springer Nature.

Xiong, M., Wang, H., Fu, Q., & Xu, Y. (2021). Digital twin–driven aero-engine intelligent predictive maintenance. *International Journal of Advanced Manufacturing Technology*, *114*(11-12), 3751–3761. doi:10.100700170-021-06976-w

Yurkevich, E. V., & Stepanovskaya, I. A. (2021). Controlling the security of the airport airspace using the digital twin. J Phys. *Conf Ser. IOP Publishing*, *1864*(1), 012128.

Chapter 7
Use Cases for Digital Twin

Imdad A Shah
School of Computer Science SC, Taylor's University, Malaysia

Quratulain Sial
Emergency Department Aga Khan University Hospital, Karachi (AKUH), Pakistan

N. Z. Jhanjhi
https://orcid.org/0000-0001-8116-4733
School of Computer Science, SCS Taylor's University, Malaysia

Loveleen Gaur
https://orcid.org/0000-0002-0885-1550
Amity University, India & Taylor's University, Malaysia & University of the South Pacific, Fiji

ABSTRACT

The "digital twin" concept creates a virtual portrayal, with the actual and virtual worlds being in perfect sync. The digitization process of a product's whole life cycle, from design to maintenance, will provide the organization with a predictive analysis of problems. Using digital representations' maximum effect of predicting issues in the development of technology would be to deliver caution in advance, avoid any disruption to the new opportunities, and design an upgraded technology. Indeed, these will have a greater impact on transmitting outstanding consumer feelings both inside and outside the company. Emerging trends of Industry 4.0, such as AI, ML, DL, and IoT play a crucial part in the creation of virtual twins, mainly used in the manufacturing, industrial IoT, and automotive industries.

INTRODUCTION

The ability to unleash various potentials of virtual product creation has increased with the use and sophistication of simulation models. While simulation software has gotten increasingly powerful, attempts to maximise the potential benefits of product simulations are increasingly centred on the input data that is now accessible. More accurate simulation models that ultimately produce better products can be created. The definition, upon which this work is based, states that "use phase data" refers to data generated

DOI: 10.4018/978-1-6684-5925-6.ch007

by the product itself during the usage phase. The term "digital twin" is frequently used to describe such integration of simulation models and the usage of phase data (Autiosalo, 2019). In this contribution, a "digital twin" is defined as "a virtual, dynamic representation of a physical system that is connected to it over the whole life cycle, enabling bidirectional data exchange (Latif, 2020) the heating and cooling systems industry partner of this case study, like many other businesses today, is having trouble changing from a "conventional" mechanical engineering firm to a forward-thinking business that fully embraces digitization. Although the goods currently in use are technically sound and frequently already supply some basic data from the usage phase, the promise of data-driven engineering and the integration of the devices on the Internet of Things are just now being realized. Some initial steps have been made, such as allowing customers to use an app to control their heating system (Tao, 2018; Beil, 2020; Bentley Systems, 2021). Digital twin technology is becoming important for digitization. Although there are many potential advantages for businesses, from predictive maintenance to the creation of new business models, there is no approach in literature or practice that fully supports businesses in introducing their digital twin, considering their unique requirements and circumstances (Biesinger, 2019; Botín-Sanabria, 2020). The digitalization of tools, procedures and products is becoming more important considering the industrial industry's significant transition and the necessity to profit from the industry 4.0 bonanza. The idea of a digital clone of a real item has been around for ages, but it is about to enter a new era (Botín-Sanabria, 2022; Briggs, 2020). Since its introduction, the digital twin has influenced product lifecycle management, driving dynamic evolution in the industrial sector. The manufacturing industry can now accept the evolving aspects of the digital twin from a variety of fresh perspectives, particularly about the asset and the product. When physical assets like equipment are digitally represented in the manufacturing sector and connected based on their functions, the equipment becomes the supply chain's and the smart factory's connection point. The connected equipment at all levels of this intelligent digital representation's connected system can send and receive data to and from it Bentley Systems (Campos-Ferreira, 2019; Carvalho, 2020). In the meanwhile, operators, maintenance experts, regulatory authorities, and other participating vendors can all read the digital depiction of the equipment, the use cases in the industry are in fig 1.

When a product has digital twins, there are additional advantages, like having complete control throughout the whole life cycle of the product and the ability to change the process if any deviations from the predesigned model occur (Conejos, 2020, Dembski, 2020). In the meantime, it is argued that while the use of digital twins in small-scale industries may initially be hindered by the associated costs and implementation difficulties, it would prove beneficial in all respects in the long term.

The manufacturing sector is now operating differently because of the digital twin. The design of items, as well as their production and upkeep, are significantly influenced by digital twins. Due to its influence, production is more proficient and enhanced, while throughput times are decreasing Erol, T. 2020. Monitoring, tracking, and regulating industrial systems digitally will be made easier by integrating digital twins with industrial enterprises. Since digital twins gather environmental data in addition to operational data, such as location, device settings, and financial frameworks, they have the potential to be powerful tools for predicting future operations and inconsistencies (Evans, 2021; Godager, 2021; Guevara, 2019). This will be an enormous help, particularly in emerging nations like India.

By supporting financial progress, ensuring effective resource management, reducing environmental impact, and increasing the overall value of a resident's life, digital twins and IoT data can improve the planning and construction of a smart city. By extracting visions from multiple sensor networks and smart technologies, the digital twin prototype can help city planners and lawmakers with the design of

Figure 1. Shows the use cases in the industry Dahmen, U.2018

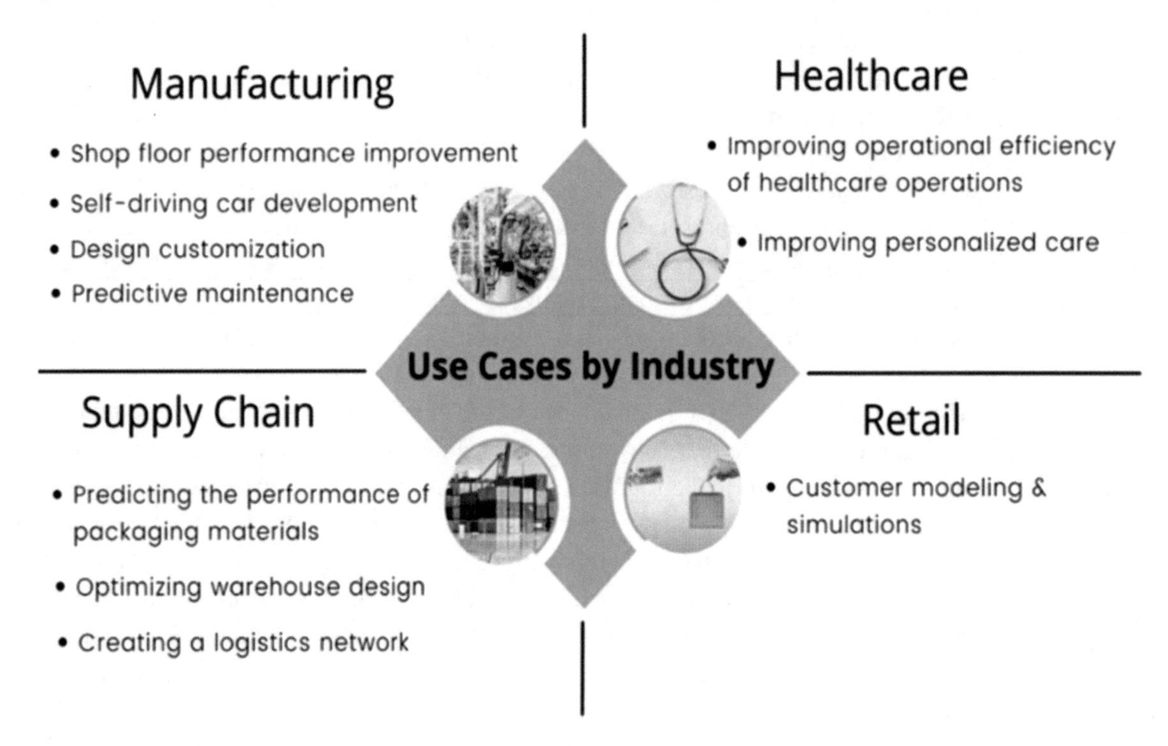

smart cities (Gutierrez-Franco, 2021). They can make informed decisions about the future because of the information the digital twins have provided.

When creating the simulated architecture of a connected vehicle, digital twins can be quite useful to the automotive industry. It obtains behavioural and functional information about the vehicle and services to assess the overall performance effectiveness of the car and the features attached to it. Additionally, Digital Twin is in favour of giving customers improved support and service. Enticing customer satisfaction is a crucial element in the field of merchandising (Haiyuan, 2021). By creating virtual twins of customers and dressing them in clothes, the use of digital twins can significantly improve the retail customer experience. The better planning of stock upkeep, safekeeping practises, and human resource management is also supported by digital twins.

LITERATURE REVIEW

Construction companies can benefit from using a digital twin since it can help them understand how a building is doing in real-time. This gives them the ability to tweak performance to maximise efficiency. The data obtained by digital twins can be utilised in the process of planning and developing new buildings in the future (He, Qiu, & Lai, 2021). The industrial business is the one that makes the most extensive use of digital twins' applications. The manufacturing industry is dependent on expensive machinery that produces a significant amount of data, which makes the creation of digital twins easier.

The current digital era has had a profound impact on both the commercial and industrial worlds. After the COVID-19 pandemic, which caused most of their activities to be disrupted, it became abundantly clear that those who had selected a digital transformation plan and had begun its execution fared better than those who hadn't (Ivanov, 2020). This was because the COVID-19 pandemic caused most of their activities to be disrupted. The ability of the digitally transformed organisation to connect was one of the benefits of the transformation (Jung, 2022; Kiran, 2021). McKinsey identified the digital technologies, tools, and processes that these organisations used to achieve their digitalization goals. (Lee, 2020) The availability of a dependable, high-performance, high-speed network connection that makes use of cutting-edge networking technology is a crucial requirement for integrating and deploying all these technologies in the process of digitization (Laubenbacher, 2021). This is one of the most important prerequisites. In addition to this, it would make it possible for users to command and initiate actions in the physical system using these interfaces even when they were not there physically. This method of deployment is referred to as a "digital twin" in the industry. To make matters even more confusing, the term "digital twin" is often used to refer to a certain technique or approach rather than a specific artefact. This shift in meaning further muddies the waters. The term "digital twin" is typically used in the manufacturing industry to refer to a certain manufacturing and testing approach rather than to a particular category of high-quality, dynamic representations (Laamarti, 2020; Laaki, 2019) one interpretation of the word holds that rather than referring to a particular artefact, it alludes to a method or an approach. Different bioinformatics applications for in silico therapy will be automatically counted as part of the digital twin paradigm, even if they do not create a digital twin (Lim, 2020; Mandolla, 2019). This will be the case regardless of whether the applications create a digital twin. Because of this, determining the current state of the shift to digital requires a lot of time and work.

The topic of these applications came up during several of our respondents' discussions, even though they do not at this time reveal digital twins in their traditional sense. The whole view of patients, with the emphasis, instead being placed on a limited number of criteria that are significant for a certain kind of diagnosis (Marcucci, 2020; Muzafar, 2020). To make matters even more confusing, the term "digital twin" is often used to refer to a certain technique or approach rather than a specific artefact. This shift in meaning further muddies the waters. In the context of manufacturing, the term "digital twin" refers to a specific manufacturing and testing strategy rather than a predetermined category of high-quality, dynamic representations. Nevertheless, this slow shift is fraught with a lot of complications. Respondents, on average, found it difficult to forecast the future of the digital twin; nevertheless, this may be an impact that is inherent to the term "digital twin" itself. Given that our respondents do not believe themselves to be taking part in a mass movement towards the digital twin, at least not in their day-to-day jobs, we may deduce that our comprehensive cross-sectoral perspective on the subject startled them a little bit. There are several industries where the application of digital twins is still in its infancy (Muzafar, 2020; Nativi, 2021). The initial step is the generalisation of applications that have already been developed. The technologies in digital twins are in fig 2.

A few decades ago, when computer simulation of the human body was restricted to specific organs or functions, there were more limitations placed on what could be copied and simulated. In the future, however, there will be fewer restrictions placed on what can be copied and simulated. Because of this, the field of "digital twins" is swiftly transitioning from a specialised effort centred, for instance, on a particular organ or physiological function, to a method that is generally accepted for diagnosis and treatment. In addition, the quality of the digital twin has significantly advanced (Pedersen, 2021; Prasad, 2019). It was agreed upon that a digital twin would continue to develop as a diagnostic and therapeutic

Figure 2. Shows the technologies used in digital twins Pan, S 2021

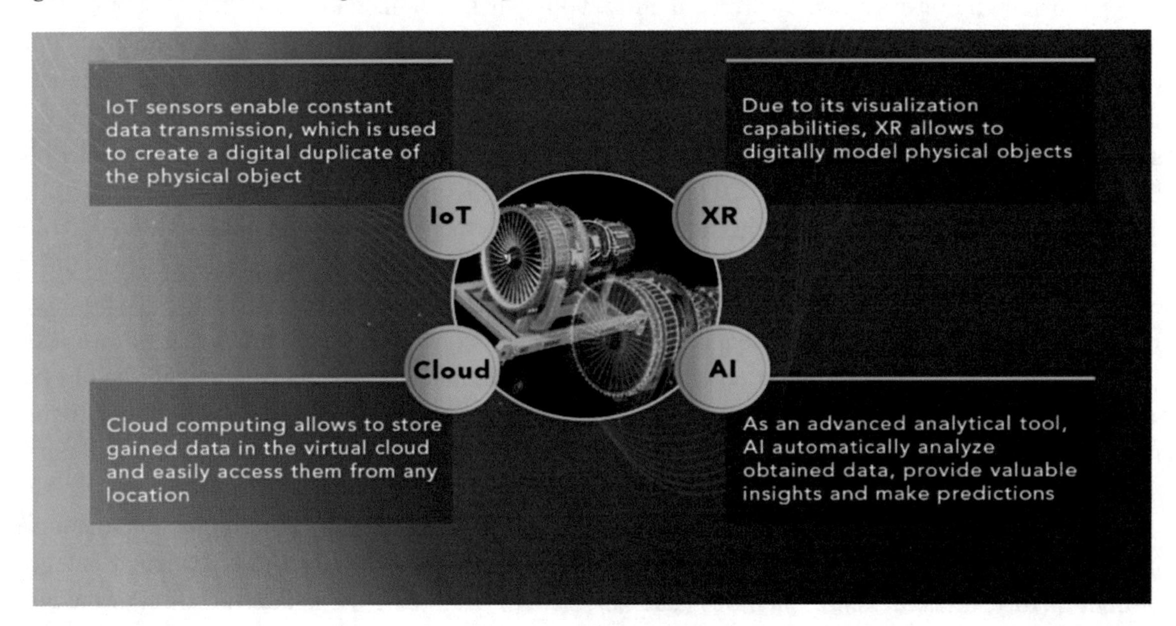

tool; nevertheless, it is sometimes questioned if the social and financial expenses that are required for this growth are worthwhile given the benefits. Despite this, there were significant gaps in the respondents' understanding of the factors that will drive this growth in certain sectors. People whose jobs involve working with models frequently focus on developing new and improved models, whereas those whose jobs involve working with data-gathering equipment (sensors) frequently focus on developing new and improved tools. On the other hand, it was either tacitly or explicitly acknowledged that "good modelling and superb data" depend on one another.

The improved digital twin will not only make therapy more effective, but it will also serve as a more effective "filtering mechanism," which will assist in lowering the burden of the disease. A variety of respondents gave contrasting forecasts regarding the sector in which the rapid advancement of digital twins is anticipated. Certain professions, such as cardiology, are thought by some to have the "advantage" of considerably boosting the demand for data and real-time optimization (Quirk, 2020; Qi, 2021; Quirk, 2020; Ran, 2019). Oncology, on the other hand, has the advantage of being able to collect data considerably more swiftly than other medical specialities since patients who have been diagnosed with cancer are less inclined to regard their comfort or privacy. In a direct imitation of this statement, one of the participants said, "Data protection is something for healthy folks", (Rathore, 2021). In keeping with the contrast, the benefits offered by organ-level replicas and implants include the fact that the conclusions they draw, and the prospective uses of their products are not necessarily limited to specific illnesses or treatments. It is difficult to forecast in which areas of the world the digital twin will "strike" hardest in the future decades because of the various advantages it offers.

Hospitals are consistently rated as one of the most difficult systems to successfully manage and consistently rank as one of the most complex systems across all categories of work and organisation contests. This is because elements in everyday life that are uncertain or highly variable interact with one another (Raes, 2021). Inside the hospital, it manifests itself in a variety of different ways, including clinical variability, flow variability, and professional variability. Real-time data entry for patients is commonly required because the hospital must provide medical care and activities centred on the prevention and treatment of diseases, the relief of pain, diagnostic procedures, and other similar things. As a result, there is a discrepancy between the actual data and the registered data, and it is the registered data that is typically used when conducting performance analysis (Sharma, 2018). New sensors that can acquire data in real-time have been made possible because of the ongoing development of technology (Sharma, 2021). The operating room is one of the most important parts of the hospital, and how it is run has a significant impact on many other aspects of the hospital's day-to-day operations, including the distribution of beds, the compilation of surgery waiting lists, the hiring of staff, and many other things.

Because of this, one of the most prevalent topics of discussion in a wide variety of scientific fields, including engineering, health, economics, and management, is the maximisation and improvement of OR efficiency (Schrotter, 2021). Repetitive and manual labour are significant issues that contribute to errors and waste of time. These problems should be avoided whenever possible. It is necessary for the medical staff to keep a record of the various times that correspond to the several phases that the patient must go through for the surgery to be successful because these acts commonly take place in the operating room. These procedures are often developed by the crew after each shift or at any other point in time when they have some spare time. Naturally, this could lead to human-caused errors and inaccuracies (Shah, 2022). In the manufacturing and construction industries, the arrival of Industry 4.0 coincided with the entrance of digital twin technology into our everyday lives. More recent research in the field of medicine has shown that it has the potential to completely revolutionise the field (Shah, 2021). The term "digital twin" refers to a digital clone of a physical asset or system that enables the modelling of the status of the asset or system. Significant progress has been made in recent years in the field of healthcare regarding the creation of digital twins of patients as well as medical equipment.

USE CASES OF THE DIGITAL TWIN IN ENGINEERING

In the past few days, I have seen several "use cases" that explain how the usage of a digitally simulated version of the product can help minimise the costs associated with product testing and prototyping when using digital twin technology. This simulated version is not an exact copy of the original in any way. In the world of engineering, digital twins are only truly helpful to engineers once their products have been deployed in the field (Shah, 2022). Following the implementation of the solution, data from the many goods that are now being used is collected and analysed to reveal unexpected strengths or weaknesses in product quality and provide insight into overall utilisation.

Application of Digital Models

Our recently published white paper focused on automotive engineers as a potential user group. Let's pretend a brand-new car line has just been unveiled, and that each model has a digital counterpart. Eventually, the engineering staff notices a persistent flaw in the tyre suspension system: one item wears out much faster than expected (Shah, 2022). Measures can be taken with varying degrees of intensity in response to the problem. If caught in time, a software update that redistributes the vehicle's weight elsewhere in the suspension system can alleviate the problem until the vehicle can be returned to service.

In many ways, recalls are extremely expensive. Assuming the recall is large enough to garner public attention, the automaker will face not only the price of repairs but also potential damage to its brand. To halt a large problem when it's still manageable, it's best to catch it early on and fix it as soon as possible.

THE USE OF DIGITAL TWINS IN SUPPLY CHAIN MANAGEMENT

Even though the manufacturing industry is where digital twins are most often applied, it is essential to keep in mind that the increasingly complex systems upon which our economy relies must be considered. The logistics business is experiencing rapid growth and cutting-edge developments. Due to the COVID-19 epidemic, the shift from a retail-based economy to a shipping-based one has intensified. Information can be a competitive advantage for businesses that are trying to get ahead (Shah, 2022). The shipping process is complex, but by using digital twins, businesses may identify areas where they can improve efficiency, reduce waste, and strengthen safety measures.

USES OF DIGITAL TWINS ON THE INTERNET OF THINGS

Digital twins can be used in many different areas, not just in one business or region. They can be used in many situations. On one side, some digital twins only model and show a single sensor inside an item (Shah, 2022). By putting sensors on machines, it's easy to get a lot of information about how they work. It's not just about figuring out how the machine works; it's also about figuring out the conditions in the processing plant. By using a "digital twin," we can link and look at these informational collections, just like a virtual copy of how production works. After some time, if the differences in how things are done are no longer clear, producers can take steps to improve their methods. A digital twin and the constructions that go with it are examples of use cases outside of production and Industry 4.0. Here, you can simulate how construction is used, considering recorded or related information, and see how changes to the plan affect the simulation (Shah, 2022). In this case, the digital twin can show areas that are using too many resources or are only used sometimes. Use-based insurance is another example of a possible use case. Instead of putting a pricey telematics unit in each new client's car, the application can now be put in the "cloud." The digital twin can be used to track the driver's driving score all the time.

GE DIGITAL TWIN

There will be signs and symptoms that indicate that the apparatus is likely to wind up having significant problems. GE makes use of digital twins to monitor and investigate the preliminary and unstable functionalities of the gadgets. Even though there are existing frameworks accessible for the detection of anomalies (Singh, 2020). An expert digital twin representation will be created by the inputs flowing from the behavioural patterns of the assets, processes, and systems, coupled with the accompanying complete domain knowledge and the incorporation of artificial intelligence. This representation may then be worked with. A normal anomaly detection forecast with a time frame of 20–30 days in advance has been altered to one with a time slot of 60 days in advance at GE when the company adopts the Digital Twin. This will aid in organising the corrective steps well in advance with all feasible appropriate inputs, and it will be of great assistance. The digital twin may also be used to provide extremely accurate projections on the amount of time a particular turbine blade will continue to function in an aircraft engine. Understanding the potential repercussions of assets is causing modifications to be made to industrial facilities (Singh, 2020). GE has also developed digital twins for businesses, which are simulations of comprehensive and composite system communications. These models simulate a variety of potential future scenarios and regulate the most significant performance parameters for those scenarios. These simulations illustrate potential circumstances that may influence a company by drawing from vast data sources, including aspects such as the weather, performance, and business operations.

CASE STUDIES OF DIGITAL TWINS IN SERVICE MANAGEMENT

Information is crucial to the success of many of us in our roles, and this is especially true in maintenance and repair. If technicians have access to a product's digital twin, they can see when, where, and by whom the product was utilised. The possibility of success on the first try is greatly increased by having this knowledge. Still, this isn't the only method by which digital twins can improve the product's service life (Singh, 2021). By understanding their products' applications and gaining deeper client insights, businesses can spot new growth prospects. Consider Celli, a leader in beverage industry machinery. Celli's original business model consisted solely of selling high-quality, simple-to-operate drink distribution equipment to customers. However, as it gathered more information about its customers, the corporation discovered it had untapped potential. Celli could offer a higher level of service to its clients and generate additional income by learning more about what its customers were purchasing and then selling that information to them.

DIGITAL TWIN ECOSYSTEM

GE's Digital Twin team includes subject matter experts, model designers, data analysts, scientists, and business innovators so that the twin can be connected in every possible way. The network brings together members of the larger community to glean the most information and spark the most creative thinking possible (Stojanovic, 2018). To manage, expand, and extend digital industrial systems, Predix serves as a comprehensive and secure application platform. There is a new digital twin ecosystem being developed by GE's partners. In 2015, Infosys became one of GE's partners to implement the digital twin methodology. This early-stage collaboration's primary goal was to create the world's first digital twin for the express purpose of providing early warnings and failure forecasts for various important components, such as landing gear, in a flight (Tao, 2018). It is possible to create a more comprehensive and advanced digital twin of the entire aircraft by combining data from the engine, airframe, and other systems. This includes things like fuel efficiency, maximisation of security, appropriateness, fuel consumption optimization, and an operational quid pro quo between these factors and the business simulation (Tagliabue, 2021). The digital twin ecosystem's ability to revolutionise industrial services through precise prediction is paired with the ecosystem's elasticity, which comes from its willingness to accommodate a variety of dimensions. Understanding how robots can talk to one another, manipulate data, and make decisions together is game-changing because of how the twins communicate and learn from each other. This will be the standard method for managing and operating digital infrastructure soon. Between 2020 and 2030, there may be more than 50 billion devices connected via IoT, and more than 7 billion internet users.

DISCUSSION

The field of healthcare is affected by variability that is caused by both natural and manmade sources. The random character of the natural variability is caused by the inherent component that is present in the administration of medical treatment. Every patient is different because of factors such as their age, the presence of other conditions, their response to treatment, and other natural differences. The variability that is produced artificially is not random and is typically linked to errors or poor choices made by organisations. An example of artificial variability is the claim made by Litvak that "the unfamiliarity with a new technology may be solved through education and certification." To put it another way, natural variability can only be observed and quantified, whereas a manager has the power to focus on the topic at hand and eradicate any variability that was artificially produced (Tao, 2018). It does a good job of illustrating these general issues, especially in the places where ANOVA analysis reveals excessive noise through SSE. The fact that only one surgical specialisation and not just one sort of surgery was selected for the sample size and the surgical procedures that were selected is a limitation of the research that was carried out. There is still a need for research into technologies that enable surgeons to better coordinate surgical activities while minimising the impact of artificial unpredictability. The application of the definition of a digital twin to the field of healthcare was carried out by (Tomin, 2020). most recently. They used equipment connected to the internet of things to caption data in real time. This information is used to provide fuel for the discrete event simulation model, which was developed by (Umrani, 2020). Software Products, Inc., employs. The approach taken by the authors recreates the efficiency of the services while also providing the decision-maker with the ability to adjust the timetable of activities, and applications of the digital twin in real estate in fig 3.

Beginning with this setting, the authors concluded that it would be beneficial to advance the use of real-time simulation by developing a tool that the surgical decision-maker could use regularly. This leads one to believe that extracting a recommendation for more effective resource distribution from the model could be possible. For instance, the model might be able to predict, based on a data warehouse of operations that are comparable to one another, the anticipated time of the conclusion of the surgical act (T4). This would enable the decision-maker to plan how to proceed most effectively considering the total amount of time that is available for operations in a single day. The immediate effect is improved management of the available resources. Dassault system and the Food and Drug Administration approved the SIMULIA Living Heart in 2014 (Yitmen, 2021). This was the first digital examination of organ–drug interactions. Validation of this DT model of human hearts was performed by medical researchers or educators. Because of this technology, medical professionals and pharmaceutical engineers can observe the intricate structure and movement of cardiac tissue, which paves the way for more effective therapy. Takeda Pharmaceuticals makes ground-breaking medicines using DT technology and distributes them all over the world. DT models streamline pharmaceutical procedures and provide more accurate predictions of the inputs and outputs of biological reactions. Atos and Siemens collaborated to develop physical DT models specifically for the pharmaceutical business to increase both production and efficiency. It is supported by the internet of things, artificial intelligence, and other advanced technologies (Zhou, 2019). Providing a quantitative measure of health and illness, the DT is expected to usher in a new era of medical

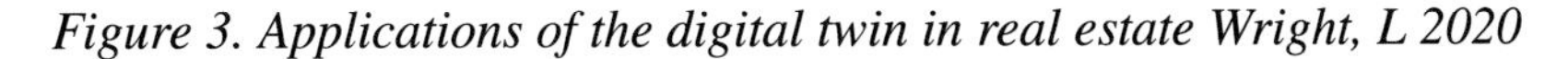
Figure 3. Applications of the digital twin in real estate Wright, L 2020

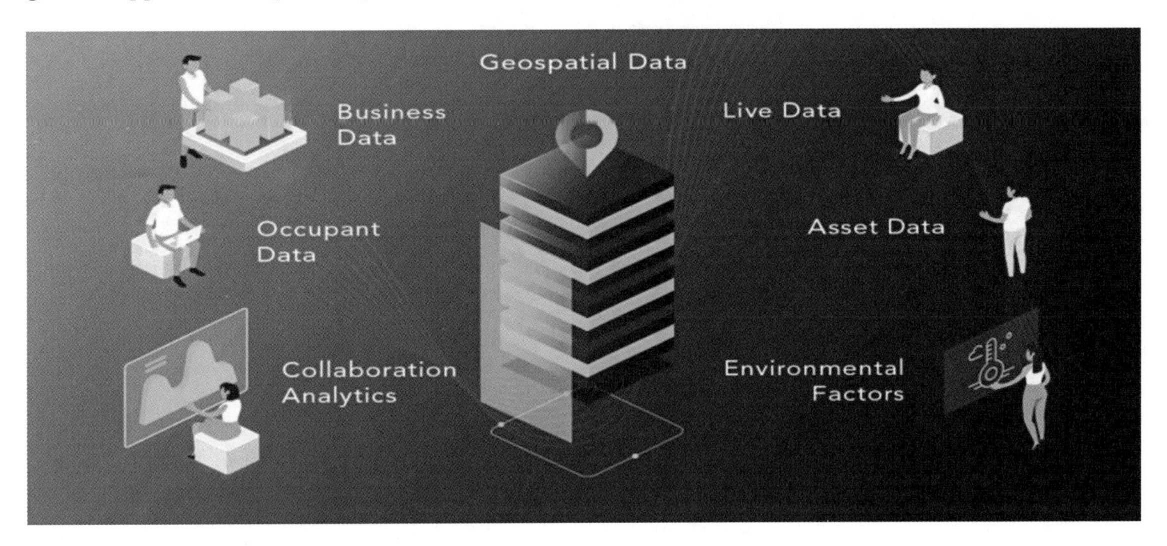

advancement. It can help with the management, design, and treatment of patients in hospitals. The DT can predict and analyse circumstances in a virtual environment, which allows for the reduction of risks as well as expenses, before arranging and implementing modifications such as the scheduling of beds and treatment alternatives. The model can also be used to verify treatment techniques and pharmaceuticals, which helps optimise treatment plans, obtain early disease diagnosis, and potentially prevent the disease altogether. Without the DT, the medical personnel at the hospital cannot schedule procedures. Several risk factors can be avoided that affect maternal health and infant mortality. Preconception care that is provided in a timely and suitable manner has the potential to improve the overall health of everyone, encourage healthier pregnancies for women, and significantly reduce the number of unfavourable outcomes for mothers and babies at the community level. Even though the preconception stage is the primary focus of this article, many other aspects are directly related to one's health throughout their entire life. Some of these aspects include leading a healthy lifestyle, improving one's diet, engaging in physical activity, preserving good mental health, and so on.

BOOK CHAPTER CONTRIBUTION AND DISCUSSION

The potential of digital twins is enormous. According to McKinsey's research, digital twin technologies can boost profits by 10% while cutting product development times in half and boosting quality by 25%. Kevin Baker, an Industry 4.0 expert with Orange Silicon Valley's Business Group, claims that digital twins have "applications in practically every sector of the industry. Any important data products can be represented and leveraged to acquire insights, improve efficiencies, and provide a more detailed view of corporate operations," regardless of industry (be it automotive, healthcare, insurance, or construction). Baker was elaborating on the significance of twins as a building block for the Fourth Industrial Revolution. He explained that processes are not excluded from the realm of coverage for the digital twin. According to Baker, having access to relevant information is the decisive factor. The ability to create a digital representation of anything in the physical world is limited only by the availability of relevant data.

Figure 4. Shows the future advantages of digital twin

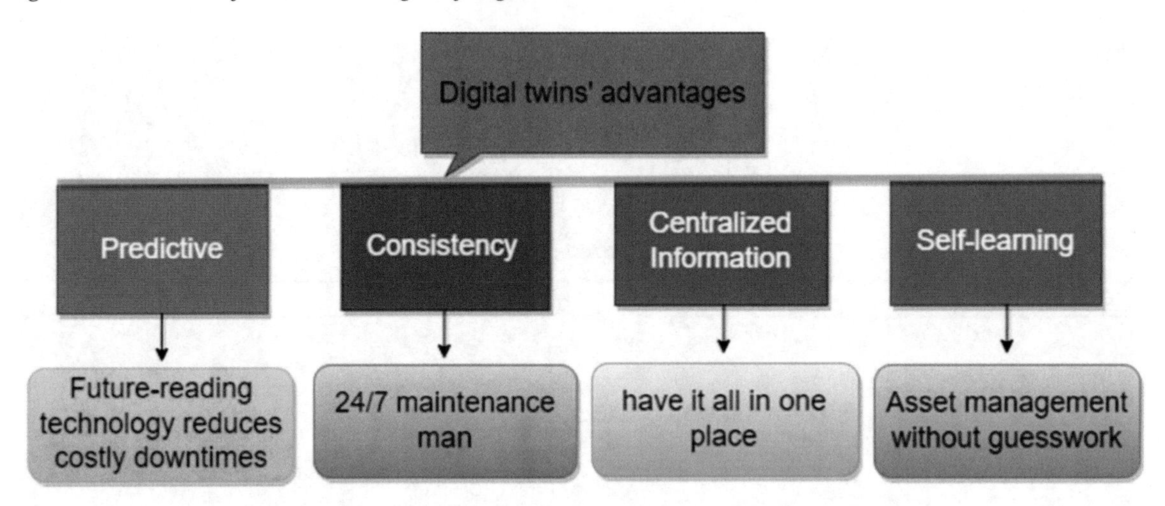

Despite these advantages, however, digital twin technology has been sluggish to gain general acceptance due to several obstacles. The panelists summed it up as up-front expenditures, a fuzzy business case, and internal divisions. Don't forget that "digital twinning" is only an idea, not a piece of hardware. Digital twins can be delivered via a wide range of technologies, from IoT sensors and platforms to edge computing and AI. According to panelist Sameer Kher, Senior Director, Product Development at Ansys, a provider of engineering simulation software, this presents an immediate challenge. The equipment you use must be sensorized, and you must have a communication protocol as well as a computing and storage infrastructure. That's a big initial outlay for many people, and the benefits of adopting digital twins may not materialise for some time. Getting buy-in from financial and policymakers can be challenging. When asked about common concerns, Dan Isaacs, CTO of the Digital Twin Consortium, noted, "Some of the regular issues that we're seeing, Isaacs attributes this worry to "a lack of meaningful value-based use cases and knowledge." In addition, many false beliefs are floating around concerning digital duplicates. Multiple participants in the consortium have noted that there are as many as ten distinct ways in which consumers are defined within their institutions. That creates walls between departments. Any implementation of a digital twin must be conducive to the ongoing functioning of the business and its existing processes.

In turn, this draws attention to the technology required to deliver the information the firm seeks. This provides a chance to achieve early success, which may then be expanded upon, the future advantages of the digital twin are in fig 4.

CONCLUSION AND FUTURE WORK

The "digital twin" concept creates a virtual representation, with the real and virtual worlds perfectly in sync. The digitization process of a product's whole life cycle, from design to maintenance, will provide the organization with a predictive analysis of problems. Using digital representations, the maximum effect of predicting issues in the development of technology would be to exercise caution in advance, avoid any disruption to the new opportunities, and design an upgraded technology. Indeed, these will have a greater impact on transmitting outstanding consumer feelings both inside and outside the company. The greatest benefit of anticipating issues in the construction of a device is that it will provide early warnings, prevent downtime, promote new prospects, and inspire the invention of improved devices or gadgets that can be used later at a lower cost. These will, without a doubt, have a broader impact on the company's ability to transmit excellent customer sentiment. The use of cutting-edge technologies such as AI, ML, DL, IoT, and big data in Industry 4.0 is critical to the success of the digital twin, which has seen widespread adoption in the fields of manufacturing, the industrial internet of things, and the automobile industry. Due to the expansion, breadth, and rapid development of the IoT in the physical world, the advantages of digital twins have become more affordable and within the grasp of a wider range of enterprises. The penetration, widespread reach, and advancement of IoT in today's world have made the power of digital twins more affordable and usable by businesses of all kinds.

REFERENCES

Autiosalo, J.; Vepsalainen, J.; Viitala, R.; Tammi, K. A (2019). Feature-Based Framework for Structuring Industrial Digital Twins. *IEEE Access 8,* 1193–1208.

Amir Latif, R. M., Hussain, K., Jhanjhi, N. Z., Nayyar, A., & Rizwan, O. (2020). A remix IDE: Smart contract-based framework for the healthcare sector by using Blockchain technology. *Multimedia Tools and Applications*, 1–24. https://ieeexplore.ieee.org/abstract/document/9214512

Ao, F., Zhang, M., Liu, Y., & Nee, A. Y. (2018). Digital twin driven prognostics and health management for complex equipment. *CIRP Annals*, *67*(1), 169–172. doi:10.1016/j.cirp.2018.04.055

Beil, C., & Kolbe, T. H. (2020). Combined Modelling of Multiple Transportation Infrastructure Within 3D City Models and its Implementation in CityGML 3.0. *ISPRS Ann. Photogramm. Remote Sens. Spatial Inf. Sci.*, *6*, 29–36. doi:10.5194/isprs-annals-VI-4-W1-2020-29-2020

Bentley Systems Incorporated. (2021). Discover OpenCities Planner–Connect The Data, People, Workflows, and Ideas Necessary to Support Today's Infrastructure Projects. *Report P-18.* https://www.bentley.com/es/products/brands/ opencities-planner .

Biesinger, F., & Weyrich, M. The Facets of Digital Twins in Production and the Automotive Industry. In *Proceedings of the 2019 23rd International Conference on Mechatronics Technology (ICMT).* IEEE. 10.1109/ICMECT.2019.8932101

Botín-Sanabria, D. M., Mihaita, A. S., Peimbert-García, R. E., Ramírez-Moreno, M. A., Ramírez-Mendoza, R. A., & Lozoya-Santos, J. D. J. (2022). Digital twin technology challenges and applications: A comprehensive review. *Remote Sensing*, *14*(6), 1335. doi:10.3390/rs14061335

Briggs, B., & Buchholz, S. (2020). Deloitte Tech Trends 2020. *Insights*, *2020*, 1–130.

Campos-Ferreira, A., Lozoya-Santos, J. J., Vargas-Martínez, A., Mendoza, R., & Morales-Menéndez, R. Digital Twin Applications: A review. In *Memorias del Congreso Nacional de Control Automático*, (pp. 606–611). Asociación de México de Control Automático.

Carvalho, A., Melo, P., Oliveira, M., & Barros, R. (2020). The 4-corner model as a synchromodal and digital twin enabler in the transportation sector. In *Proceedings of the 2020 IEEE International Conference on Engineering, Technology and Innovation (ICE/ITMC)*, IEEE. 10.1109/ICE/ITMC49519.2020.9198592

Conejos, P., Martínez, F., Hervas, M., & Alonso, J. C. (2020). Building and Exploiting a Digital Twin for the Managmenet of Drinking Water Distribution Networks. *Urban Water Journal, 17*(8), 704–713. doi:10.1080/1573062X.2020.1771382

Dembski, F., Wossner, U., Letzgus, M., Ruddat, M., & Yamu, C. (2020). Urban Digital Twins for Smart Cities and Citizens: The Case Study of Herrenberg, Germany. *Sustainability, 12*(6), 2307. doi:10.3390u12062307

Dahmen, U., & Rossmann, J. Experimentable Digital Twins for a Modeling and Simulation-based Engineering Approach. In *Proceedings of the 2018 IEEE International Systems Engineering Symposium (ISSE)*. IEEE. 10.1109/SysEng.2018.8544383

Erol, T., Mendi, A. F., & Doğan, D. (2020, October). The digital twin revolution in healthcare. *2020 4th International Symposium on Multidisciplinary Studies and Innovative Technologies (ISMSIT)* (pp. 1-7). IEEE. https://ieeexplore.ieee.org/abstract/document/9255249

Evans, S., Savian, C., Burns, A., & Cooper, C. (2019). Digital Twins for the Built Environment: An Introduction to the Opportunities, Benefits, Challenges and Risks. *Built Environmental News*. https://www.theiet.org/impact-society/ sectors/built-environment/built-environment-news/digital-twins-for-the-built-environment/.

Godager, B.; Onstein, E.; Huang, L. (2021). The Concept of Enterprise BIM: Current Research Practice and Future Trends. *IEEE, 9,* 42265–42290.

Guevara, N., Diaz, C., Sguerra, M., Martinez, M., Agudelo, O., Suarez, J., Rodriguez, A., Acuña, G., & Garcia, A. (2019). Towards the design and implementation of a Smart City in Bogotá, Colombia. Rev. Fac. DeIng. *Univ. Antioq., 93*(93), 41–45. doi:10.17533/udea.redin.20190407

Gutierrez-Franco, E., Mejia-Argueta, C., & Rabelo, L. (2021). Data-Driven Methodology to Support Long-Lasting Logistics and Decision Making for Urban Last-Mile Operations. *Sustainability, 13*(11), 6230. doi:10.3390u13116230

Haiyuan, Y., Dachuan, W., Mengcha, S., & Qi, Y. (2021). Application of Digital Twins in Port System. *Journal of Physics: Conference Series*, 1846.

He, X., Qiu, Y., Lai, X., Li, Z., Shu, L., Sun, W., & Song, X. (2021). Towards a shape-performance integrated digital twin for lumbar spine analysis. *Digital Twin., 1*, 8. doi:10.12688/digitaltwin.17478.1

Ivanov, S., Nikolskaya, K., Radchenko, G., Sokolinsky, L., & Zymbler, M. Digital Twin of City: Concept Overview. In *Proceedings of the 2020 Global Smart Industry Conference (GloSIC)*. IEEE.. 10.1109/GloSIC50886.2020.9267879

Jung, A., Gsell, M. A. F., Augustin, C. M., & Plank, G. (2022). An integrated workflow for building digital twins of cardiac electromechanics-a multi-fidelity approach for personalising active mechanics. *Mathematics, 10*(5), 823. doi:10.3390/math10050823 PMID:35295404

Kiran, S. R. A., Rajper, S., Shaikh, R. A., Shah, I. A., & Danwar, S. H. (2021). Categorization of CVE Based on Vulnerability Software By Using Machine Learning Techniques. *International Journal (Toronto, Ont.), 10*(3).

Lee, S., Jain, S., Zhang, Y., Liu, J., & Son, Y. J. (2020). A Multi-Paradigm Simulation for the Implementation of Digital Twins in Surveillance Applications. In *Proceedings of the 2020 IISE Annual Conference*. IISE.

Laubenbacher, R., Sluka, J., & Glazier, J. (2021). Using digital twins in viral infection. *Science, 371*(6534), 1105–1106. doi:10.1126cience.abf3370 PMID:33707255

Laamarti, F., Badawi, H., Ding, Y., Arafsha, F., Hafidh, B., & El Saddik, (2021). An ISO/IEEE 11073 Standardized Digital Twin Framework for Health and Well-Being in Smart Cities. *IEEE Access, 8*, 105950–105961.

Laaki, H., Miche, Y., & Tammi, K. (2019). Prototyping a Digital Twin for Real Time Remote Control Over Mobile Networks: Application of Remote Surgery. *IEEE Access, 7*, 20325–20336.

Lim, K., Zheng, P., & Chen, C. (2020). A state-of-the-art survey of Digital Twin: Techniques, engineering product lifecycle management and business innovation perspectives. *Journal of Intelligent Manufacturing, 31*(6), 1313–1337. doi:10.100710845-019-01512-w

Mandolla, C., Petruzzelli, A. M., Percoco, G., & Urbinati, A. (2019). Building a digital twin for additive manufacturing through the exploitation of blockchain: A case analysis of the aircraft industry. *Computers in Industry, 109*, 134–152. doi:10.1016/j.compind.2019.04.011

Marcucci, E., Gatta, V., Le-Pira, M., Hansson, L., & Brathen, S. (2020). Digital Twins: A Critical Discussion on Their Potential for Supporting Policy-Making and Planning in Urban Logistics. *Sustainability, 12*(24), 623. doi:10.3390u122410623

Muzafar, S., & Jhanjhi, N. Z. (2020). Success stories of ICT implementation in Saudi Arabia. In *Employing Recent Technologies for Improved Digital Governance* (pp. 151–163). IGI Global. https://www.igi-global.com/chapter/success-stories-of-ict-implementation-in-saudi-arabia/245980 doi:10.4018/978-1-7998-1851-9.ch008

Nativi, S., Mazzetti, P., & Craglia, M. (2021). Digital Ecosystems for Developing Digital Twins of the Earth: The Destination Earth Case. *Remote Sensing, 13*(11), 2119. doi:10.3390/rs13112119

Pan, S., Zhou, W., Piramuthu, S., Giannikas, V., & Chen, C. (2021). Smart city for sustainable urban freight logistics. Int. J. Prod. Res. 2021, 59, 2079–2089. 51. Shengli, W. Is Human Digital Twin possible? . *Comput. Methods Programs Biomed. Update, 1*, 100014.

Pedersen, A., Brup, M., Brink-Kjaer, A., Christiansen, L., & Mikkelsen, P. (2021). Living and Prototyping Digital Twins for Urban Water Systems: Towards Multi-Purpose Value Creation Using Models and Sensors. *Water (Basel), 13*(5), 592. doi:10.3390/w13050592

Prasad, R. B., & Groop, L. (2019). Precision medicine in type 2 diabetes. *Journal of Internal Medicine, 285*(1), 40–48. doi:10.1111/joim.12859 PMID:30403316

Quirk, D., Lanni, J., & Chauhan, N. (2020). Digital twins: Answering the hard questions. *ASHRAE Journal, 62*, 22–25.

Ran, Y., Lin, P., Zhou, X., & Wen, Y. A (2019). Survey of Predictive Maintenance: Systems, Purposes and Approaches. *Comput. Sci. Eng.* http://xxx.lanl.gov/abs/1912.07383 .

Rathore, M.; Shah, S.; Shukla, D.; Bentafat, E.; Bakiras, S. (2021). The Role of AI, Machine Learning, and Big Data in Digital Twinning: A Systematic Literature Review, Challenges, and Opportunities. *IEEE Access, 9*, 32030–32052.

Raes, L., Michiels, P., Adolphi, T., Tampere, C., Dalianis, T., Mcaleer, S., & Kogut, P. (2021). DUET: A Framework for Building Secure and Trusted Digital Twins of Smart Cities. *IEEE Internet Computing*.

Sharma, M., & George, J. P. (2018). *Digital Twin in the Automotive Industry: Driving Physical-Digital Convergence; TCS White Papers*. Tata Consultancy Services Limited.

Sharma, A., Kosasih, E., Zhang, J., Brintrup, A., & Calinescu, A. (2021). *Digital Twins: State of the Art Theory and Practice*. Challenges, and Open Research Questions.

Juarez, M., Botti, V., & Giret, A. (2021). Digital Twins: Review and Challenges. *Journal of Computing and Information Science in Engineering, 21*, 030802.

Schrotter, G., & Hurzeler, C. (2021). The Digital Twin of the City of Zurich for Urban Planning. *J. Photogramm. Remote Sens. Geoinf. Sci., 88*, 99–112.

Sakdirat, K., Rungskunroch, P., & Welsh, J. (2019). A Digital-Twin Evaluation of Net Zero Energy Building for Existing Buildings. *Sustainability, 11*, 159.

Sujatha, R., Chatterjee, J. M., Jhanjhi, N. Z., & Brohi, S. N. (2021). Performance of deep learning vs machine learning in plant leaf disease detection. *Microprocessors and Microsystems, 80*, 103615. doi:10.1016/j.micpro.2020.103615

Shah, I. A., Wassan, S., & Usmani, M. H. (2022). E-Government Security and Privacy Issues: Challenges and Preventive Approaches. In Cybersecurity Measures for E-Government Frameworks (pp. 61-76). IGI Global.

Shah, I. A., & Rajper, S., & ZamanJhanjhi, N. (2021). Using ML and Data-Mining Techniques in Automatic Vulnerability Software Discovery. *International Journal (Toronto, Ont.), 10*(3).

Shah, I. A. (2022). Cybersecurity Issues and Challenges for E-Government During COVID-19: A Review. *Cybersecurity Measures for E-Government Frameworks*, 187-222.

Shah, I. A., Jhanjhi, N. Z., Amsaad, F., & Razaque, A. (2022). The Role of Cutting-Edge Technologies in Industry 4.0. In *Cyber Security Applications for Industry 4.0* (pp. 97–109). Chapman and Hall/CRC. doi:10.1201/9781003203087-4

Shah, I. A., Jhanjhi, N. Z., Humayun, M., & Ghosh, U. (2022). Health Care Digital Revolution During COVID-19. In *How COVID-19 is Accelerating the Digital Revolution* (pp. 17–30). Springer. doi:10.1007/978-3-030-98167-9_2

Shah, I. A., Jhanjhi, N. Z., Humayun, M., & Ghosh, U. (2022). Impact of COVID-19 on Higher and Post-secondary Education Systems. In *How COVID-19 is Accelerating the Digital Revolution* (pp. 71–83). Springer. doi:10.1007/978-3-030-98167-9_5

Shah, I. A., Habeeb, R. A. A., Rajper, S., & Laraib, A. (2022). The Influence of Cybersecurity Attacks on E-Governance. In *Cybersecurity Measures for E-Government Frameworks* (pp. 77–95). IGI Global. doi:10.4018/978-1-7998-9624-1.ch005

Singh, M., Fuenmayor, E., Hinchy, E. P., Qiao, Y., Murray, N., & Devine, D. (2021). Digital Twin: Origin to Future. . *Appl. Syst. Innov.*, *4*(2), 36. doi:10.3390/asi4020036

Singh, A. P., Pradhan, N. R., Luhach, A. K., Agnihotri, S., Jhanjhi, N. Z., Verma, S., Kavita, Ghosh, U., & Roy, D. S. (2020). A novel patient-centric architectural framework for blockchain-enabled healthcare applications. *IEEE Transactions on Industrial Informatics*, *17*(8), 5779–5789. https://ieeexplore.ieee.org/abstract/document/9259231. doi:10.1109/TII.2020.3037889

Singh, M., Fuenmayor, E., Hinchy, E. P., Qiao, Y., Murray, N., & Devine, D. (2021). Digital Twin: Origin to Future. *Appl. Syst. Innov.*, *4*(2), 36. doi:10.3390/asi4020036

Stojanovic, N., & Milenovic, D. (2018, December). Data-driven Digital Twin approach for process optimization: An industry use case. In *2018 IEEE International Conference on Big Data (Big Data)* (pp. 4202-4211). IEEE. 10.1109/BigData.2018.8622412

Tao, F., Zhang, H., Liu, A., & Nee, A. Y. (2018). Digital twin in industry: State-of-the-art. *IEEE Transactions on Industrial Informatics*, *15*(4), 2405–2415. https://ieeexplore.ieee.org/abstract/document/8477101. doi:10.1109/TII.2018.2873186

Tagliabue, L., Cecconi, F., Maltese, S., Rinaldi, S., Ciribini, A., & Flammini, A. (2021). Leveraging Digital Twin for Sustainability Assessment of an Educational Building. . *Sustainability*, *13*(2), 480. doi:10.3390u13020480

Tao, F., Cheng, J., Qi, Q., Zhang, M., Zhang, H., & Sui, F. (2018). Digital twin-driven product design, manufacturing and service with big data. *International Journal of Advanced Manufacturing Technology*, *94*(9-12), 3563–3576. doi:10.100700170-017-0233-1

Tomin, N., Kurbatsky, V., Borisov, V., & Musalev, S. (2020). Development of Digital Twin for Load Center on the Example of Distribution Network of an Urban District. *Energy*, *209*, 02029.

Umrani, S., Rajper, S., Talpur, S. H., Shah, I. A., & Shujrah, A. (2020). Games based learning: A case of learning Physics using Angry Birds. *Indian Journal of Science and Technology*, *13*(36), 3778–3784. doi:10.17485/IJST/v13i36.853

Wright, L., & Davidson, S. (2020). How to tell the difference between a model and a digital twin. . *Advanced Modeling and Simulation in Engineering Sciences*, *7*(1), 13. doi:10.118640323-020-00147-4

Yitmen, I., Alizadehsalehi, S., Akiner, I., & Akiner, M. (2021). An Adapted Model of Cognitive Digital Twins for Building Lifecycle Management. *Applied Sciences (Basel, Switzerland)*, *11*(9), 4276. doi:10.3390/app11094276

Zhou, M., Yan, J., & Feng, D. (2019). Digital Twin Framework and Its Application to Power Grid Online Analysis. *CSSE J. Power Energy Syst.*, *5*, 391–398.

Chapter 8
An Advanced Lung Disease Diagnosis Using Transfer Learning Method for High-Resolution Computed Tomography (HRCT) Images:
High-Resolution Computed Tomography

Sreelakshmi D.
Institute of Aeronautical Engineering, India

V. Sitharamulu
Institute of Aeronautical Engineering, India

Sarada K.
Koneru Lakshmaiah Education Foundation, India

Muniraju Naidu Vadlamudi
Institute of Aeronautical Engineering, India

Saikumar K.
Koneru Lakshmaiah Education Foundation

ABSTRACT

In the past decades, medical image technologies have been rapidly growing. The x-rays, ultrasound (US), MRI scan, and CT scan are the pulmonary techniques to examine human diseases, and CT techniques have more resolution images than other techniques. HRCT is another advanced technology derived from the CT family and working in 3D to capture the images. High-resolution computed tomography techniques are used to examine all humankind's problems like heart, brain, breast, lung, kidney, etc. The diagnosis accuracy depends on expert doctors, radiologists, or pathologists, and wrong judgment leads to wrong treatment or diagnosis. To overcome this, a computer-based technology is introduced instead of manual operation because of its higher efficiency, accuracy, and achieved by transfer learning methods.

DOI: 10.4018/978-1-6684-5925-6.ch008

INTRODUCTION

Medical-based research was supported by the analysis of medical images. Before going to diagnosis, a large amount of research (in terms of research) was conducted in the laboratory (Haas et.al., 2008). Day-to-day development of medical technology has led to a variety of medical images emerging. The commonly available methods that are available nowadays are Magnetic resonance imaging (MRI), X rays, Computer tomography (CT), and Ultrasound (UT) (Shen et.al., 2017). The first technique used in medical imaging is X-rays. They are simple to examine, and the cost is lower. Compared to all the techniques, CT provides higher density, higher resolution images, but it depends on the doctor's skill. These two techniques are harmful to the human body and should not be used too often (Inoue et.al., 2021). MRI does not emit radiation and provides a clear image, but it takes longer to investigate, and some patients may suffer due to the longer time it takes to investigate the patients (Duan et.al., 2015).

High-resolution computed tomography (HRCT) image is an advanced technology used to capture images in 3D technology and is driven by the CT family, to enhance image resolution. The spatial resolution method is used to enhance imaging parameters, and the speed of the scan is also enhanced to minimize the size of each pixel. All the techniques have their own characteristics, and the doctor needs to prefer one based on a patient diagnosis.

The transfer learning-based methods are non-invasive class-type techniques, not harmful to the patient's system and applied to several parts of the human body, such as the brain, lung, kidney, heart, etc. This type of medical analysis is done by an expert doctor's team to identify the problem, and a wrong judgment will lead to a wrong diagnosis. To overcome this, scientists and doctors are studying and performing research to introduce computer-based technology instead of manual operation because of its more efficiency and accuracy. The growth of the transfer learning method is shown in Figure 1, and data is taken from the web of science journal on transfer learning methods.

In this manuscript, a HRCT image is described in Section 2. The review of interstitial lung diseases (ILD) is explored in Section 3. Section 4 will give a little overview of the transfer learning methods. Finally, Section 5 gives a clear overview of this review paper that is conclusive and followed by references.

HIGH RESOLUTION COMPUTED TOMOGRAPHY (HRCT)

HRCT image is a cutting-edge CT technique that collects images in 3D to improve image clarity by improving image resolution. It makes use of the spatial resolution concept to increase scan speed by reducing pixel size. HRCT images can reveal disease features and use visual patterns to aid in differential diagnosis and narrowing (Hussein et.al., 2017).

Surgery for lung biopsy has decreased as a result of HRCT's influence on clinical treatment. Clinical practise recommendations for diagnosis and treatment have been updated in recent years in light of new data provided by the ATS/ERS consensus statement from 2002 (Raghu et.al., 2011). Although the cellular infiltration and architectural deformation with honeycombing indicative of a process like UIP are not clearly seen in the HRCT images (Peikert et.al., 2008). HRCT is still a valuable non-invasive approach for revealing aberrant parenchymal densities caused by microscopic morphological changes (Misumi & Lynch, 2006). It can provide direction for the best spot to get a biopsy of a characteristic or active disease (Costabel et.al., 2007).

Figure 1. Papers published on web of science journals on transfer learning method

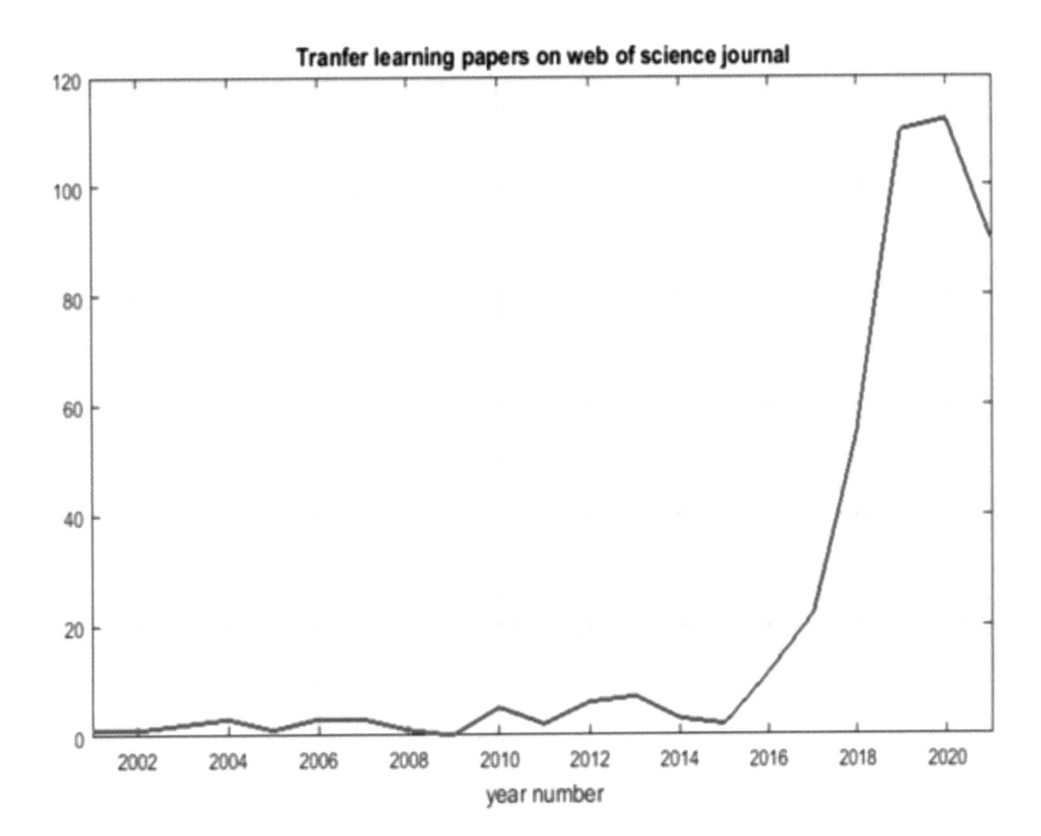

Consequently, Widely acknowledged that the level of visual-abnormalities correlates with the extent of pathogenic participation as well as the brutality of physiologic abnormalities (Saketkoo et.al., 2011), and hence longitudinal-HRCT image is suitable to monitor the therapy response and disease progression (Collard et.al., 2007).

Interstitial Lung Diseases

The An ILDs are developed jointly by the European Respiratory and the American Thoracic Society and fall into a heterogeneous group, resulting in various forms of lung disorders (Travis et.al., 2013), and ILDs classifications are shown in Figure. 2 (Olson et.al., 2011). The lungs are blocked for inhalation in ILDs, which are classified as pulmonary illnesses such as emphysema and COPD. In some circumstances, the patient is unable to take a full breath due to a blockage of airflow in their lungs. ILDs are also caused by pollution in the environment (Ryerson et.al., 2013). Some cases of ILD do not satisfy the particular definitions for any ILD and are thus classified as 'unclassifiable' (Raghu et.al., 2006).

use of HRCT in identifying and categorising ILD has increased in recent years. The characteristic imaging features may be diagnostic for several pathologic conditions, including idiopathic pulmonary fibrosis (IPF) and typical interstitial pneumonitis (UIP). During inpatient treatment, the ability of radiologic examination to discriminate between illnesses such as UIP, which has a death rate of roughly 75%

five years after diagnosis, and other diseases with a less concerning prognosis has proven critical (Ley et.al., 2011). A number of non-specific interstitial lung diseases (ILDs), such as desquamative interstitial pneumonia, hypersensitivity pneumonitis, respiratory bronchiolitis-associated interstitial lung disease, lymphoid interstitial pneumonia, and cryptogenic organising pneumonitis (COP), have distinct HRCT characteristics. These separate disease processes, on the other hand, may share a clinical phototype and can have indeterminate radiographic and pathologic manifestations. Furthermore, some individuals, such as those with combined pulmonary fibrosis and emphysema syndrome (Cottin et.al., 2011), can have both restrictive/fibrotic and destructive/obstructive processes, which can confound physiologic testing and cause biopsy results to fluctuate widely depending on the location of sampling. The fundamental clinical problems of detecting, characterizing, and differentiating the many ILDs continue to be diagnostic hurdles. Nonetheless, each of the major ILD and mixed parenchymal illnesses has a markedly different prognosis and treatment options (Flaherty et.al., 2007), and it is becoming increasingly obvious that targeting a specific pathogenic process will be critical for modifying the development of these often incurable diseases. Some other ILDs are nonspecific interstitial pneumonitis, hypersensitivity pneumonitis, desquamative interstitial pneumonitis, acute interstitial pneumonitis, respiratory bronchiolitis associated interstitial lung disease, lymphoid interstitial pneumonia, and cryptogenic organising pneumonitis, can all have distinct HRCT features (Watadani et.al., 2013). A same clinical phenotype can be seen in both the pathology and the radiological findings of several distinct disease processes.

It may be difficult to judge ILD's complex morphological patterns, which may change in size and appearance over time. The manual categorization and assessment of extent is also a time-consuming and inaccurate method of data collection. The diagnosis of ILD is hampered by high inter-and intra-observer variation (Kundel, 2006, pp 402-408). Even if advances in imaging technology or a physician's training can improve his or her ability to accurately describe and characterise the disease, there are still inherent differences in interpretation, perception of visual disease features, and reader error that may not be overcome (Sverzellati et.al., 2011).

It has also been shown that the final clinical diagnosis of ILD may be affected by radiologists, clinicians, and pathologists working alone or in a multidisciplinary examination of illness even in a well-controlled trial with well defined participants. Academic and community health centre doctors from a variety of disciplines are more likely to encounter these differences in real-world patient care (Galbán et.al., 2012). Even if a diagnosis is reached by the consensus of several specialists and the application of methodologies for continuous learning, these do not guarantee reliable outcomes (Depeursinge et.al., 2010).

There is an opportunity to automate, computer-aided identification and quantitative image analysis because of the variability in clinical assessments of ILD. By using current image processing technologies, it is possible to maximise the detection of anomalies recognised to signify pathogenic changes on HRCT and to allow reliable quantification and characterisation of ILD symptoms. Quantitative results may be employed as biomarkers, leading in better diagnosis and better disease monitoring and prognosis determination (Sawada & Kozuka, 2015). Over the last several decades, numerous efforts have been made to robustly identify observable patterns in chest CT scans and x-rays using a variety of different methodologies. As a general rule, the evaluation of data from certain early texture based analysis is the same: "interstitial lung disease is difficult to classify and quantify, and even expert chest radiologists frequently struggle with differential diagnosis (Shouno et.al., 2015). Automated systems that identify the percentage of afflicted lungs or the likelihood of developing a certain disease would undoubtedly be beneficial, but would require significantly more research" (Christodoulidis et.al., 2016).

Figure 2. ILDs classification

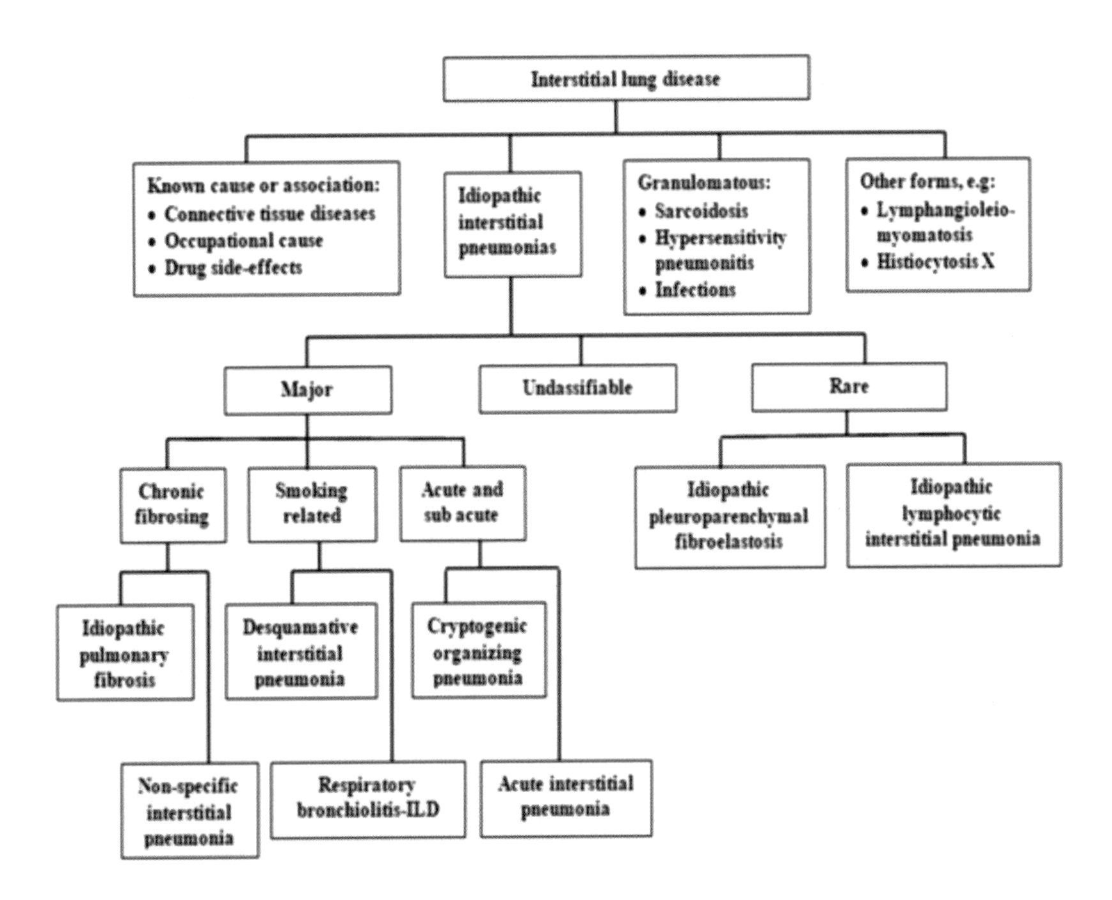

Fortunately, quantitative approaches for assessing the severity of emphysema and other aspects of COPD on CT images have become additional tough over last two decades, as numerous techniques have evolved and been optimised. These quantitative analytical results may be useful as biomarkers for diagnosing COPD symptoms, monitoring the disease development, and predicting prognosis (Paul et.al., 2016).

Although CT-based measurements have shown to be more challenging, the findings have been less encouraging. First-order features like density masks, pixel counting and several higher-order features or texturing approaches such as continuous learning with a physician in the loop are only partly effective at assessing particular illnesses and even differentiating normal vs abnormal areas (Seelan et.al., 2016). Additionally, many of the approaches now utilised to evaluate ILD interms of research are computationally intensive and require hours or even days of processing. Due to these practical constraints, it is difficult to translate those ideas into everyday clinical practise (Shen et.al., 2016).

Transfer Learning

It is incredibly expensive and difficult to maintain and develop a database on medical images. As a result, maintaining the sample data is difficult, and another approach is to learn from previous tasks before moving on to new ones. This is accomplished by transfer learning, which initializes the target from the existing source domain. The generalized diagram of transfer learning is given in figure 3, and the most widely used transfer learning methods are instant based, parameter-based, feature relying, and relation based.

Figure 3. Working principle of transfer learning

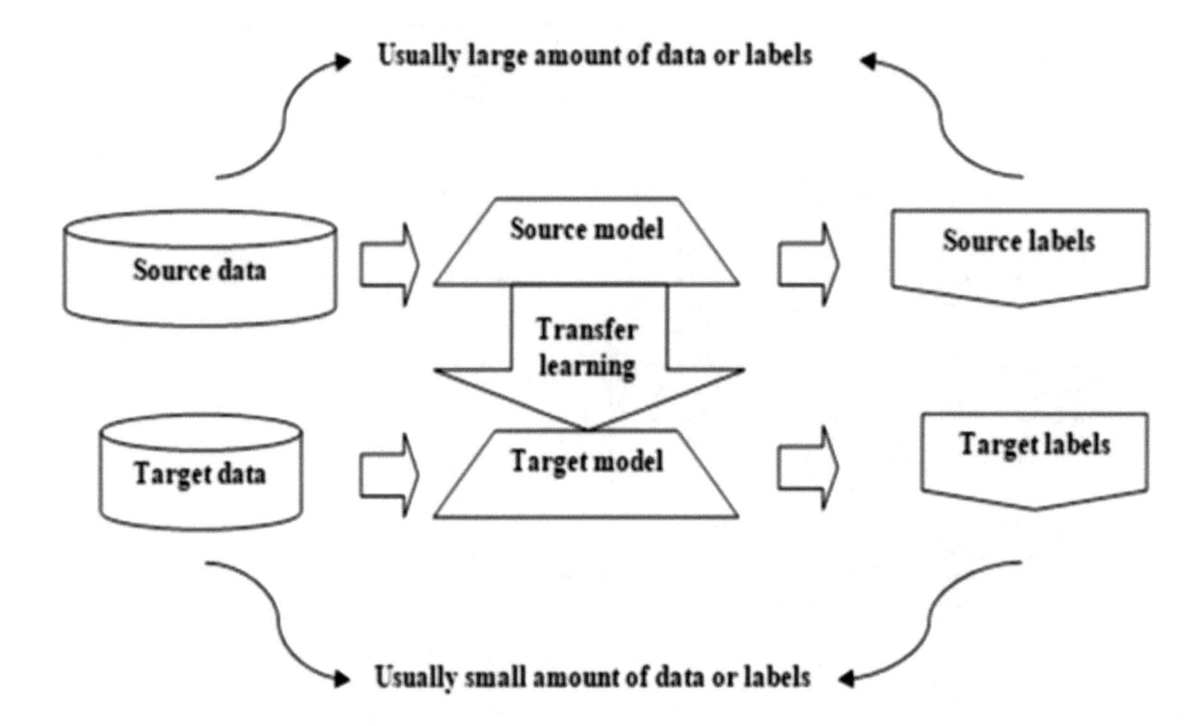

- **Instant based Transfer-learning**

This procedure is similar to filtering through the data in the source domain to find the most relevant information for the destination domain and matching it to the target domain. As a result, this technique has a higher degree of uncertainty, is less stable, and does not always have a subset of data in the source domain that is particularly comparable to the destination domains.

- **Parameter based transfer learning**

Initialize the retraining process using parameters from the source domain and give them a higher priority weighting. Using a pre-trained model, it is much easier to train new neural networks at a high pace than it is to start from scratch

- **Feature relying transfer learning**

The premise behind this method is that the two domains those are target and source domain can share some overlapping properties. Using feature transformation may combine the two domains into a single space. As a result, we may apply machine learning to complete the remaining tasks. The strength of the method is to work effectively, but the weakness is frequently not easy to compute.

- **Relation based-transfer learning.**

Here, the source and destination domains are compared to find the logical relation between them to share some kind of information. In this strategy, the key idea is to transmit logical connections from the input space to the destination domain.

The table 1 reveals the data of transfer learning methods applied to lung disease. In the source domain, (Nibali et.al., 2017) introduced the concept of multi-prediction deep boltzman machines to satisfy database requirements and convert them into tuned networks. The x-ray images to identify the lung disease are based on the concept of fine tuning. (Shan et.al., 2017) used a deep convolution network, which is a pre-trained network, applied to non medical images to extract lung diseases. Better performance is achieved by training the natural images first and then applying the transfer learning method to HRCT images.

Table 1. Transfer learning method on lung disease

Ref. No.	Disease Name	Transfer Method
(Wang et.al., 2017)	Lung CT/ Diffuse lung disease	Fine-tuning
(Da Nóbrega et.al., 2018)	Lung CT/ Survival prediction of lung adenocarcinoma VGG / Lung Lesion / lung cancer prediction	Feature extractor
(Hosny et.al., 2018)	Pulmonary nodule classification	Finetuning on ResNet
(Dey et.al., 2018)	Lung nodule classification / Lung cancer prognostication	Feature extractor
(Fang, 2018, pp. 286-290)	Lung cancer	Feature extractor
(Nishio et.al., 2018)	Lung-nodule classification	Finetuning on DenseNet / Fine-tuning on GoogLeNet / VGG-16 as feature extractor
(Hussein et.al., 2019)	Lung-nodule detection	Finetuning / Fine-tuning on VGG-16 / Fine-tuning on LeNet-5 / Extreme learning applied after feature extraction

The extracting low level feature using CNN was introduced by (Li et.al., 2019) and used six public texture databases. The CT scanning image database is used in this model and increases the accuracy by 2%. (Sreelakshmi & Inthiyaz, 2021) extract deep features of lung diseases using a pre trained CNN network, too different classifiers be utilized towards achieve the most excellent results in predicting the survival-time of humans with lung diseases (Sreelakshmi & Inthiyaz, 2021). The doctor and researches are finally concluded that, transfer learning methods are better solution to extract the deep features on lung images.

(Saikumar & Rajesh V, 2020) proposed model for lung nodule recognition and the model used here is a three-dimensional CNN network, which acquires the deep features more efficiently. This method is first pre trained on nonmedical images before applying it to CT images. Transfer learning methods are popular nowadays to extract the features in lung images (Saikumar & Rajesh V, 2020). (Raju et.al., 2022) introduced algorithms like Dense-Net, Google-Net, and VCG-16 feature extractor for lung nodule classification, and three-dimensional CT scan images are used in these models. The literature models like (Sankara Babu et.al., 2022) are supporting deep learning medical diagnosis process.

CONCLUSION

This paper, reviewed the classifications of Interstitial Lung Diseases using HRCT images. Firstly, we will discuss the overview of general imaging techniques like CT scan, MRI etc. HRCT is one class of the CT family and provides a higher resolution image because of 3D capturing. The accuracy of the diagnosis depends on expertise in that field, which otherwise leads to the wrong judgment of diseases. To avoid that, transfer learning methods were introduced, predicting the target domain from source data. These can be varied by instant-based or parameter based or feature-based or relation based and finally ended with a discussion of different transfer learning methods used in lung diseases. Furthermore, extend this work with pixel mapping for feature extraction and then followed by transfer learning techniques for better accuracy.

REFERENCES

Christodoulidis, S., Anthimopoulos, M., Ebner, L., Christe, A., & Mougiakakou, S. (2016). Multisource transfer learning with convolutional neural networks for lung pattern analysis. *IEEE Journal of Biomedical and Health Informatics*, *21*(1), 76–84.

Collard, H. R., Tino, G., Noble, P. W., Shreve, M. A., Michaels, M., Carlson, B., & Schwarz, M. I. (2007). Patient experiences with pulmonary fibrosis. *Respiratory Medicine*, *101*(6), 1350–1354.

Costabel, U., Du Bois, R. M., & Egan, J. J. (Eds.). (2007). *Diffuse parenchymal lung disease* (Vol. 36). Karger Medical and Scientific Publishers.

Cottin, V., Nunes, H., Mouthon, L., Gamondes, D., Lazor, R., & Hachulla, E., & Groupe d'Etudes et de Recherche sur les Maladies "Orphelines" Pulmonaires. (2011). Combined pulmonary fibrosis and emphysema syndrome in connective tissue disease. *Arthritis and Rheumatism*, *63*(1), 295–304.

Da Nóbrega, R. V. M., Peixoto, S. A., da Silva, S. P. P., & Rebouças Filho, P. P. (2018, June). Lung nodule classification via deep transfer learning in CT lung images. In *IEEE 31st international symposium on computer-based medical systems (CBMS)* (pp. 244-249). IEEE.

Depeursinge, A., Iavindrasana, J., Hidki, A., Cohen, G., Geissbuhler, A., Platon, A., ... Müller, H. (2010). Comparative performance analysis of state-of-the-art classification algorithms applied to lung tissue categorization. *Journal of Digital Imaging*, *23*(1), 18–30.

Dey, R., Lu, Z., & Hong, Y. (2018, April). Diagnostic classification of lung nodules using 3D neural networks. In *2018 IEEE 15th international symposium on biomedical imaging (ISBI 2018)* (pp. 774-778). IEEE.

Duan, Y., Coatrieux, G., & Shu, H. Z. (2015, August). Computed tomography image source identification by discriminating CT-scanner image reconstruction process. In *37th Annual International Conference of the IEEE Engineering in Medicine and Biology Society (EMBC)* (pp. 5622-5625). IEEE.

Fang, T. (2018, August). A novel computer-aided lung cancer detection method based on transfer learning from GoogLeNet and median intensity projections. In *2018 IEEE international conference on computer and communication engineering technology (CCET)* (pp. 286-290). IEEE.

Flaherty, K. R., Andrei, A. C., King, T. E. Jr, Raghu, G., Colby, T. V., Wells, A., & Martinez, F. J. (2007). Idiopathic interstitial pneumonia: Do community and academic physicians agree on diagnosis? *American Journal of Respiratory and Critical Care Medicine*, *175*(10), 1054–1060.

Galbán, C. J., Han, M. K., Boes, J. L., Chughtai, K. A., Meyer, C. R., Johnson, T. D., & Ross, B. D. (2012). Computed tomography–based biomarker provides unique signature for diagnosis of COPD phenotypes and disease progression. *Nature Medicine*, *18*(11), 1711–1715.

Haas, B., Coradi, T., Scholz, M., Kunz, P., Huber, M., Oppitz, U., André, L., Lengkeek, V., Huyskens, D., van Esch, A., & Reddick, R. (2008). Automatic segmentation of thoracic and pelvic CT images for radiotherapy planning using implicit anatomic knowledge and organ-specific segmentation strategies. *Physics in Medicine and Biology*, *53*(6), 1751–1771. doi:10.1088/0031-9155/53/6/017 PMID:18367801

Hosny, A., Parmar, C., Coroller, T. P., Grossmann, P., Zeleznik, R., Kumar, A., & Aerts, H. J. (2018). Deep learning for lung cancer prognostication: A retrospective multi-cohort radiomics study. *PLoS Medicine*, *15*(11), e1002711.

Hussein, S., Cao, K., Song, Q., & Bagci, U. (2017, June). Risk stratification of lung nodules using 3D CNN-based multi-task learning. In *International conference on information processing in medical imaging* (pp. 249-260). Springer, Cham.

Hussein, S., Kandel, P., Bolan, C. W., Wallace, M. B., & Bagci, U. (2019). Lung and pancreatic tumor characterization in the deep learning era: Novel supervised and unsupervised learning approaches. *IEEE Transactions on Medical Imaging*, *38*(8), 1777–1787.

Inoue, A., Johnson, T. F., Voss, B. A., Lee, Y. S., Leng, S., Koo, C. W., & Fletcher, J. G. (2021). A Pilot Study to Estimate the Impact of High Matrix Image Reconstruction on Chest Computed Tomography. *Journal of Clinical Imaging Science, 11*. 10.25259/JCIS_143_2021

Kundel, H. L. (2006). History of research in medical image perception. *Journal of the American College of Radiology*, *3*(6), 402–408.

Ley, B., Collard, H. R., & King, T. E. Jr. (2011). Clinical course and prediction of survival in idiopathic pulmonary fibrosis. *American Journal of Respiratory and Critical Care Medicine*, *183*(4), 431–440.

Li, Y., Zhang, L., Chen, H., & Yang, N. (2019). Lung nodule detection with deep learning in 3D thoracic MR images. *IEEE Access: Practical Innovations, Open Solutions*, *7*, 37822–37832.

Misumi, S., & Lynch, D. A. (2006). Idiopathic pulmonary fibrosis/usual interstitial pneumonia: Imaging diagnosis, spectrum of abnormalities, and temporal progression. *Proceedings of the American Thoracic Society*, *3*(4), 307–314. doi:10.1513/pats.200602-018TK PMID:16738194

Nibali, A., He, Z., & Wollersheim, D. (2017). Pulmonary nodule classification with deep residual networks. *International Journal of Computer Assisted Radiology and Surgery*, *12*(10), 1799–1808.

Nishio, M., Sugiyama, O., Yakami, M., Ueno, S., Kubo, T., Kuroda, T., & Togashi, K. (2018). Computer-aided diagnosis of lung nodule classification between benign nodule, primary lung cancer, and metastatic lung cancer at different image size using deep convolutional neural network with transfer learning. *PLoS One*, *13*(7), e0200721.

Olson, A. L., Swigris, J. J., Sprunger, D. B., Fischer, A., Fernandez-Perez, E. R., Solomon, J., & Brown, K. K. (2011). Rheumatoid arthritis–interstitial lung disease–associated mortality. *American Journal of Respiratory and Critical Care Medicine*, *183*(3), 372–378.

Paul, R., Hawkins, S. H., Balagurunathan, Y., Schabath, M., Gillies, R. J., Hall, L. O., & Goldgof, D. B. (2016). Deep feature transfer learning in combination with traditional features predicts survival among patients with lung adenocarcinoma. *Tomography*, *2*(4), 388–395.

Peikert, T., Daniels, C. E., Beebe, T. J., Meyer, K. C., & Ryu, J. H. (2008). Assessment of current practice in the diagnosis and therapy of idiopathic pulmonary fibrosis. *Respiratory Medicine*, *102*(9), 1342–1348. doi:10.1016/j.rmed.2008.03.018 PMID:18621518

Raghu, G., Collard, H. R., Egan, J. J., Martinez, F. J., Behr, J., Brown, K. K., Colby, T. V., Cordier, J.-F., Flaherty, K. R., Lasky, J. A., Lynch, D. A., Ryu, J. H., Swigris, J. J., Wells, A. U., Ancochea, J., Bouros, D., Carvalho, C., Costabel, U., Ebina, M., & Schunemann, H. J. (2011). An official ATS/ERS/JRS/ALAT statement: idiopathic pulmonary fibrosis: evidence-based guidelines for diagnosis and management. *American Journal of Respiratory and Critical Care Medicine*, *183*(6), 788–824. doi:10.1164/rccm.2009-040GL PMID:21471066

Raghu, G., Weycker, D., Edelsberg, J., Bradford, W. Z., & Oster, G. (2006). Incidence and prevalence of idiopathic pulmonary fibrosis. *American Journal of Respiratory and Critical Care Medicine*, *174*(7), 810–816.

Raju, K., Chinna Rao, B., Saikumar, K., & Lakshman Pratap, N. (2022). An Optimal Hybrid Solution to Local and Global Facial Recognition Through Machine Learning. In P. Kumar, A. J. Obaid, K. Cengiz, A. Khanna, & V. E. Balas (Eds.), A Fusion of Artificial Intelligence and Internet of Things for Emerging Cyber Systems. Intelligent Systems Reference Library (Vol. 210). Springer. https://doi.org/10.1007/978-3-030-76653-5_11.

Ryerson, C. J., Urbania, T. H., Richeldi, L., Mooney, J. J., Lee, J. S., Jones, K. D., & Collard, H. R. (2013). Prevalence and prognosis of unclassifiable interstitial lung disease. *The European Respiratory Journal*, *42*(3), 750–757.

Saikumar, K., & Rajesh, V. (2020). Coronary blockage of artery for Heart diagnosis with DT Artificial Intelligence Algorithm. *Int J Res Pharma Sci*, *11*(1), 471–479.

Saikumar, K., & Rajesh, V. (2020). A novel implementation heart diagnosis system based on random forest machine learning technique International. *Journal of Pharmacy Research, 12*, 3904–3916.

Saketkoo, L. A., Matteson, E. L., Brown, K. K., Seibold, J. R., & Strand, V. (2011). Developing disease activity and response criteria in connective tissue disease-related interstitial lung disease. *The Journal of Rheumatology, 38*(7), 1514–1518.

Sankara Babu, B., Nalajala, S., Sarada, K., Muniraju Naidu, V., Yamsani, N., & Saikumar, K. (2022). Machine Learning Based Online Handwritten Telugu Letters Recognition for Different Domains. In P. Kumar, A. J. Obaid, K. Cengiz, A. Khanna, & V. E. Balas (Eds.), A Fusion of Artificial Intelligence and Internet of Things for Emerging Cyber Systems. Intelligent Systems Reference Library (Vol. 210). Springer. https://doi.org/10.1007/978-3-030-76653-5_12.

Sawada, Y., & Kozuka, K. (2015, May). Transfer learning method using multi-prediction deep Boltzmann machines for a small scale dataset. In *14th IAPR International Conference on Machine Vision Applications (MVA)* (pp. 110-113). IEEE.

Seelan, L. J., Suresh, L. P., & Veni, S. K. (2016, October). Automatic extraction of Lung lesion by using optimized toboggan based approach with feature normalization and transfer learning methods. In *2016 International Conference on Emerging Technological Trends (ICETT)* (pp. 1-10). IEEE.

Shan, H., Wang, G., Kalra, M. K., de Souza, R., & Zhang, J. (2017, June). Enhancing transferability of features from pretrained deep neural networks for lung nodule classification. In *Proceedings of the 2017 International Conference on Fully Three-Dimensional Image Reconstruction in Radiology and Nuclear Medicine*.

Shen, D., Wu, G., & Suk, H. I. (2017). Deep learning in medical image analysis. *Annual Review of Biomedical Engineering, 19*(1), 221–248. doi:10.1146/annurev-bioeng-071516-044442 PMID:28301734

Shen, W., Zhou, M., Yang, F., Dong, D., Yang, C., Zang, Y., & Tian, J. (2016, October). Learning from experts: developing transferable deep features for patient-level lung cancer prediction. In *International conference on medical image computing and computer-assisted intervention* (pp. 124-131). Springer.

Shouno, H., Suzuki, S., & Kido, S. (2015, November). A transfer learning method with deep convolutional neural network for diffuse lung disease classification. In *International Conference on Neural Information Processing* (pp. 199-207). Springer.

Sreelakshmi, D., & Inthiyaz, S. (2021). Fast and denoise feature extraction based ADMF–CNN with GBML framework for MRI brain image. *International Journal of Speech Technology, 24*(2), 529–544.

Sreelakshmi, D., & Inthiyaz, S. (2021). A pervasive health care device computing application for brain tumors with machine and deep learning techniques. *International Journal of Pervasive Computing and Communications*.

Sverzellati, N., Devaraj, A., Desai, S. R., Quigley, M., Wells, A. U., & Hansell, D. M. (2011). Method for minimizing observer variation for the quantitation of high-resolution computed tomographic signs of lung disease. *Journal of Computer Assisted Tomography, 35*(5), 596–601.

Travis, W. D., Costabel, U., Hansell, D. M., King, T. E. Jr, Lynch, D. A., Nicholson, A. G., & Valeyre, D. (2013). An official American Thoracic Society/European Respiratory Society statement: Update of the international multidisciplinary classification of the idiopathic interstitial pneumonias. *American Journal of Respiratory and Critical Care Medicine*, *188*(6), 733–748.

Wang, C., Elazab, A., Wu, J., & Hu, Q. (2017). Lung nodule classification using deep feature fusion in chest radiography. *Computerized Medical Imaging and Graphics*, *57*, 10–18.

Watadani, T., Sakai, F., Johkoh, T., Noma, S., Akira, M., Fujimoto, K., & Sugiyama, Y. (2013). Interobserver variability in the CT assessment of honeycombing in the lungs. *Radiology*, *266*(3), 936–944.

Chapter 9
Geospatial Information Based Digital Twins for Healthcare

Pradeep K. Garg
https://orcid.org/0000-0002-7126-3698
Indian Institute of Technology Roorkee, India

ABSTRACT

A digital twin refers to a virtual model of a process, product, or service. It is a bridge between the physical world and digital world. Due to its obvious benefits, more organizations are adopting it, particularly in medicines and healthcare. The big data can be collected through wearable sensors, GPS, images, and IoT, and analysed with AI and machine learning that can be very helpful in various aspects of health sector. The GIS improves data capture and integration, leads to better real-time visualisation, offers detailed analysis and automation of future projections, and facilitates communication and cooperation. Digital twins are very helpful in personalised healthcare, monitoring the treatment. There are, however, many challenges associated with the digital data of patients, such as digitization of health records, security of data, and real-time analysis and predication to provide efficient and economical healthcare services.

INTRODUCTION

Our world is changing very fast and becoming high-tech. It is anticipated that by 2050, 2/3rd of the world's population would be living in the major cities. As the technology grows, it has the potential to improve the comfort and quality of lives of people living in the cities. The 4th Industrial Revolution (IR) is rapidly changing the way we live, we think, we work and we interact; creating a visible impact on our cities. This dramatic change is possible only through the adoption of latest digital technologies, such as the digital twin, internet of things (IoT), sensors, artificial intelligence (AI), machine learning (ML), autonomous vehicles, big data analytics, cloud computing, blockchain, virtual reality (VR), augmented reality (AR), building information modeling (BIM), and many others. Geospatial technology is considered as a powerful tool for transformation of digital information into actions (Garg, et.al., 2022).

A digital twin is called a virtual model which replicates the 3-D framework, physical properties and environmental conditions of a process, product or service. It works as a bridge between the physical

DOI: 10.4018/978-1-6684-5925-6.ch009

world and the digital world. The digital twin model allows us to examine the input-output factors, and thus it enhances the learning which then can be applied to its physical counterpart. Digital twins can represent current, past, or even future states of assets that may not exactly represent what exists in the real-world (Mostak, 2021). The state of art digital twins provide information beyond the current state of Earth and its objects and infrastructure.

Since 1960s, the concept of digital twins is being used. The NASA has been creating digital twins of its physical space mission systems to test the equipment in a complete virtual environment. In 1990s, the idea of digital twins emerged in David Gelernter's book (Gelernter, 1993). The digital twin idea has originally emerged in the product manufacturing sector (Arun, 2017). Since then, the digital twin technology has received much attention both in industry and research, and is being used in a large number of industrial applications (Kamel Boulos & Zhang, 2021). For example, precise digital models of complex structures, e.g., aeroplanes, can used for testing their performances. With digital twins, integration of additional layers is possible; each incrementally improving the representation and analysis (Mostak, 2021). In recent years, the integration of geospatial technology, BIM, and interactive 3D model have enhanced the use of digital twins. Digital twins deploy automated techniques to enhance the business processes, reduce the risk involved, maximise the output, and fasten the decision-making by predicting outcomes. geographic information system (GIS) technology provide the basic framework for the creation of any digital twin model.

Digital twins are already being developed in engineering and manufacturing, but researchers are now exploring the same principles to apply to the medical world to improve the clinical and public health outcomes. Earlier, it was not common to see digital twins beyond industrial manufacturing because they were very expensive to build. Today, digital twins can help researchers and doctors to detect the diseases and study the effects of medicines through simulation. Affordable new technologies have now given the flexibility in making digital twins more accessible and applicable. The digital twin technology is creating a revolution in the healthcare and biotechnology to create a revolution in the lives of the people. It can help identifying useful symptoms for chronic diseases, and make a comparison of various treatment methods of similar types of patients. This kind of analysis will be very useful for medical doctors to actually perform the tests with the patients (Ghazanfari, 2022). Digital twin has the capabilities to enhance the processes of clinical treatments, as it can be used to ask questions and get possible answers, and use these answers to derive into actions without actually experimenting straightaway on patients.

ELEMENTS OF A DIGITAL TWIN

There are four broad elements as given below:

1. **Data Capture:** Digital twins are providing opportunities to organizations to devise approaches for capturing and visualizing the data. In addition, it is important to use the techniques to integrate the data and analyze information, such as data modelling, feature creation & extraction, and workflow & business systems
2. **Real-Time Analysis:** It helps selecting the right decisions, discovering the new patterns, and revealing the future trends with real-time information. It includes dashboards, reporting, real-time IoT integration, analytics, and visualization of data.

3. **Share:** Digital twins supported by GIS technology help the organizations and people by sharing information, eliminating the shortage of data, and increasing the accuracy of outcome. It also includes visual display of information and communication, enhances engagement and collaboration, and transparency in information.
4. **Analyze and Predict:** Digital twins can be used to carry out modelling, simulation and scenario building. In addition, it is helpful in faster analysis and making accurate predictions using various statistical, machine learning (ML), deep learning (DL), and AI methods.

GEOSPATIAL DATA

Data is the key to unlock the future of medicines. More data into the digital twin system would result in more discoveries and more optimised treatment. The "big" health data, such as electronic health records (EHR), digitised medical images, test reports, etc., are all inputs for developing digital twins. Digital twins help pooling the data of similar patients that otherwise would be difficult in real-life scenario (Ghazanfari, 2022). In 2019, with the threat of Covid-19, it has become evident that the data plays an integral role in decision making. During Covid-19, data charts published daily and real-time data analysis derived important decisions on restrictions to our everyday life. It is clear that the location or geospatial element of data is also very important, in the context of popular phrase in geography "everything happens somewhere". To build a geospatial digital twin which is geospatially ecentric, it has to be refined through analyzing the volume of data being collected and that data has to be integrated geospatially. Building and leveraging such digital twins will be transformational in healthcare (Mostak 2021).

Geospatial data involves collecting photos/images, locational data of the Earth surface and its objects using photogrammetry, remote sensing, Global Positioning System (GPS), GIS and Unmanned Aerial Vehicles (UAVs)/drones (Garg, 2019). The contributions of these data have given a mass awareness to utilize the geospatial technology in responding to disease outbreaks. The use of geospatial data has seen a rise during 2020 in response to Covid-19 pandemic. The impact of the decisions made using the data demanded the need for trusted and good quality data. To overcome with this greater demand for good quality geospatial data, and increasing demands on budgets, there is a need to implement innovative ways to collect and share the geospatial data to a larger community. Digital twins are reliant on a good quality 3D dataset as their backbone which is reliable, current and accurate. In an increasingly data-driven world, health planners and decision makers are relying heavily on geospatial data to manage, simulate various scenarios and support evidence-based decision making. Digital twins are supporting this decision making process and get a true understanding of the potential impact of decisions made (Foster, 2021).

Digital twin offers a secure environment for experimenting the impact of change. It will be particularly critical to understand the effects of Covid-19 pandemic and completely recover from it. The pandemic has given us unexpected challenges by leveraging digital twins to help the affected people (Ghazanfari, 2022). Digital twins have the potential to understand this prior unknown situations, and finding answers of key questions, (such as people at most risk, the most common symptoms and most effective treatment). The digital twin technology developed to recover from the Covid-19 can also be utilised to create high-resolution, disease-specific digital twin that doctors and health professional can use for many other applications in the healthcare sector.

Hippocrates firstly established a relationship between the geographical characteristics of a region with its people health (Fradelos, et. al., 2014). Over a period of time, it has been proved that mapping the diseases and their geographic location is extremely vital not only for medical research but also studying various processes involved in spread of diseases. The mapping technology using geospatial data reproduced the world accurately in digital environment. In digital age, it is important to know the activities at a geographical location. This information is required in several sectors, including agriculture, military, energy, food, transport, urban, health, and many more. High resolution images from satellites and UAVs/drones, digitally-enabled devices and sensors, including both cell phones and IoT sensors provide geospatial data (Garg, 2020). Photogrammetry or LiDAR data can be used to create digital twins, with an accuracy to a few meters or less, while GPS can provide the locational geospatial data. All these data can be used to represent every building, hospitals, roads, power pole and trees in an area (Mostak 2021). GIS and its spatial analysis capabilities can support the construction of accurate digital twin models.

A number of gadgets are available today, such as diet monitors, tracking devices and telemedicine services, and their demand is continuously increasing which is further encouraging the development of more digital twins to improve medical diagnosis, treatments and healthcare of patients (Kamel Boulos and Zhang, 2021). Smart sensors can gather useful real-time data about the working condition, or position, which can be connected to a cloud-based system that would process all the data. From the analysis of input data along with the other useful data, opportunities may be identified and lessons are learnt within the virtual environment (Paul, 2018). In modern healthcare system, digital devices play a significant role in helping both service providers as well as patients, from data collection to disease control & management.

Data scientists can analyze the huge data which is required to run iterative models to generate actionable insights. They study the changes in physical objects captured by the attached sensors, and can use the data to develop an algorithmic model. The model can simulate the physical objects to study the performance and problems in near real-time. It is important to understand that huge datasets are required to support the outcome of digital twins. As the volume and frequency of data increase, the digital twin models generate results closer to reality. For effective digital twinning, this massive data is required to be processed at a very high speed. The technology to process such data is changing very fast as the condition of analysis is changing. With the right kind of analytics technology, decision-makers can analyse and explore data at a faster pace.

The conceptual model of digital twin comprises of three components (Kamel Boulos and Zhang, 2021): the (source) product in the physical space, digital representation of the product, and connections between the physical and digital products (Figure 1). A digital thread shown in the figure is a digital twin's temporal data pipeline (i.e., data pipeline over time), e.g., from a person's or cell's lifecycle (birth to death), enabling tracking, asking questions, and discovering useful relations between various temporal data. The digital twin model may have three types of data; past data, present data, and future data. Past data comprises the historical performance data of the system while present data covers the real-time data output received from the system. Future data refers to the machine learning part. It uses all sets of data to simulate an exact digital model of the real-world system. Digital twin also generates higher quantity and quality of data required in making better decisions. It also leads to better management and maintenance of assets. Creation of a digital twin has several advantages, and it is due to that it is gaining popularity in medical sciences.

Figure 1. Composition of a digital twin (bidirectional link between the real world (human body and its component parts) and the corresponding digital twin) (Kamel Boulos and Zhang, 2021)

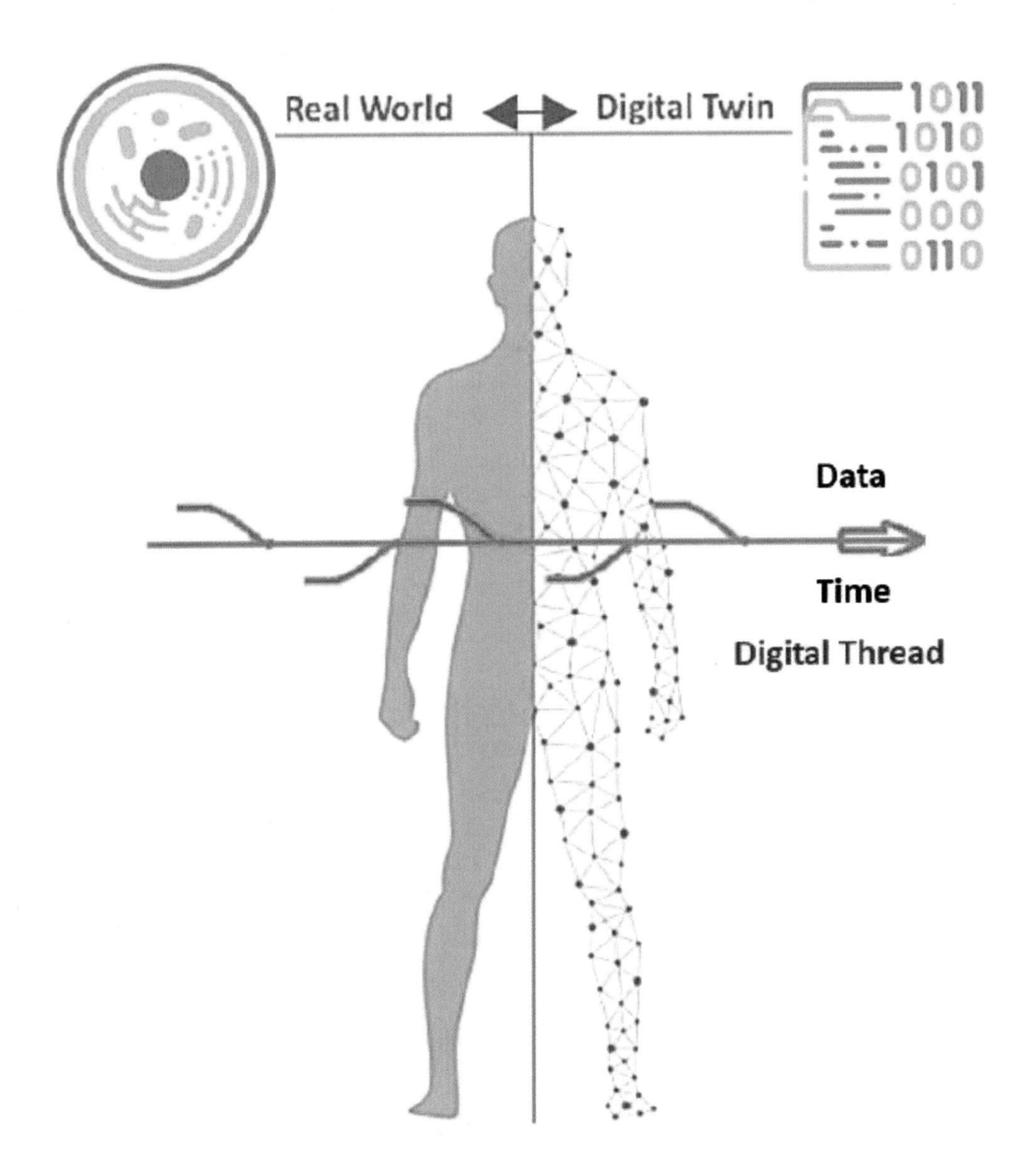

EMERGING TECHNOLOGIES

Employing the digital twin technology, medical professionals use genetic data and medical history, and details of long-term effects to create individualised treatment simulations. It leads to identification of best therapy option, without risking the patients. The technology eliminates the need to use real-life objects due to associated risks. In healthcare sector, it enables health professionals to determine optimum treatment, improve patient outcomes, leading to economical treatment in hospitals (Ghazanfari, 2022).

With increasing complexity within healthcare system, digital twin can take up complex tasks, such as personalized care, prediction of health outcomes, and taking proper care of the patients. For example, a digital twin may be used to convert medical images into visualisation model that would help to engage their patients. In addition, it can be effectively used before the operation and after the operation of patients to create better health plans for the patients. It is an important tool for healthcare service providers in order to analyze real-time data and taking correct decisions. Integration with IoT and sensors may further enhance the simulation process, disease predictions, and correct diagnosis to enhance the quality of life (Mostak, 2021)

A digital twin leverages the latest technologies, such as smart sensors, data analytics, AI, ML, and IoT, so as to detect the defects and prevent in advance the system failure, thus enhancing the efficiency. Figure 2 presents the modern technologies used in constructing the digital twins. Digital technology has helped making the latest data available, diagnosing the processes, remote monitoring the patients, and generating the reports of the patients. The core 'digital thread' tracking feature (see Figure 1) plays a major role in using the AI (Kamel Boulos & Zhang, 2021). The AI, machine learning and cloud computing offer advanced data analytics, which provide not only on-demand networked computational resources, but also process large quantities of data in real-time and offer new knowledge discovery.

Figure 2. Various technologies used for construction of digital twins

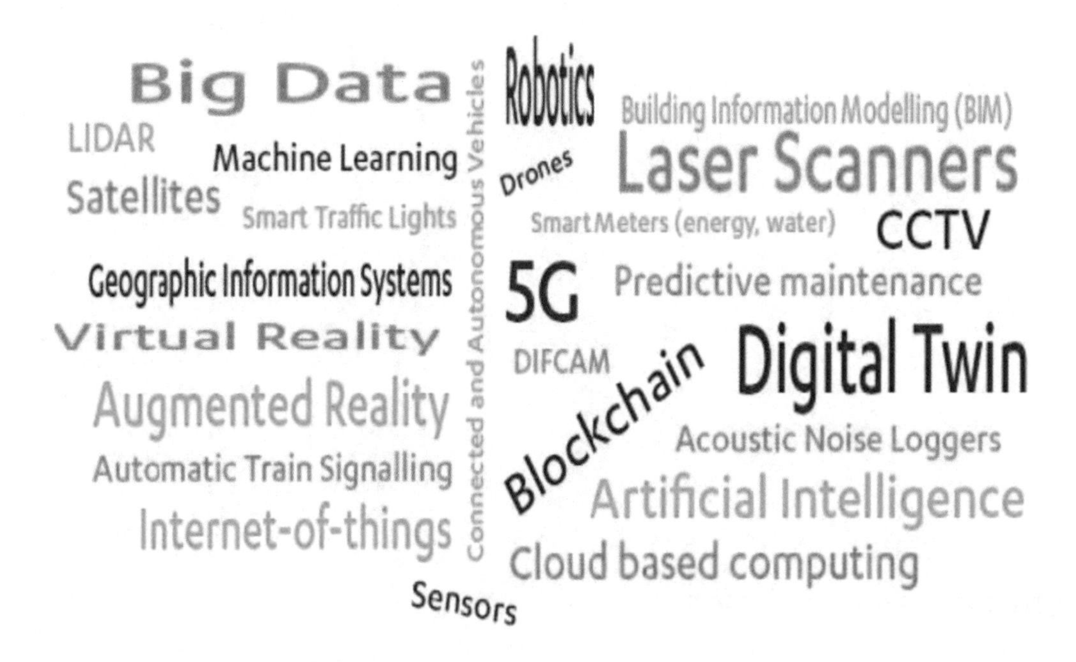

The growth in sensors and wireless networks have enhanced the utility of IoT in digital twin technology. With the integration of AI and advanced analytics, the digital twin has the ability to accurately predict the performance of a process. The predicted results can be shared to gather the information feedback to original entity, which in turn would encourage to use this technology for creating complex digital structures of the physical entity. It would thus enhance the decision-making criteria without affecting the original product. Digital twins can carry out in-depth analyses using big data, IoT and AI. In addition, one can get immediate feedbacks about the results, and apply necessary corrections immediately (Choudhary, 2020). With latest technologies, a cost-effective twin system may be developed. A virtual model would allow planning scenario and testing these against the huge data collected by various sensors. With IoT, edge computing and AI, the data collection and their analysis for creating digital twins are easily approachable for most of the industries (Stevens, 2021).

Geospatial technology has been used for epidemiological studies of vector-borne infections; restricted by environmental factors, such as the ambient temperature (Garg et.al., 2022). Big data, combined with geospatial technology, can be utilised not only for visualization, but also for dissemination of epidemic information. In addition, these will be helpful in tracking of virus source and its spreads, developing priorities for prevention and control, as well as prediction of disease. Remote sensing technology using time-series images can be used for monitoring infectious disease outbreaks and providing information about possible disease-carrying vectors (Zolli, 2020). The use of UAV/drone technology has proved to be enormously helpful for the management of Covid-19 pandemic (Bora, 2020). During Covid-19, drones have greatly helped the administration to monitor the people, disinfect the areas, delivery of goods and medicines and broadcasting the important messages (Garg, 2020). Using GPS technology, a medical staff from his/her room could use real-time location trackers to monitor the movement of patients to different departments of a hospital. Similarly, an administrator could make use of such information for taking real-time decisions on the number of staff and resources required, thus making care delivery systems efficient.

The GIS technology is considered as foundation for creating any digital twin. It integrates many types of digital data and models to create digital twins of objects on Earth. Creating the physical objects in digital form would require a more realistic 3D model of physical systems, particularly in an urban setup. It is therefore important that digital twin applications are created on digital terrain model (DTM) by integrating satellite images, GPS, and BIM in GIS, which can represent real-life objects, such as structures, trees, people etc. Furthermore, these 3D representations will provide different perspectives from planning point of view (Park and Yang, 2020).

The GIS enhances the data acquisition and data analysis, visualization, and future predictions. In addition, it allows for quick information sharing and collaboration (Garg, 2019). The digital twins of real-world assets or natural systems in GIS, can make the best decisions, explore new patterns, and unleash the power of data (Arun, 2017). The GIS could be used to derive new visual representations of the real-life assets (Garg, 2019). It helps organisations with increased information sharing, increased public and private interaction, through activities, such as visualisation, and data access.

Geospatial-based digital twins can bring together geospatial knowledge and real-time data to create better results (Stevens, 2019). Digital twins can be utilised to prepare and respond to risks involved, e.g., a terrorist attack in an area. Insurance companies are using it in a big way to cope up with the risk. Thus, better decisions can be taken by public health planners to revisit policies for well-being of public (Kamel Boulos and Zhang, 2021). A deep understanding of all the variables as well as understanding the place is critical that will make it possible to derive the best response (Stevens, 2019).

APPLICATIONS IN HEALTH SECTOR

The digital twin technology has been used widespread in several sectors. There is a huge potential in these areas. In general, the digital twin technology allows real-time monitoring of assets, products, or systems and enables predictive maintenance, waste reduction, product enhancements, and operational efficiency. Digital twins can also shorten yje production time. It introduces endless opportunities, like mass customization and small-batch manufacturing and also establishes efficient supply and delivery chains. Virtual troubleshooting is another area where digital twins can support by eliminating the need for physical presence at a location. The technology also works autonomously, proposes solutions, and even puts them into action.

Digital twin application in healthcare along with the IoT plays a crucial role in health sector. Digital twin solutions are needed to health professionals to improve the processes, decrease operating costs, and support healthcare. In addition, the applications can be enhanced with the geo-location technologies, like GPS, which provides a powerful data source for identifying the objects. The healthcare services for patients to track a variety of health indicators can be enhanced through the use of digital twins. The organizations can develop innovative solution to minimize the possibility of arising risks.

With advanced algorithms and simulation capabilities, digital twins can be created to model various parts of a human body. It can be used to assess the drug reactions, impact of treatment, procedural safety, etc. By assessing the medical records of individual, digital twin technology can also be used to strengthen personalised health research (Kamel Boulos and Zhang, 2021). It helps in systematic scheduling of maintenance routine of medical devices to provide continuity of care as well as save time, efforts and money. Another advantage is that the simulation of outcome can be created before developing a prototype medical device which can reduce iterations and development time & expenditure. The other benefits are presented in Figure 3.

Some of the applications are briefly described below:

1. Environmental Factors Related to Health

The climate of Earth changing fast, primarily due to various human activities. The change in climate has made a wider impact across various regions. Several environmental factors have an adverse impact on human health. Models incorporating the environmental factors can be developed and used for better planning of health decisions. The European Space Agency (ESA) Copernicus Sentinel-5P satellite mission has provided key information about the changes in concentrations of atmospheric pollutants globally, such as Nitrogen Dioxide (NO_2) during complete lockdown of Covid-19 (Kumar, 2020). The NO_2, a precursor of ozone and particulate matter, is considered as a key air pollutant factor which affects health. High resolution satellite images can offer details of environment and its surroundings. Organisation can use the capabilities of GIS to develop new initiatives that would improve health at workplace.

2. Real-Time and Visualization

Using real-time data, individuals can make the best decisions, as well as explore new patterns. Digital twins with real-time IoT integration, insights and analytics, can be used for reporting the information on dashboards, and its visualization in 2D and 3D. With augmented reality/virtual reality, it is rapidly growing to provide training and education required to healthcare practitioners.

Figure 3. Benefits of using digital twins in healthcare

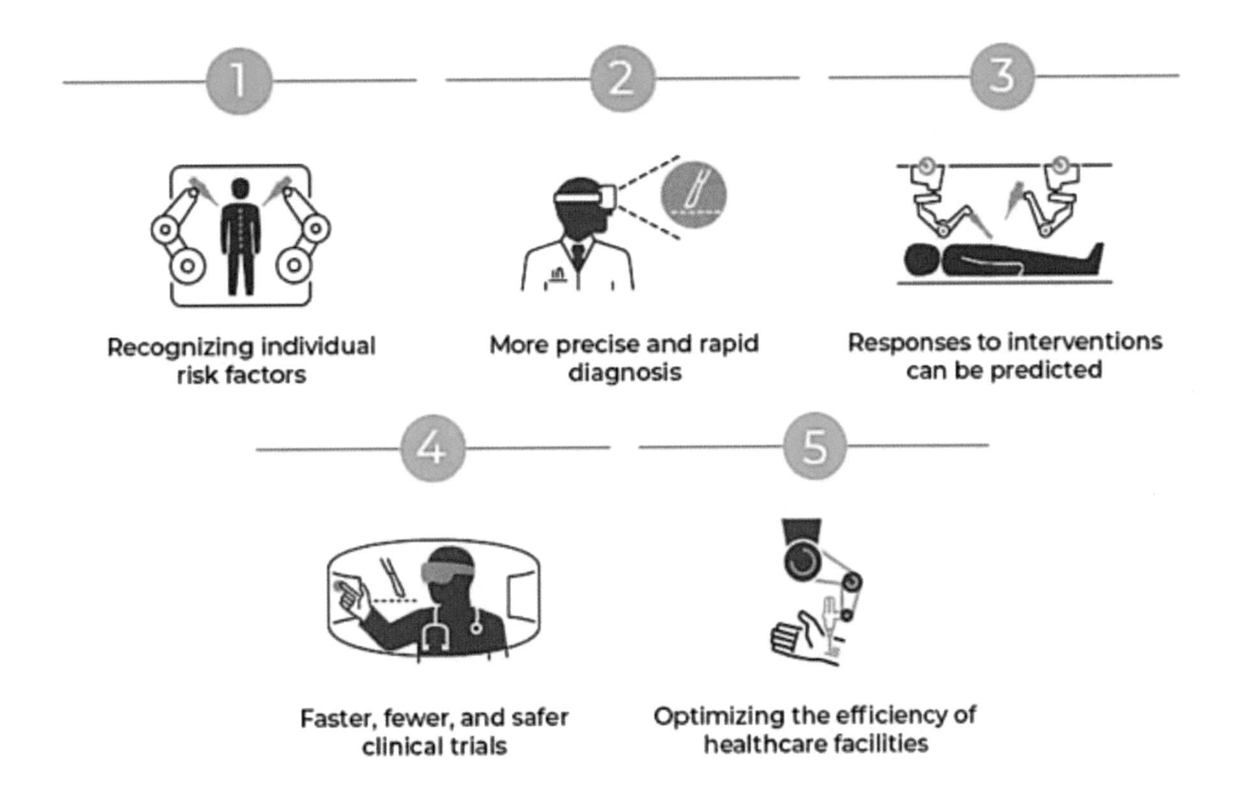

3. **Disaster Management**

In many areas, fires, flood, drought, landslides, earthquake and drought occur frequently. The digital twins can be employed to build smart building, smart infrastructure, utility networks, and emergency response action plans, to minimise the losses during a disaster (Stevens, 2019). In case of flood, digital twin can provide useful information in real-time about the areas that affected by flood, about the infrastructure that will be shut down, about the nearest hospitals, and thus allowing rescue workers to take immediate steps. Digital twin technology in GIS can provide real-time decision support system for public health planners in applications of smart cities; from traffic management (e.g., to reduce traffic congestion, air and noise pollution, and accidents) to providing immediate services during flood. Digital twins can create simulations to reduce the damages caused during disasters, and thus allowing citizens to lead a safer life (Paul, 2018). Digital twins can be used to develop utility networks, and emergency services response from disasters, such as landslide, flooding, and drought, which can offer guidance to governments and organizations to respond quickly to disasters.

4. **Patient Surgery**

The digital twins help to select the treatment through prediction of outcome by simulating the clinical procedure. It can be used effectively for the selection of medical devices. Digital twins help doctors to study a particular patient's organ and test it with different approaches to prevent its deterioration that is likely to occur in future. It also enables patient-specific surgery training to prepare for complex invasive procedures. The virtual model of a patient can be utilised to plan surgical operation in an effective manner, and assess the likely risks. In some cases, the models can assist to have the treatment done without for surgery. Digital twin models of brains of sports persons can help to accurately assess trauma from likely brain injuries, as such analysis offers additional benefits in saving time during the surgical procedures and recovery plans, in case a player receives brain injury.

5. **Patient Monitoring**

The digital twins of patients greatly help the doctors in monitoring the patients, remotely. It uses fast algorithm to produce precise results as a result of continuous data being collected from sensors. The patients can be monitored through smart wearables, sensors and IoT (Garg et.al., 2022). Sensors-based smaller and comfortable wearables can be used to provide real-time input data in the cloud-based system. With the growth of diseases and continuous patient data collection through biometric, digital twin system can be used to develop models that detect the symptoms at an early stage, providing flexibility to doctors to diagnose the patient much earlier. In addition, during treatment, it is possible to monitor and analyse if the treatment is effective. Real-time monitoring, and post-operation care of patients is a complicated process. The digital twin could also be used to assess the risk areas by studying the epidemiology data to keep a track on an infection. The digital twin has simplified the monitoring and evaluation of patient's health, thus providing effective outcomes.

6. **Personalized Healthcare**

Personalised medicine is growing in medicines and healthcare that aims at providing treatment of diseases and their prevention, e.g., genetic composition, lifestyle, and surrounding environment, that make each patient different from others (Kamel Boulos and Zhang, 2021). Digital twin is capable to model every single patient with varying habits and genetic structure. It is aimed at personalization with precision to implement personalized medicine without long-waiting times for screening/diagnostic results. It can help to provide treatment of disorders, and solution for prevention.

A digital twin model can be applied to the hospital and administrators to get real-time information of patients, and suggest them a suitable time-schedule. It may help in reducing waiting time for the patients while monitoring appointments and accurate inventory procedures & maintenance. Using AI, it can assist doctors in making a better diagnosis as to how different medicines might affect each patient (Garg et. al, 2022). The combination of AI, machine learning and IoT technologies have enormous effect to produce data for individual patients, and thus helping the doctors to take better decisions. These technologies along with digital twin can surely serve as a strong backbone for shifting the focus of healthcare more on preventive and high quality care of individuals.

7. **Developing Drug Therapy Model**

Digital twins are also utilised by several pharmaceutical industries in large applications, e.g., for drug development (Canzoneri, et al., 2021). A virtual twin with several drugs can be used to figure out the best one for a particular case. It can be used to create a database of real patients, with same symptoms, and test new drugs to assess the most useful drug and its optimum dosage which has cured many patients in shortest time. Digital twin technologies can be used to characterize the disease of individual so as to automate the choice of drugs. It helps doctors manage large number of patients quickly, effectively and remotely, while reducing the expenses.

8. **Medical Imaging**

As there is a high demand for medical imaging facilities, diagnosing the medical imaging is a challenging area around the globe. Digital twin technologies are updating the records of the patient from check-in to discharge details. A patient-centric workflow can be created where the health organization can provide the best practices and quality care.

9. **Predicting Outcome**

Today, patient care information related to genetic, physiological, and behavioral aspects of each patient is captured to create personalized digital twin. It can predict and analyze the health outcome as well as help in reducing the healthcare costs. Digital twins can reduce the time of patients and healthcare staff in optimizing the output from the extracted data/information of patient-specific as well as scheduling the visits.

10. **Decision Support for Diagnosis and Treatment**

Digital twin captures continuous data from the individual throughout its life. Its solutions provide more effective care by helping the doctors to know more about the patient. Digital twin solutions depend on health data sources, like imaging records, laboratory reports, etc., which help health staff during the diagnosis. The twin model predicts the health status of a patient from available clinical data and deriving the missing values statistically.

CHALLENGES & OPPORTUNITIES

Digital twin has been recognised as the most demanding technological innovation (Mostak 2021). The digital twin is creating a digital revolution to improve the quality of life of mankind. For successful implementation of digital twins, optimization, prediction, and simulations are essential. Figure 4 shows how various stakeholders in health sector are making use of digital twin to offer quality services.

As per the Gartner Hype Cycle in 2018, digital twins are one of five emerging technologies. Gartner mentioned that hundreds of millions of things would use digital twins within next five years (Grieves, 2014). The fast growing digital twin market points out that further demand for digital twins will continue to rise, while many digital twins are already being used by several industries. A recent Markets & Markets report estimated that the market of Digital Twin would grow from US$ 3.1 billion in 2020 to US$ 48.2 billion per year by 2026, at an annual CAGR growth of 58% (Ghazanfari, 2022).

There are several benefits of creating a digital twin, but still all the benefits have not been fully explored, as there are a few bottlenecks for its successful implementation (Kamel Boulos and Zhang, 2021). Implementation of digital twins will have several challenges as faced by the AI and big data analytics,

Figure 4. Various stakeholders in the healthcare sector utilizing the digital twin to deliver quality healthcare services

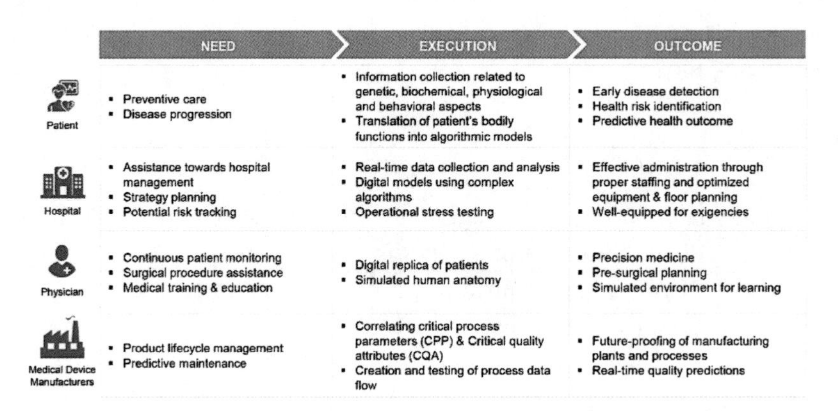

i.e., data availability, data quality; data integration, data and interoperability; data sharing; data privacy and security across platforms and systems; etc. Good quality data is the heart of a modern AI/machine learning algorithm. Not just the big data, but data sample of all sizes are important. The bias reduction in data for digital twins can be done by using a well-represented sample of population. The AI-based digital twins are expected to provide support to hospitals world-wide, to advance health, education and economy for one billion people by year 2030. It is important to have significant computational storage, as well as AI and ML-based algorithm to design proper actions; while at the same time keeping the privacy and data security of the patient (Ghazanfari, 2022). The other challenges include, requirement of accurate and up-to-date data, integration of geospatial data from various sources, and creating a geospatial data infrastructure for multiple uses (Stoter et al., 2021).

Digital twin needs to be created for each patient, which is time-consuming and expensive, so a proper mechanism must be developed for creating virtual models. Voluminous information is required to be processed regularly for creating the updated database and continuously upgrading the twin models; which makes it a cumbersome and time-taking process. In addition, healthcare organizations may not have sufficient storage and processing facility to handle big data sets. Digital twins may need complex data structures and algorithms, so patient's data safety is required to be ensured. In addition, privacy and security are big concerns with digital technologies. As the digital data has associated risks, the organisations need to assess their security protocols to safeguard the health data of individuals. Data integrity and availability of trained manpower to develop complex models for digital twins can cause hindrance to the advancement of digital twins in healthcare, however the regulations, like the General Data Protection Regulation (GDPR) will ensure a smooth development of digital twin models in healthcare (Mostak 2021).

CONCLUSION

A geospatial digital twin model of an object is extrapolated from different data types, such as, sensors, images, and GPS data. There are a number of possibilities for the applications of geospatial twins. Geospatial technology integrates the data, systems, and models to create digital representations of features/

objects. It harnesses GIS data into usable information. Integrating GIS with big geospatial data will allow a deep knowledge about the digital twin system for taking intelligent decisions and actions.

Digital twins, combining huge data and AI algorithms, are expected to change the services provided by the public health sector. These technologies will be useful to keep a track on electronic health/medical records of individuals to be utilised in medicine and public health. The IoT has been providing extensive support in the healthcare sector, collecting real-time clinical and health data to facilitate effective communications between equipment, machines, and humans. In future, digital twins will play important role in delivering highly specialised personal treatment (Kamel Boulos and Zhang, 2021).

Digital twins could be useful to fight against the pandemic and other diseases, which combine the experience, knowledge and skills. Over the next five years, several organisations/industries would rely on digital twins to perform their processes, through a distributed, hybrid, multicloud environment. For this purpose, there is a need of using right technology that can offer the appropriate hardware, and software services, while protecting the data it represents (Ghazanfari, 2022). The application of digital twins in future are limitless, as the increasing amount of cognitive power is constantly being developed. Digital twins are evolving new skills to make the products and services better in healthcare sector.

REFERENCES

Arun, S. (2017), Digital Twin - An Emerging Technology for Geospatial World. *Satpalda Geospatial Services*. https://www.satpalda.com/blogs/digital-twin-an-emerging-technology-for-geospatial-world

Bora, G. (2020). https://economictimes.indiatimes.com/small-biz/startups/features/covid-19-in-the-times-of-touch-me-not-environment-drones-are-the-new-best-friends/articleshow/74924233.cms?utm_source=contentofinterest&utm_medium=text&utm_campaign=cppst

Canzoneri, M., de Luca, A., & Harttung, J. (2021). Digital twins: A general overview of the biopharma industry. *Advances in Biochemical Engineering/Biotechnology*, *177*, 167–184. doi:10.1007/10_2020_157 PMID:33604707

Choudhary, M. (2020), What are use cases of Digital Twin? *Geospatial World*. https://www.geospatial-world.net/blogs/what-are-use-cases-of-digital-twin/

Foster, L. (2021), Authoritative Geospatial Data and Digital Twins. *techUK*. https://www.techuk.org/resource/authoritive-geospatial-data-and-digital-twins-denmark-in-3d.html

Fradelos, E. C., Papathanasiou, I. V., Mitsi, D., Tsaras, K., Kleisiaris, C. F., & Kourkouta, L. (2014). Health Based Geographic Information Systems (GIS) and their Applications. *Acta Inform Med., 22*(6), 402-405, . doi:10.5455/aim.2014.22.402-405

Garg, P. K. (2019). *Theory and Principles of Geoinformatics*. Khanna Book Publishing, Co. Ltd.

Garg, P. K. (2020). *Introduction to UAV*. New Age International Pvt Ltd.

Garg, P. K., & Tripathi, N. K., Kappas, M., & Gaur, L. (2022) Geospatial Data Science for Healthcare in Society 5.0. Springer Nature.

Gelernter, D. (1993). *Mirror Worlds: Or the Day Software Puts the Universe in A Shoebox. How It Will Happen and What It Will Mean*. Oxford University Press.

Ghazanfari, A. (2022), How digital-twin technology could revolutionise the healthcare industry. *Computer Weekly*. https://www.computerweekly.com/opinion/How-Digital-Twin-Technology-Could-Revolutionise-the-Healthcare-Industry

Grieves, M. (2014) *Digital Twin: Manufacturing Excellence through Virtual Factory Replication (Digital Twin White Paper-2014)*, https://www.researchgate.net/publication/275211047_Digital_Twin_Manufacturing_

Kamel Boulos, M. N., & Zhang, P. (2021). Digital Twins: From Personalised Medicine to Precision Public Health. *Journal of Personalized Medicine*, *2021*(11), 745. doi:10.3390/jpm11080745 PMID:34442389

Kumar, A. (2020). Bonus benefit! Satellite data shows significant decrease in NO2 emissions in India due to Covid-19 lockdown. India Today.

Mostak, T. (2021). The Future of Geospatial Analytics Is In Digital Twins. *Forbes*. https://www.forbes.com/sites/forbestechcouncil/2021/11/18/the-future-of-geospatial-analytics-is-in-digital-twins/?sh=168ffc7dd590

Park, J., & Yang, B. (2020). GIS-Enabled Digital Twin System for Sustainable Evaluation of Carbon Emissions: A Case Study of Jeonju City, South Korea. *Sustainability*, *2020*(12), 9186. doi:10.3390u12219186

Paul, S. (2018), Digital twins – connecting information and insights through the entire project lifecycle. *Geospatial World*. https://www.geospatialworld.net/blogs/digital-twins-connecting-information-and-insights-through-the-entire-project-lifecycle/

Stevens, L. (2019), Geospatial Digital Twins. *The Medium*. https://medium.com/@linda_29745/geospatial-digital-twins-a8e2bc886fd4

Stoter, J., Ohori, K. A., & Noardo, F. (2021), Digital Twins: A Comprehensive Solution or Hopeful Vision? *GIM Internationjal*. https://www.gim-international.com/content/article/digital-twins-a-comprehensive-solution-or-hopefulvision?utm_source=newsletter&utm_medium=email&utm_campaign=Newsletter+%7C+GIM+%7C+17-03-2022++&sid=34800

Zolli, A. (2020). How Satellite Data Can Help With COVID-19 And Beyond. *Planet*. https://www.planet.com/pulse/how-satellite-data-can-help-with-covid-19-and-beyond/

Chapter 10
Healthcare for the Elderly With Digital Twins

Rita Komalasari
https://orcid.org/0000-0001-9963-2363
Yarsi University, Indonesia

ABSTRACT

Assistive technology for the elderly was the focus of the literature review that would help support the elderly's healthcare. This chapter discusses the potential of assistive technology in general to offer a cost-effective way of assisting healthcare services for the elderly; no systematic research on the expenses of these technologies for this population has been carried out. Throughout the process of evaluation, evidence of significance is considered. This chapter explains the methods and conclusions of the literature review. As a result of this chapter, the elderly will have better access to health care.

INTRODUCTION

Assistive technology is discussed and evaluated in this chapter, which focuses mainly on the elderly. Another benefit is that it aids in discovering metrics by which we may assess the potential implications and social effects of elderly treatment. The promising benefit is that it aids AI in sustainable health care, precision medicine, and privacy concerns (Santosh & Gaur, 2022). The economic and educational systems rely heavily on public health, which demands particular care. One such epidemic is COVID-19, a genuine case of an infectious illness. Health protection, illness prevention, and health promotion are at the heart of WHO's mission to provide public health systems that can meet the aforementioned critical challenges. For example, deep convolution neural networks, with their AI and machine learning capabilities, can positively affect public health in several areas (e.g., existing medical image-based detection of COVID-19) (Gaur et al., 2021). If we examine resource-constrained places, they are invaluable instruments not only for diagnosing and analyzing pathology but also for speeding up the decision-making process (e.g., infectious diseases: pneumonia and tuberculosis) (Mahbub et al., 2022).

Assistive technology for the elderly was the focus of the literature review that would contribute to supporting healthcare services for the elderly. In this chapter, the relationship between "Telecare and the

DOI: 10.4018/978-1-6684-5925-6.ch010

elderly," we used a comprehensive definition of assistive technology for this evaluation (Van Der Roest et al., 2017). Using telecommunication and automated systems, 'in-home healthcare and social services for those unable to leave their homes. This chapter reviews nursing homes and sheltered housing where people live in groups. The evaluation looked at both types of technology for official and personal usage. The features of care at home and assistance for informal caregivers are crucial in a legislative environment that is more oriented toward personalized services. Early on, the evidence base was fragmented; cost-effectiveness techniques were variable, and the outcome measures employed included many things (Edney et al., 2018). During the review process, this wide range of data and methods were found and looked at seeing if they should be included.

There is mixed information on assistive technology, including telehealth care, telemedicine, and Telecare. Even in the face of an aging population, assistive technology is a solution that could be efficient compared to how services are currently delivered. The Indonesian National Telehealth and Telecare Delivery Plan state as much. We cannot continue providing our services in their current form (Durrani & Khoja, 2009). Schröders (2021) reported that the breadth and quality of the reviews had been restricted. Cost and cost-effectiveness data were relatively lacking in reliability. It largely ignored the aging population in academic and policy literature, at least in Indonesia. They account for only 33% of the 21 million people who receive technology-based services. Rather than looking at a broader body of work, we narrowed our scope to devices geared towards the elderly.

METHOD

In terms of the method, refined search keywords were developed after initial searches to establish a compromise between specificity (identifying all-important studies but with a significant volume of irrelevant stuff) and sensitivity (more relevant research, but the risk of missing some important ones). It was around this time that the words were first introduced. They included assistive technology and any other expense consideration in the thorough, methodical evaluation of costs. With so much information accessible and little time, the study concentrated on articles published in recent years. Because this is a rapidly growing subject, implementation evidence rather than pilot studies is more important. I judged more recent articles more relevant. I reviewed more than half of the items during the previous five years. After the relevance of the abstracts was verified, fifty-nine texts were evaluated. Thirty-three of the fifty-nine candidates were discarded following a comprehensive text review.

The following were the exclusion and inclusion criteria:

A researcher read over each item in great detail. It was determined whether they were relevant enough to the research to warrant further evaluation using our proforma review method. Use this tool to collect information on each item's substance and conclusions and an attribute evaluation. As a result, the evaluation process thoroughly evaluated the research's overall quality (Komalasari et al., 2022).

RESULTS

This section presents the result of the literature discussing "advanced" technology, such as ICT and electrical parts. Applications that could be transferred from location to location comprised one-third of the applications, while those that could not be relocated comprised the other third. More than half of the solutions are portable, permanent, or otherwise difficult to categorize since they lack a physical form (for example, an ICT-based support intervention). It is possible that the technology is pre-the user may control programmed. This technology includes the devices' "users," demonstrating just how broadly targeted the devices were: many of them were used by many groups.

There are still a few gadgets that fall into over one category, since they are multi-functional. As we will see in the next section, analyzing cost-effectiveness may be difficult because of the wide variety of functions. We look at various potential outcomes, psychological or functional results, and those connected to the relationships between individuals and service providers. These are the kinds of objectives that technology providers want to achieve in certain situations. In other cases, the researchers themselves choose the results. Much of the research considers several outcomes. Cost-effectiveness may be assessed in various ways, and we will cover this in more detail below.

The publications used various methods of weighing costs and advantages. I considered a wide variety of stakeholders while calculating the costs and benefits. There are three categories of evidence in Bayer et al.'s (2021) categorization of healthcare innovations: first, low-risk, universally applicable technology; First, there is the utility and cost-effectiveness of the technologies in question; second, there are affordable technological innovations for some users (referred to as "home run" technologies). There are no detailed cost-effectiveness analyses in these general assessments. Instead, it summarizes how much reading this article persuaded many people of the validity of the claims stated (for example, avoiding a fall saves money on medical expenses). There is a need to evaluate the prospective advantages (for example, caregivers who get more significant assistance may continue caring for their loved ones for a more extended period). This assistance prevents costly institutional care.

The quality of the research was evaluated across all studies based on a set of criteria tailored to each study's method. However, only a small percentage of studies were of good quality, while around 20% were found to be of poor quality. Reliable information on assistive technology costs and advantages continues to be scarce. Our discussion will touch on the strength of the evidence and the higher quality of the research we address throughout the article. Our research includes a Cochrane study (Kachouie et al., 2014) that found high-quality randomized controlled trial (RCT) evidence is needed, including for elderly home care. However, none of the studies satisfied the inclusion criterion. This lack of evidence highlights the necessity of incorporating studies of various sorts. We draw on the same criterion. Our evaluation would have only found two papers, one of high quality (Boockvar et al., 2020) and one of medium quality (Marcantonio et al., 2010). McKenna et al. (2018) conducted a high-quality CCT (Controlled Clinical Trial). Two studies found economic assessments only in Greene et al. (2022) and Johansson et al. (2022). However, many other investigations have considered costs and benefits more widely. Research by Hirsch et al. (2000) and Esfandiari et al. (2009) was judged to be of poor quality because of their small size and unclear findings, respectively. Throughout, we will discuss the weight of the evidence in our deliberations. This lack of evidence underlines the better quality of the study. Here, we emphasize the need to include a wide range of studies: No papers matched the inclusion criteria for the Cochrane review (Yusif et al., 2016) that we used when examining high-quality Randomized Controlled Trials (RCTs) on senior home care.

DISCUSSION

This section discusses the cost-benefit analysis of assistive technology for the elderly as an arduous task, as seen by the research cited above. There are a variety of reasons this is so difficult. It is important to remember that the phrase "assistance technology" encompasses many gadgets and configurations. It is common for studies to focus on a particular area, focusing on a specific component of technology. Second, the results that are considered are pretty diverse. The intended effects of technology may be to reduce costs, enhance services, enhance the well-being of the elderly, improve helper assistance, or any other consequence for various stakeholder groups and groups. Telecare, for example, may allow patients the right to stay in their residences, saving hospitalization money. Materials focusing on exercise and remembrance can enhance the quality of life, and telemedicine can improve QALY results (quality-adjusted life years). It is also important to note that the aged population is diverse, and the issues faced by those with the disease might alter. It is also essential to consider how assistive technology affects the elderly. This technology affects both costs and advantages for both the individual and society. The topics that emerged from our qualitative literature study are now discussed. Most of the evidence we use comes from sources rated medium to high quality.

Low-Quality Evidence Is Singled Out for Special Attention

In-depth studies on the practical use of commercially available technology and the technological maturity, new advancements, and consequences for the elderly are discussed in this section of the paper.

'Off-The-Shelf' Technology

Existing 'off-the-shelf' technologies are discussed in particular literature, frequently focusing on cheap costs. Substantial evidence is that nurses can communicate with the elderly and their caregivers at home using free Skype (Cutler et al., 2015). According to their findings, there is "inadequate" evidence of the costs and benefits of the system. They point out that despite the technology's availability for free, the potential problems of inadequate connection have not been considered when comparing it to other low-cost solutions like landline telephones. People who purchase off-the-shelf technologies fail because they cannot integrate them into their daily routines. From an individual's point of view, it is not cost-effective, according to Gibson et al. (2019). Roberts (2009) examines the same difficulties in additional care housing established Telecare systems (mature technology). However, although there is firm evidence devices may successfully help the elderly, they are seldom used. There may be some concerns when the user handles the installation cost.

Technology's Level of Maturity

Rapid technological advancements have contributed to a lack of research on the economic benefits of using assistive technology. New technologies and small-scale pilot projects are the subjects of most academic literature. A few exceptions to this rule are critical to understanding how assistive technology for the elderly will be implemented. Technology and systems that have been around longer should be prioritized. According to Barnard et al. (2013), there has been an extensive study of pilots and new gadgets. They believe products employed in real-world service-providing settings should be considered.

The case of Indonesia has received vast amounts of focus, as it has been employing Telecare technologies to serve the elderly in their own homes since 2001 and has a long track record in this area. According to Morato (2021), the Telecare system in Indonesia has resulted in lower costs and more satisfied service consumers. Central Jakarta included Telecare in a major reform of local services, including the closure of half of the region's care homes and the construction of dozens of new housing units with on-site healthcare facilities. Antarsih et al. (2021), economists, conducted an early study of the system and discovered that it had reduced the quality of health and social care services while keeping costs low.

Assistive technology delivery at scale is an ongoing problem. As an additional example, with long-term diseases like heart failure, COPD, and diabetes eligible for Medicaid, they participated in Whole System Demonstrator (WSD) programs (not dementia). Three thousand two hundred thirty participants from 179 general practitioners' offices participated in a cluster-randomized study using telehealth technology to transport data between patients and professionals during diagnosis and treatment. As Lyth et al. (2021) reported, telehealth reduced hospitalizations and deaths during the 12 months. According to cost-effectiveness research (Delgoshaei et al., 2017), telehealth was not a cost-effective in the care regime. At first glance, because of fewer hospitalizations (the informal care that may be provided), telemedicine expenses from secondary healthcare providers are being shifted to themselves.

The study did not include these goods since they do not specifically target the elderly. In this chapter, we present the results of their importance to the area of assistive technology.

Twenty-nine different technologies were studied by Beneito et al. (2018) for 25 older people who were living at home. There were just a few in this situation, researchers who made any effort to do economic research of any kind.

The absence of a control group is one of the study's limitations, and the authors' inability to fully account for all the expenses of using technology to aid with everyday life in the community. An average length of stay in technologically aided communities is eight months, despite the inferior quality of the study.

For the aged, there are several new advances and consequences. The expense of developing assistive technology may be a barrier to its widespread use. I found some of these in the literature review. If the elderly are included, it's costly to provide older people with the support they need when developing assistive technology. This report points out that it is critical to find more resources to guarantee that the elderly can be appropriately assisted.

Wolters and colleagues (2016) tested the COACH cognitive assistance system for the elderly with actors. However, acknowledging that they would need further the elderly in the process, they demonstrated that this considerably cheaper way might influence development expenses. They found that the technique proved promising in another of their tests (Mihailidis et al., 2008) that included COACH-supported older people cleaning their hands. In the literature, new technologies that are not ready for deployment are widespread. COACH is no exception.

Older people were engaged in developing new items (Day & Hitchings, 2011). They say that making things together might help eliminate some negative stereotypes about the elderly.

Potential Cost-Cutting Measures Are Possible

I often refer cost savings to in the literature, with varying degrees of proof. While Robinson et al. (2014) found a wide variety of commercially accessible technology gadgets that they believe have the potential to cut healthcare costs, they also found that additional studies into cost-effectiveness are required, particularly for the elderly. Page (2014) studied ten research papers that used technology to enhance cognitive performance and assist memory. For example, memory aids, telemedicine monitoring, and GPS trackers can enhance cognitive performance. They believe these devices have possible savings as a reduction in customer support costs, notwithstanding the modest size of the research evaluated. It is possible to save money by keeping the elderly in their homes longer with improved nighttime assistance, according to Riemersma et al. (2008, a shoddy investigation) when looking at nighttime care technology. Chang et al. (2012) discuss memory prompts for the elderly. They suggest that this method has the potential to save expenses since individuals will need less assistance from services. As the prices of ICT technologies continue to fall, Elsy (2020) concludes that these technologies will become more cost-effective. According to Mostaghel (2016), these technologies are trustworthy enough to assist older people released from hospitals, resulting in significant cost savings. Cognitively impaired individuals may benefit from memory-supporting devices. Nevertheless, Mason et al. (2012) note that although some are already in use, others are pricey and not yet developed enough to be widely used. Some suggest that an electronic platform for aiding the elderly at home might postpone admission to an institution, saving both time and money (Memon et al., 2014). HOPE's three-country research by Ware et al. (2017) raises whether individuals will pay for comprehensive electronic monitoring, communication, and rehabilitation systems. Research by Broadbent et al. (2009) examines whether people's own houses may serve as a "multisensory habitat." There is no relief from caring for those in their care, despite the technology used to make them calmer and more comfortable. This one is another intervention regarded as "promising" but needing additional study. With the elderly, Sugarhood et al. (2014) are confident in their assertion that Telecare saves money and will be widely embraced in years to come. Technology-aided care and ethics are their primary focus. Are considered, and healthcare practitioners exercise prudence because older people may get isolated because of the widespread use of technology. Like Sugarhood (2014) also raises how much money individuals should be paid—those prepared to pay for their technical support. This study supports Kaswan et al. (2021), who suggest that prediction error and system bias are critical to AI's widespread acceptance in any technology treatment technique. For example, the identification of breast cancer risk factors and assessments of these variables. Machine learning segmentation and 3D MRI mammography are regarded as promising methods for detecting breast cancer at an early stage (Saeed et al., 2022).

CONCLUSION

In conclusion, I have found an alarming lack of research in the literature on the expenses of elderly care technologies. While indirect evidence suggests cost-effectiveness, there are obvious signs of this in several areas. Many people believe that in-home care costs less than in-patient treatment. Only a few studies have considered the total societal cost of caring for the elderly, including the expenditures of caregivers who can no longer work. There will be less demand for institutional care, such as hospitals and care homes if informal caregivers can help the elderly stay in their homes. Good evidence of how effective caregiver support systems show they are cost-effective in both direct and indirect ways.

On the other hand, institutional care is regarded as more costly than home care provided by official care agencies. In order to help the elderly remain at home, assistive technology, memory aids, telemedicine monitoring, and GPS trackers, for example, may be cost-effective options. In places where informal care is readily accessible, they may also serve as a stand-in for more formalized care critical to AI's widespread acceptance in elderly treatment. The unique study of AI for the elderly makes this chapter highly relevant to supporting healthcare services for the elderly.

REFERENCES

Antarsih, N. R., Setyawati, S. P., Ningsih, S., Sulaiman, E., & Pujiastuti, N. (2022, January). *Telehealth Business Potential in Indonesia.* In *International Conference on Social, Economics, Business, and Education (ICSE 2021)* (pp. 73-78). Atlantis Press.

Barnard, Y., Bradley, M. D., Hodgson, F., & Lloyd, A. D. (2013). Older adults' learning to use new technologies: Perceived difficulties, experimentation behavior, and usability. *Computers in Human Behavior, 29*(4), 1715–1724. doi:10.1016/j.chb.2013.02.006

Bayer, S., Kuzmickas, P., Boissy, A., Rose, S. L., & Mercer, M. B. (2021). Categorizing and rating patient complaints: An innovative approach to improve patient experience. *Journal of Patient Experience, 8*, 2374373521998624. doi:10.1177/2374373521998624 PMID:34179397

Beneito-Montagut, R., Cassián-Yde, N., & Begueria, A. (2018). *What do we know about the relationship between internet-mediated interaction and social isolation and loneliness in later life?* Quality in Aging and Older Adults. doi:10.1108/QAOA-03-2017-0008

Boockvar, K. S., Judon, K. M., Eimicke, J. P., Teresi, J. A., & Inouye, S. K. (2020). Hospital Elder Life Program in Long-Term Care (HELP-LTC): A Cluster Randomized Controlled Trial. *Journal of the American Geriatrics Society, 68*(10), 2329–2335. doi:10.1111/jgs.16695 PMID:32710658

Broadbent, E., Stafford, R., & MacDonald, B. (2009). Acceptance of healthcare robots for the older population: Review and future directions. *International Journal of Social Robotics, 1*(4), 319–330. doi:10.100712369-009-0030-6

Chang, W. Z. D., & Bourgeois, M. (2012). Effects of memory aids on the conversations of elderly Chinese persons. *Asia Pacific Journal of Speech, Language and Hearing, 15*(4), 245–263. doi:10.1179/136132812804731767

Cutler, N. E. (2015). Will the Internet Help Your Parents to Live Longer? Isolation, Longevity, Health, Death, and Skype™. *Journal of Financial Service Professionals, 69*(2).

Day, R., & Hitchings, R. (2011). 'Only old ladies would do that': Age stigma and older people's strategies for dealing with winter cold. *Health & Place, 17*(4), 885–894. doi:10.1016/j.healthplace.2011.04.011 PMID:21606000

Delgoshaei, B., Mobinizadeh, M., Mojdenar, R., Afzal, E., Arabloo, J., & Mohamadi, E. (2017). Telemedicine: A systematic review of economic evaluations. *Medical Journal of the Islamic Republic of Iran, 31*(1), 113. doi:10.14196/mjiri.31.113 PMID:29951414

Durrani, H., & Khoja, S. (2009). A systematic review of the use of telehealth in Asian countries. *Journal of Telemedicine and Telecare, 15*(4), 175–181. doi:10.1258/jtt.2009.080605 PMID:19471028

Edney, L. C., Haji Ali Afzali, H., Cheng, T. C., & Karnon, J. (2018). Estimating the reference incremental cost-effectiveness ratio for the Australian health system. *PharmacoEconomics*, *36*(2), 239–252. doi:10.100740273-017-0585-2 PMID:29273843

Elsy, P. (2020). Elderly care in society 5.0 and kaigo rishoku in Japanese hyper-aging society. *Jurnal Studi Komunikasi*, *4*(2), 435–452.

Esfandiari, S., Lund, J. P., Penrod, J. R., Savard, A., Mark Thomason, J., & Feine, J. S. (2009). Implant overdentures for edentulous elders: Study of patient preference. *Gerodontology*, *26*(1), 3–10. doi:10.1111/j.1741-2358.2008.00237.x PMID:18498362

Gaur, L., Bhatia, U., Jhanjhi, N. Z., Muhammad, G., & Masud, M. (2021). Medical image-based detection of COVID-19 using deep convolution neural networks. *Multimedia Systems*, 1–10. doi:10.100700530-021-00794-6 PMID:33935377

Gibson, G., Dickinson, C., Brittain, K., & Robinson, L. (2019). Personalisation, customisation and bricolage: How people with dementia and their families make assistive technology work for them. *Aging and Society: An Interdisciplinary Journal*, *39*(11), 2502–2519. doi:10.1017/S0144686X18000661

Greene, A. J. (2022). Elder financial abuse and electronic financial instruments: Present and future considerations for financial capacity assessments. *The American Journal of Geriatric Psychiatry*, *30*(1), 90–106. doi:10.1016/j.jagp.2021.02.045 PMID:33781661

Hirsch, T., Forlizzi, J., Hyder, E., Goetz, J., Kurtz, C., & Stroback, J. (2000, November). The ELDer project: social, emotional, and environmental factors in the design of eldercare technologies. In *Proceedings on the 2000 conference on Universal Usability* (pp. 72-79). ACM. 10.1145/355460.355476

Johansson-Pajala, R. M., & Gustafsson, C. (2022). Significant challenges when introducing care robots in Swedish eldercare. *Disability and Rehabilitation. Assistive Technology*, *17*(2), 166–176. doi:10.1080/17483107.2020.1773549 PMID:32538206

Kachouie, R., Sedigheh Deli, S., Khosla, R., & Chu, M. T. (2014). Socially assistive robots in elderly care: A mixed-method systematic literature review. *International Journal of Human-Computer Interaction*, *30*(5), 369–393. doi:10.1080/10447318.2013.873278

Kaswan, K. S., Gaur, L., Dhatterwal, J. S., & Kumar, R. (2021). AI-based natural language processing for the generation of meaningful information electronic health record (EHR) data. In Advanced AI Techniques and Applications in Bioinformatics (pp. 41-86). CRC Press.

Komalasari, R., Nurhayati, N., & Mustafa, C. (2022). Enhancing the Online Learning Environment for Medical Education: Lessons From COVID-19. In Policies and Procedures for the Implementation of Safe and Healthy Educational Environments: Post-COVID-19 Perspectives (pp. 138-154). IGI Global.

Lyth, J., Lind, L., Persson, H. L., & Wiréhn, A. B. (2021). Can a telemonitoring system lead to decreased hospitalization in elderly patients? *Journal of Telemedicine and Telecare*, *27*(1), 46–53. doi:10.1177/1357633X19858178 PMID:31291794

Mahbub, M. K., Biswas, M., Gaur, L., Alenezi, F., & Santosh, K. C. (2022). Deep features to detect pulmonary abnormalities in chest X-rays due to infectious diseases: Covid-19, pneumonia, and tuberculosis. *Information Sciences*, *592*, 389–401. doi:10.1016/j.ins.2022.01.062 PMID:36532848

Marcantonio, E. R., Bergmann, M. A., Kiely, D. K., Orav, E. J., & Jones, R. N. (2010). Randomized trial of a delirium abatement program for post-acute skilled nursing facilities. *Journal of the American Geriatrics Society*, *58*(6), 1019–1026. doi:10.1111/j.1532-5415.2010.02871.x PMID:20487083

Mason, S., Craig, D., O'Neill, S., Donnelly, M., & Nugent, C. (2012). Electronic reminding technology for cognitive impairment. *British Journal of Nursing (Mark Allen Publishing)*, *20*(14), 855–861. doi:10.12968/bjon.2012.21.14.855 PMID:23252168

McKenna, G., Allen, P. F., Hayes, M., DaMata, C., Moore, C., & Cronin, M. (2018). Impact of oral rehabilitation on the quality of life of partially dentate elders in a randomized controlled clinical trial: 2 year follow-up. *PLoS One*, *13*(10), e0203349. doi:10.1371/journal.pone.0203349 PMID:30307966

Memon, M., Wagner, S. R., Pedersen, C. F., Beevi, F. H. A., & Hansen, F. O. (2014). Ambient assisted living healthcare frameworks, platforms, standards, and quality attributes. *Sensors (Basel)*, *14*(3), 4312–4341. doi:10.3390140304312 PMID:24599192

Mihailidis, A., Boger, J. N., Craig, T., & Hoey, J. (2008). The COACH prompting system to assist older adults with dementia through handwashing: An efficacy study. *BMC Geriatrics*, *8*(1), 1–18. doi:10.1186/1471-2318-8-28 PMID:18992135

Morato, J., Sanchez-Cuadrado, S., Iglesias, A., Campillo, A., & Fernández-Panadero, C. (2021). Sustainable technologies for older adults. *Sustainability*, *13*(15), 8465. doi:10.3390u13158465

Mostaghel, R. (2016). Innovation and technology for the elderly: Systematic literature review. *Journal of Business Research*, *69*(11), 4896–4900. doi:10.1016/j.jbusres.2016.04.049

Page, T. (2014). Touchscreen mobile devices and older adults: A usability study. International. *Journal of Human Factors and Ergonomics*, *3*(1), 65–85. doi:10.1504/IJHFE.2014.062550

Riemersma-Van Der Lek, R. F., Swaab, D. F., Twisk, J., Hol, E. M., Hoogendijk, W. J., & Van Someren, E. J. (2008). Effect of bright light and melatonin on cognitive and noncognitive function in elderly residents of group care facilities: A randomized controlled trial. *Journal of the American Medical Association*, *299*(22), 2642–2655. doi:10.1001/jama.299.22.2642 PMID:18544724

Roberts, C., & Mort, M. (2009). Reshaping what counts as care: Older people, work and new technologies. *Alter*, *3*(2), 138–158. doi:10.1016/j.alter.2009.01.004

Robinson, H., MacDonald, B., & Broadbent, E. (2014). The role of healthcare robots for older people at home: A review. *International Journal of Social Robotics*, *6*(4), 575–591. doi:10.100712369-014-0242-2

Saeed, S., Jhanjhi, N. Z., Naqvi, M., Humyun, M., Ahmad, M., & Gaur, L. (2022). Optimized Breast Cancer Premature Detection Method With Computational Segmentation: A Systematic Review Mapping. *Approaches and Applications of Deep Learning in Virtual Medical Care*, 24-51.

Santosh, K. C., & Gaur, L. (2022). *Artificial Intelligence and Machine Learning in Public Healthcare: Opportunities and Societal Impact*. Springer Nature, Sugarhood, P., Wherton, J., Procter, R., Hinder, S., & Greenhalgh, T. (2014). Technology as system innovation: a key informant interview study of the application of the diffusion of innovation model to telecare. *Disability and Rehabilitation. Assistive Technology*, *9*(1), 79–87.

Schröders, J. (2021). *Diversity, dynamics, and deficits: the role of social networks for the health of aging populations in Indonesia* [Doctoral dissertation, Umeå University, Sweeden].

Van der Roest, H. G., Wenborn, J., Pastink, C., Dröes, R. M., & Orrell, M. (2017). Assistive technology for memory support in dementia. *Cochrane Database of Systematic Reviews*, *2017*(6), 6. doi:10.1002/14651858.CD009627.pub2 PMID:28602027

Ware, P., Bartlett, S. J., Paré, G., Symeonidis, I., Tannenbaum, C., Bartlett, G., & Ahmed, S. (2017). Using eHealth technologies: Interests, preferences, and concerns of older adults. *Interactive Journal of Medical Research*, *6*(1), e4447. doi:10.2196/ijmr.4447 PMID:28336506

Wolters, M. K., Kelly, F., & Kilgour, J. (2016). Designing a spoken dialogue interface to an intelligent cognitive assistant for people with dementia. *Health Informatics Journal*, *22*(4), 854–866. doi:10.1177/1460458215593329 PMID:26276794

Yusif, S., Soar, J., & Hafeez-Baig, A. (2016). Older people, assistive technologies, and the barriers to adoption: A systematic review. *International Journal of Medical Informatics*, *94*, 112–116. doi:10.1016/j.ijmedinf.2016.07.004 PMID:27573318

ADDITIONAL READING

Komalasari, R. (2022). A Social Ecological Model (SEM) to Manage Methadone Programmes in Prisons. In Handbook of Research on Mathematical Modeling for Smart Healthcare Systems (pp. 374-382). IGI Global.

Komalasari, R. (2022). Pemanfaatan Kecerdasan Buatan (Ai) Dalam Telemedicine: Dari Perspektif Profesional Kesehatan. *Jurnal Kedokteran Mulawarman*, *9*(2), 72–81.

Komalasari, R. (2023). Telemedicine in Pandemic Times in Indonesia: Healthcare Professional's Perspective. In N. Vajjhala & P. Eappen (Eds.), *Health Informatics and Patient Safety in Times of Crisis* (pp. 138–153). IGI Global.

Komalasari, R. (2023). Designing Health Systems for Better, Faster, and Less Expensive Treatment. In *Exploring the Convergence of Computer and Medical Science Through Cloud Healthcare*. IGI Global.

Komalasari, R. (in press). History and Legislative Changes Governing Medical Cannabis in Indonesia. In *Medical Cannabis and the Effects of Cannabinoids on Fighting Cancer, Multiple Sclerosis, Epilepsy, Parkinsons and Other Neurodegenerative Diseases*. IGI Global.

Komalasari, R. (in press). The ethical consideration of using Artificial Intelligence (AI) in medicine. In *Advanced Bioinspiration Methods for Healthcare Standards, Policies, and Reform*. IGI Global.

Komalasari, R. (in press). Postnatal mental distress, exploring the experiences of mothers navigating the health care system. In *Perspectives and Considerations on Navigating the Mental Healthcare System*. IGI Global.

Komalasari, R. (in press). Treatment of menstrual discomfort in young women and a cognitive behavior therapy (CBT) program. In *Perspectives on Coping Strategies for Menstrual and Premenstrual Distress*. IGI Global.

Komalasari, R. (in press). Literature Review: Health Aspects and Legal Protection for Children in Scotland and Indonesia. *Buana Gender: Jurnal Studi Gender dan Anak.*

Komalasari, R. (in press). Manfaat Positif Allium Sativum L. (Bawang Putih) Dalam Kaitannya Dengan Berbagai Penyakit. [JFM]. *Jurnal Farmasimed.*

Komalasari, R. (in press). Pelatihan Kesehatan dan Pengembangan Profesional Berkelanjutan untuk Pendidik Olah Raga. *Jurnal Ilmiah STOK Bina Guna Medan.*

Komalasari, R. (in press). Persepsi Hakim tentang Rehabilitasi Pengguna Narkoba:Tantangan dan Peluang. *Arena Hukum.*

Komalasari, R., & Mustafa, C. (2021). Meningkatkan Pelayanan Administrasi Publik di Indonesia. *PaKMas: Jurnal Pengabdian Kepada Masyarakat, 1*(1), 20–27. doi:10.54259/pakmas.v1i1.29

Komalasari, R., & Mustafa, C. (2021). Pendidikan Profesi dan Pengabdian Masyarakat di Indonesia. *PaKMas: Jurnal Pengabdian Kepada Masyarakat, 1*(1), 28–36. doi:10.54259/pakmas.v1i1.30

Komalasari, R., & Mustafa, C. (2022). Empowerment of Women with Narcotic Cases. *Buana Gender: Jurnal Studi Gender dan Anak, 7*(1).

Komalasari, R., Nurhayati, N., & Mustafa, C. (2022). Insider/Outsider Issues: Reflections on Qualitative Research. *Qualitative Report, 27*(3), 744–751. doi:10.46743/2160-3715/2022.5259

Komalasari, R., Nurhayati, N., & Mustafa, C. (2022). Enhancing the Online Learning Environment for Medical Education: Lessons From COVID-19. In Policies and procedures for the implementation of safe and healthy educational environments: Post-COVID-19 perspectives (pp. 138-154). IGI Global.

Komalasari, R., Nurhayati, N., & Mustafa, C. (2022). Kebijakan Penanganan Penyintas HIV/AIDS Di Lembaga Pemasyarakatan. *Jurnal Kesehatan Kartika, 17*(1), 19–27.

Komalasari, R., Nurhayati, N., & Mustafa, C. (2022). Professional Education and Training in Indonesia. In *Public Affairs Education and Training in the 21st Century* (pp. 125–138). IGI Global. doi:10.4018/978-1-7998-8243-5.ch008

Komalasari, R., Wilson, S., & Haw, S. (2021). A systematic review of qualitative evidence on barriers to and facilitators of the implementation of opioid agonist treatment (OAT) programmes in prisons. *The International Journal on Drug Policy, 87*, 102978. doi:10.1016/j.drugpo.2020.102978 PMID:33129135

Komalasari, R., Wilson, S., & Haw, S. (2021). A social ecological model (SEM) to exploring barriers of and facilitators to the implementation of opioid agonist treatment (OAT) programmes in prisons. *International Journal of Prisoner Health, 17*(4), 477–496. doi:10.1108/IJPH-04-2020-0020

Komalasari, R., Wilson, S., Nasir, S., & Haw, S. (2020). Multiple burdens of stigma for prisoners participating in Opioid Antagonist Treatment (OAT) programmes in Indonesian prisons: A qualitative study. *International Journal of Prisoner Health.*

Mustafa, C. (2021). The Challenges to Improving Public Services and Judicial Operations: A unique balance between pursuing justice and public service in Indonesia. In Handbook of research on global challenges for improving public services and government operations (pp. 117-132). IGI Global. doi:10.4018/978-1-7998-4978-0.ch007

Mustafa, C. (2021). Key finding: result of a qualitative study of judicial perspectives on the sentencing of minor drug offenders in Indonesia: Structural inequality. *Qualitative Report*, *26*(5), 1678–1692. doi:10.46743/2160-3715/2021.4436

Mustafa, C. (2021). The view of judicial activism and public legitimacy. *Crime, Law, and Social Change*, *76*(1), 23–34. doi:10.100710611-021-09955-0

Mustafa, C. (2021). Qualitative method used in researching the judiciary: Quality assurance steps to enhance the validity and reliability of the findings. *Qualitative Report*, *26*(1), 176–186. doi:10.46743/2160-3715/2021.4319

Mustafa, C. (2021). The News Media Representation of Acts of Mass Violence in Indonesia. In Mitigating Mass Violence and Managing Threats in Contemporary Society (pp. 127-140). IGI Global. doi:10.4018/978-1-7998-4957-5.ch008

Mustafa, C., Malloch, M., & Hamilton Smith, N. (2020). Judicial perspectives on the sentencing of minor drug offenders in Indonesia: Discretionary practice and compassionate approaches. *Crime, Law, and Social Change*, *74*(3), 297–313. doi:10.100710611-020-09896-0

Suhariyanto, B., Mustafa, C., & Santoso, T. (2021). Liability incorporate between transnational corruption cases Indonesia and the United States of America. *Journal of Legal, Ethical and Regulatory Issues*, *24*(3). .

Suhariyanto, B., & Mustafa, C. (2022). Analysis And Evaluation Of Legal Aid In The Indonesian Court. *Jurnal Hukum dan Peradilan*, *11*(2), 176-194.

KEY TERMS AND DEFINITIONS

COACH: Caring for Older Adults and Caregivers at Home
CCT: Controlled Clinical Trial
COPD: Chronic obstructive pulmonary disease
GPS: The Global Positioning System
HOPE: Home for Elderly People
ICT: Information and Communication Technologies
WSD: Whole System Demonstrator
QALY: Quality-Adjusted Life Years
RCTs: Randomized Controlled Trials

Chapter 11
Healthcare Multimedia Data Analysis Algorithms Tools and Applications

Sheik Abdullah A.
https://orcid.org/0000-0001-8707-9927
Vellore Institute of Technology, India

Selvakumar S.
Visvesvaraya College of Engineering and Technology, India

Suguna M.
Vellore Institute of Technology, India

Priyadarshini R.
Vellore Institute of Technology, India

ABSTRACT

In the domain of information retrieval, there exists a number of models which are used for different sorts of applications. The extraction of multimedia is one of the types which specifically deals with the handling of multimedia data with different types of tools and techniques. This chapter provides a complete insight into the audio, video, and text semantic descriptions about the multimedia data with the following objectives: i) methods ii) data summarization iii) data categorization and its media descriptions. Upon considering this organization, the entire chapter has been dealt with a case study depicting feature extraction, merging, filtering, and data validation.

INTRODUCTION

The domain of information retrieval is considered to be as an important paradigm in the different sorts of real-time applications. The advancement in the process of data retrieval techniques has been established more than five thousand years ago. In practice, the intent of the data retrieval to that of information retrieval

DOI: 10.4018/978-1-6684-5925-6.ch011

has been raised with the accordance of model development, process analysis, and data interpretation and evaluation. One of the major forms of data which has multiple supportable formats is multimedia data. This data utilizes different sorts of information retrieval models to establish a particular decision support system. At certain context the aspect of feature based analysis plays a significant role in data prediction and validation. The only advent is it must adapt to that of the particular database community and the modular applications in which it deals with the formats.

The process of research practice and its supporting culture has become blooming with the process of handling different types of data. The supporting types are having different issues with the data processing platforms which are suited for analysis. Also, the utilization of data driven models is getting increased day by day with its available metrics. Metric based data validation and extraction is found to be one of the tedious task in this which then certainly make the data to be variant suitably for analysis. The algorithmic models may vary certainly but the aspect that has to be considered should be quite easy. In the present stages of study the designers choose their own way of representing and handling the data to a certain extent, especially:

- Design of decision support systems to provide a complete service
- To utilize the system effectively in order to communicate with the professionals this states the expectations behind the system.
- To enhance the researchers to effectively utilize the model in terms of data integration, analysis and spotting of relevant multimedia data.

The extraction of multimedia data sources are analyzed with efficient forms of data analysis and linguistic process. These methods can be efficiently organized into three such groups:

1. Methods suitably used for the process of summarizing the media data which is specifically the result of feature extraction process.
2. Methods and techniques for filtering out the media content and its sub processes.
3. Methods that are suitable for categorizing the media into different sorts of classes and functions.

Techniques for Summarizing Media Data

Feature extraction is motivated by innumerably large multimedia object, their redundancy and possibly nosiness. By feature extraction two goals can be achieved.

- Data summary generation
- Data correlation analysis with specific autocorrelation and comparison

Techniques for Filtering Out Media Data

The process of MIR emphasise the channels that are locally visible and executable for the different forms of IR models that are suitably supported. The results are merged into one description per media content. Descriptions are classified into two based on their size. They are of two types,

- Fixed-size

- Variable size

The process of merging takes place through the process of simple concatenation, especially in the form of fixed and variable size lengths. Size has to be normalized to fixed size before merging. They most often occur as motion description. The most commonly used filtering mechanisms are

- Factor analysis
- Single value decomposition
- Kalman filter

Techniques for Media Description Categorization - Classes

The main concept of machine learning is applied to categorization of multimedia descriptions. The list of applicable classifiers is as follows:

- Metric based model development
- Nearest neighbour based model development
- Minimization of risk in estimation models
- Density-based evaluation/approaches
- Feedforward neural network
- Simple heuristic analysis

The main objective of this model is to minimize the overhead of user needed information. Some of the major application areas include: Bio-information analysis, face recognition, speech recognition, video browsing, Bio-signal processing etc.

Literature Survey

1) Aditi and Durgar stated that to reduce the time complexity during the video retrieval, it is better to search a video based on its metadata description. According to the journal, the video is firstly searched based on its content and then video's two main features is considered: one is visual screen which is nothing but text and the other one is audio tracks which is nothing but speech.

This process started from the process of video segmentation in which video one has to classify moving objects of a lecture video sequence. Followed by the second step, in which the transition of the actual slide is captured. This process is repeated to completely reduce the content's redundancy.

The next step is to create a video OCR for the characters in the text. An OCR is a system which can process an image and according to the similarity of the loaded image and the image model, the image is recognized.

In the next step, ASR (automatic speech recognition) technology helps to identify the words spoken by a person and then it is converted to text. Its ultimate goal is to recognize speech in real-time with full accuracy. Finally after applying OCR and ASR algorithms on those keyframes, the results are stored in the database with a unique identifier and timestamp. When a user searches for content, if it matches the content in the database, then the video search is successful. So this is called the content based video retrieval.

2) The work by the author Vaishali et al., proposed an mechanism for the analysis of retrieval based on the multimodal fusion which includes the component of textual and visual data. They have used data clustering and association rule mining techniques for evaluation to explicitly retrieve the content modality and analysis. They have utilized the possible way of three-mode data segregation and analysis.

The proposed model involves a multimodal analysis of three way combination of data retrieval platform. Here the relevant image which is supposed to be retrieved is taken with subsequent forms of model extraction. The fusion subsystem and the LBP pattern is used for the next level of data analysis and retrieval.

Experimental results justifies that, when visual data is fed into the system based on which textual data is entered into the system, after searching relevant image comparison is done between the two data using the LBP. Finally, the images that are matched are retrieved. After when the images are mapped with the model to extract the suitable patterns from the test set of data.

2) Xaro Benavent, Ana Garcia-Serrano proposed an idea for the retrieval of both textual and visual features through multimedia fusion method to increase the accuracy of the retrieved results based on the existing levels of fusion such as, early fusion which is based on the extracted features from different information sources, late fusion or hybrid which combines the individual decision got by the momomodel feature extraction process and the model development metrics.

In the developed environment, a system involves some steps like: Extraction of textual information, and textual preprocessing which includes three steps like elimination of ascents and stopwords and stemming. Then indexation is done using the White Space Analyzer. Finally, searching is done to obtain the textual results.

Content-Based Information Retrieval subsystem involves two steps: Feature Extraction and a similarity module which is specifically allotted to extract the data similarity content from the contextual part of the data.

The process of late fusion algorithm is segregated into two types of categories:

1. Relevant score
2. Re-ranking the score normalization process.

The work by the authors Lew et al., proposed a novel idea for the mechanism of content based retrieval process in extracting the multimedia image contents. They have also analyzed the phenomenon of text annotations and incomplete data transformations. Media items including text, annotated contents, multimedia and browsing contents are also used for analysis.

Rationale Behind the Proposed Work

The impact of data-driven decision-making has rapidly increased with the availability of data in different formats. Each of the data has to be carefully examined to discover new patterns from it. Different processing steps exist to format the raw data into a suitable model format, making the insights interpretable and justifiable. The challenge lies at the stage of analyzing the raw data and making it suitable for processing and model development. Among all types of data formats, the most promising arena is multimedia data which needs to be carefully evaluated along with the data patterns. Multiple techniques exist for summarizing, filtering, and merging multimedia data contents at varying levels. Identifying and understanding the relevant form of multimedia data with suitable techniques is the most challenging part of medical data analysis. This research focuses on the best utilization of the available techniques with the varying nature of data patterns.

Table 1. Summary of literature review

S.No	Year	Authors	Methods used	Dataset used	Improvements / Accuracy
1.	2018	Ankit et al.,	Naive Bayes, Random Forest, SVM and Logistic Regression Classifiers, Ensemble classifier	Stanford - Sentiment140 corpus, Health Care Reform (HCR)	Ensemble models perform well for sentiment analysis than other classification algorithms.
2.	2019	Araque et al.,	Sentiment Classification	Twitter data	Statistical significance proves the validation of text analysis process for all classification schemes.
3.	2018	Doaa et al.,	Sentiment Analysis & Text Analysis	Tweet Dataset	The authors conclude this paper by comparing papers and provide an overview of challenges in sentiment analysis related to sentiment analysis approaches and techniques.
4.	2018	MahaHeikal et al.,	Ensemble method	Twitter data (Arabic)	The performance has been tested and evaluated with an F1-score of 64.46%,
5.	2018	Abdulmohsen et al.,	Sentiment Analysis	SauDiSenti, AraSenTi	The proposed model using AraSenTi performs well than the other models, and the same can be used for analyzing different categories of sentiments.
6.	2018	NaaimaBoudad et al.,	SVM, NB, MNB	Arabic Tweets	SVM and NB classifier works well for binary classification with highest performance in accuracy, precision and recall and Multinomial Naive Bayes works for Multi-way classification
7.	2018	Prabhsimran Singh et al	Sentiment Analysis	Twitter Data	Results conclude that only 30% of people are unhappy with the demonetization policy introduced by the Indian Government.
8.	2018	Murugan Anandarajan et al.,	Lexicon Based Sentiment Analysis	Movie Reviews	Built-in lexicons can be used well for categorical sentiments.
9.	2018	Koyel Chakraborty et al.,	Google's algorithm Word2Vec	Movie Reviews	Comparing different types of clustering algorithms and types of clusters.
10.	2018	Swastika Pandey et al.,	Sentiment classification	Movie Reviews	Precision- 92.02%

METHODOLOGY

Now, let's discuss in detail about the methods available to perform retrieval based on multimedia information retrieval.

I) Techniques for Data Summarization:

The domain of feature extraction and analysis lies at the extent of data processing and analysis. In order to remove the noise and redundancy in the given dataset, we have to check for the nature of data with its available transformation and the consistency levels. This can be got by the set of derived values and procedures suitable for facilitating the learning and the analysis process. In healthcare big data platform, the intent of analyzing the data lies at the possible states of complete data security and redundancy. This comes under the platform of dimensionality reduction and process generalization. From the observed data in various formats supporting the healthcare data analysis, it should be noted that the features should be explicitly classified under one constraint and correction phenomenon which describes the original dataset. An example for this method is depicted in Figure 1.

If the input algorithm is found to be more robust, then the data can be certainly analyzed into different variations with a reduced feature set for subsequent feature extraction and quantization process. Image analysis and image based data segmentation lies at the quality of the data, which explicitly relies on the pixels generated with the video stream. The shapes may vary, but the exact realm lies in the analysis of image data segmentation with the robust machine learning algorithms. It specifically involves:

- Low detection rate analysis
- Edge-based data segmentation with reduced level of noise in digital images
- Facilitating automated recovery of data segments

The rate of low level edge detection involves certain sub-tasks for analysis as follows:

1. Edge detection with mathematical methods determining the brightness and the level of point of segmentation during analysis with mild and high effects.
2. Corner analysis with the determination of the missed feature contents at certain edges with panorama effects during 3D editing, modelling and object recognition.
3. Blob segment with different imaging properties at the curvature points determining the similar cases with image analysis properties.
4. Ridge analysis making the functions of two variables to determine the set of curvature points at least at one single dimension.

II) Merging and Filtering Method

According to this model, in order to understand the content of the media, multiple channels are employed. Media specific feature transformation describes these channels. At last these annotations have to be merged with a single description per object. As already explained merging is of two types:

- Fixed-size merging
- Variable sized merging

Figure 1. Process of summarizing the media content

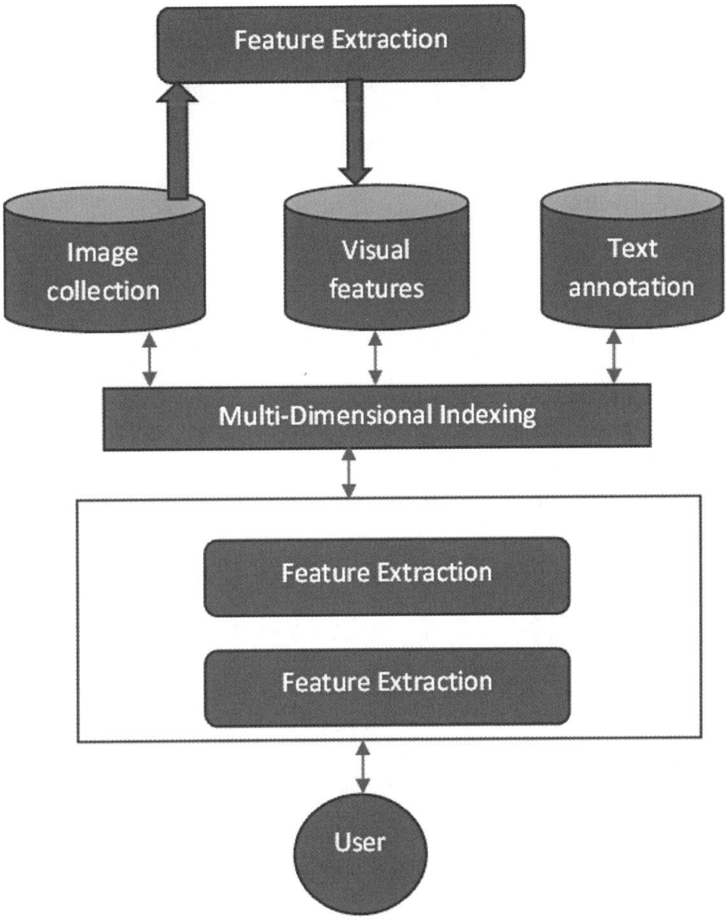

Feature Extraction

Image collection

Visual features

Text annotation

Multi-Dimensional Indexing

Feature Extraction

Feature Extraction

User

Figure 2. Multimedia content extraction process and Analysis

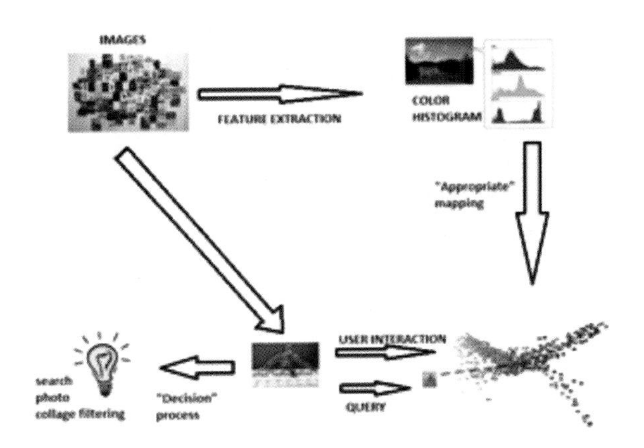

If the description is of a fixed size, then simple concatenation is done to merge two or more descriptions. For variable sized descriptions, the descriptions have to be normalized to fixed size, and they most commonly occur in motion description.

Commonly used filtering methods are as follows:

- Factor analysis
- Singular value decomposition
- Extraction and testing of statistical moments
- Kalman filter

FACTOR ANALYSIS

This technique is adopted to reduce a larger number of variables into a smaller number of factors. These techniques most probably extract the common variances from all the all variables and place them into a common score.

TYPES OF FACTORING

- **Principal Component Analysis –** it extracts a large number of variables and put them into single first factor
- **Common Factor Analysis** – it extracts common variables and put them into a single factor.
- **Image Factoring** – this method is based on a correlation matrix which determines exact correlation.
- **Maximum Likelihood Method** – this is also based on correlation matrix.

SINGULAR VALUE DECOMPOSITION

The process of singular value decomposition involves a set matrix A which has an factorization value with A=UDV T in which the column values are assigned to be ortho-normal and the matrix D is said to be as the diagonal with real positive values. The process of singular value decomposition is used in different sorts of applications which specifically includes ranking of data esteeming the low and high rank levels.

In medical data analysis, the multimedia content is of many forms of representation. A simple example includes the analysis of doctors' textual description needs a text to audio conversion then into structured forms of representation. In this context, there exist variations and complicated structures for analyzing the data into different sorts of manipulations.

Some of the practical examples include:

- Nearest orthogonal matrix
- The kabsch algorithm
- Signal processing
- Total least-square minimization

Extraction and Testing of Statistical Moments

In this process there are unscented transformations with the process following moment generating functions. This is more popular in the field of electromagnetic computation for large scale data analysis. At certain stages Monte Carlo approach is used. This method represents the combination of the Unscented Transform (UT) with the Method of Moments (MoM). This combination allows the modelling of uncertainty in electromagnetic computations. The procedure shows results with high accuracy which is similar to the Monte Carlo approach but using a much smaller number of simulations. This work uses standard MoM based solvers.

There are various steganalysis methods that have emerged as means to deter covert communication by terrorists. Steganalysis is the scientific technology to decide if a medium carries some hidden messages or not and also to determine what the hidden messages are. In addition to that, preventing secret communication among terrorists, steganalysis serves as a way to judge the security performance of steganography techniques. A good steganographic method should be imperceptible not only to human vision systems, but also for computer analysis.

III) **Categorization Methods:**

Lots of forms of machine learning can also be employed for the categorization of multimedia descriptions though some of the methods are frequently used in one area than another. hidden Markov models are state-of-the-art in speech recognition, while dynamic time wrapping, a semantically related method is state-of-the-art in gene sequence alignment. The list of applicable classifiers includes the following:

1. Metric Approaches

Cluster Analysis:

Cluster Analysis is one of the processes that includes of clustering of a set of objects in a way that things in the same one group are more similar to each other than to those ones in other groups.

Vector Space Model:

Vector space model is also a algebraic model that is used for representing the text documents as vectors of identifiers given, for example, index terms.

2. Nearest Neighbor methods

K-Nearest Method Algorithm:

In pattern recognition, the *k closest* neighbors algorithm is also a non parametric method used for classification and regression of the objects risk minimization.

Support Vector Machine:

They are supervised learning multi models used for regression processes

Linear Discriminate Analysis:

Linear discriminate analysis is also a generalization of the Fisher's linear discriminate and also uses pattern recognition for learning the objects

3. Density-Based Methods:-

Figure 3. Dataset description

Your Data

age	sex	cp Type	trestbps	chol	fbs	restecg	thalach	exang	oldpeak	slope	ca	thal	class label
63	1	1	145	233	1	2	150	0	2.3	3	0	6	Zero
67	1	4	160	286	0	2	108	1	1.5	2	3	3	Two
67	1	4	120	229	0	2	129	1	2.6	2	2	7	One
37	1	3	130	250	0	0	187	0	3.5	3	0	3	Zero
41	0	2	130	204	0	2	172	0	1.4	1	0	3	Zero

Markov Process:

A Markov Chain is a stochastic model that describes a sequence of possible events in which the probability of each event depends on the states attained in the previous event.

4. Neural Networks

Perception:

It is one of the major algorithms primarily used for a supervised learning and skilled working of specific classes

5. Heuristics

Decision Tree:

It is a decision support tool that uses a more tree like models of decisions and their conditions and also their possible consequences, which combines event outcomes and utility. It is one of the ways to display an algorithm which only contains conditional control statements.

SAMPLE ILLUSTRATION: CASE STUDY

The illustration can be considered with the analysis of considering the predictive maintenance using medical data for analysis. This involves the analysis of benchmark data from the UCI machine learning repository which concerns about the heart disease of signified patients. The following Figure 3 describes the data description:

At each stages of the disease the influencing factors is observed and the analysis is made accordingly. In order to overcome with these factors the weight level can be introduced and can be increased or decreased at certain levels. The following Figure 4 provides the incorporation of weight with the influencing rates.

Figure 4. Factors influencing the rate of analysis

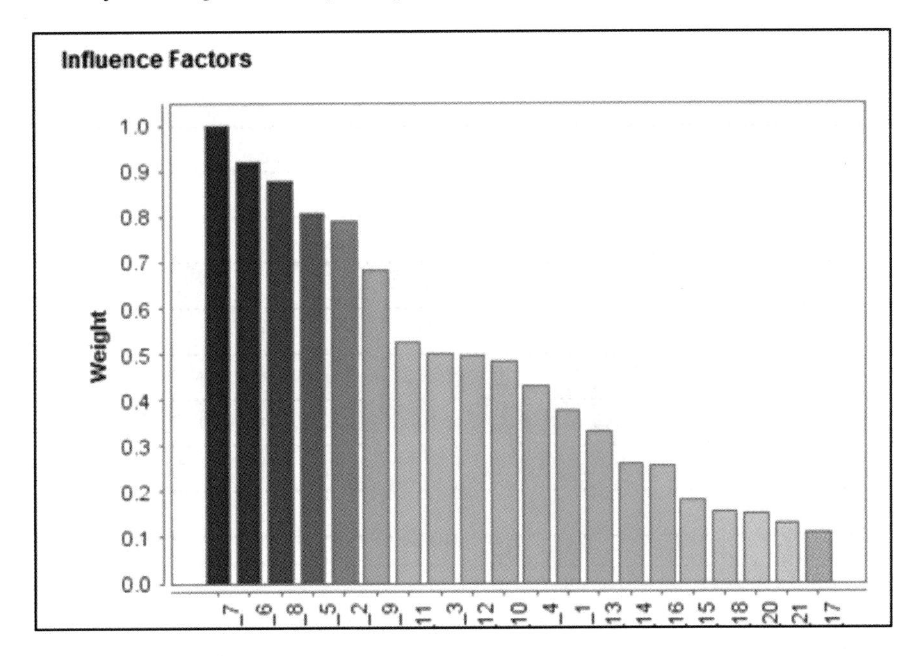

The patients at certain stages can be varied in accordance to the number of situations leveraging the factors to be considered. This provides a scenario for data curation, and it should be overcome by introducing confidence levels for the situation-based analysis.

Finally, in each situation the risk level can be determined with the count of the patients who have utterly suffered and recovered from illness. Figure 7 provides the risk level estimations with different conditions and scenarios of understanding levels.

Figure 5. Detection curve over the observed situations of the disease

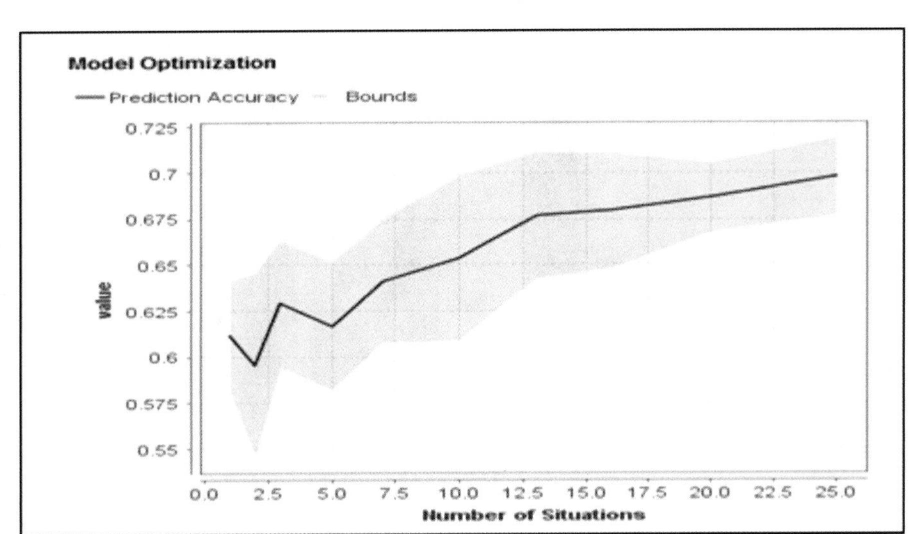

Figure 6. Confidence level and failure rate

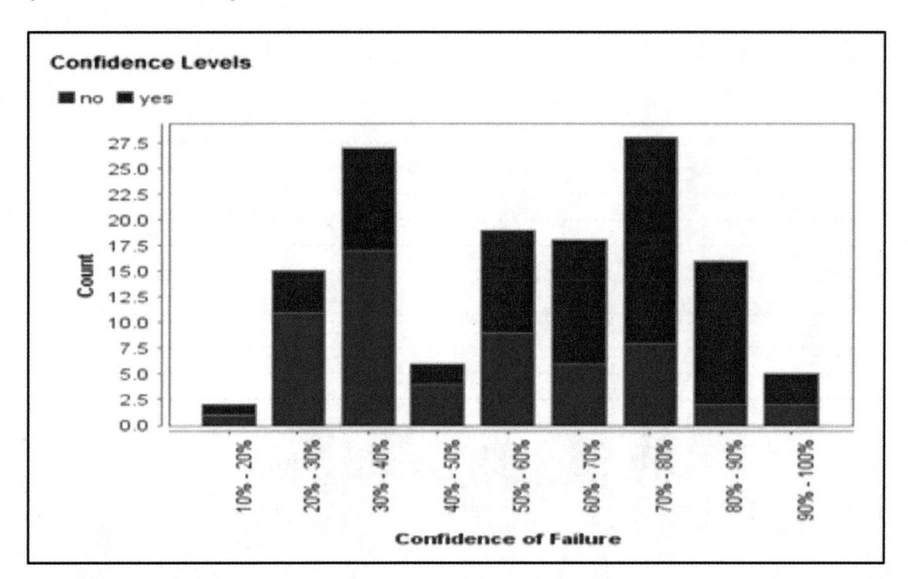

APPLICATIONS

The variants of text-based models are significantly used in different sectors for conceptual analysis of text design and extraction. Significant analysis has to be made in making the data to be exact and confirming to a decision at the best level [9]. Applications include bioinformatics, signal processing, content-based retrieval, and speech recognition platforms.

Figure 7. Risk levels and its failure rate

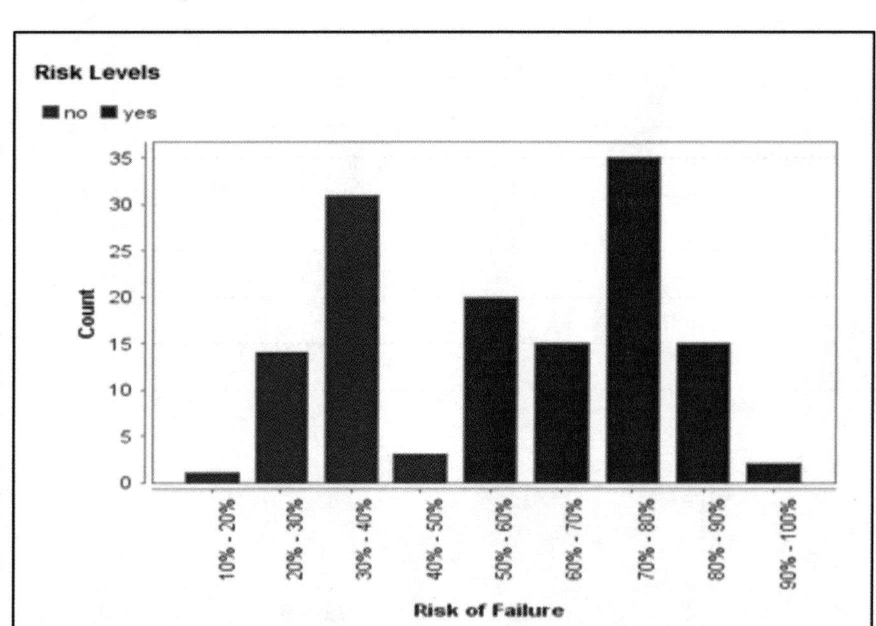

1. **Bio-Informatics:** this is concerned with the arena of biological data analysis with complete model extraction and analysis. The data may be of semi or in an unstructured format.
2. **Bio-Signal Processing:** it is concerned with the signals concerned with the living beings in a given environment.
3. **Content-Based Image Retrieval**: it deals with the search of digital images for the given environment of large data collection.
4. **Facial Recognition System:** It concern with the activity recognition for the given platform in the sequence of data frames.
5. **Speech Recognition System:** The process of transformation of speech to text as recognized by the computers.
6. **Technical Chart Analysis**: market data analysis usually falls under this category of concern. This can be of type chart and visual perception analysis.

CONCLUSION

The healthcare technology domain ultimately focuses on incorporating ICT in practice with advanced tools and techniques. The availability of the data varies by the formats in the medical domain. Managing and providing fruitful information from diverse data representation plays a significant role in the medical informatics decision-making process. This research provides varying techniques for summarizing media data with its descriptive parameters. Also, significant data summarization and data filtering methods are discussed with statistical inference. An illustration has been made along with a case study depicting the nature of data associated with multimedia content with the significance in IR modeling and its illustrative aspects. Most of the modeling in multimedia data follows significant IR-based modeling to bring out the essential facts and truths behind it. In this chapter, we have discussed the different forms of IR models, tools, and applications with an example case study illustrating the flow of medical data analysis during the modeling process stages. In the future, the aspects of different strategies can be discussed following the level of data that can be monitored with various tools and applications.

REFERENCES

A. S. Abdullah, A. Manoj and S. Selvakumar. (2021). A Hybrid Data Analytic Approach to Evaluate the Performance of Stirling Engine using Machine Learning Techniques. *2021 IEEE Bombay Section Signature Conference (IBSSC)*, 2021, pp. 1-4. IEEE. doi: 10.1109/IBSSC53889.2021.9673219. doi:10.1109/IBSSC53889.2021.9673219

A Sheik Abdullah, Manoj A, Selvakumar S. Assessment and Evaluation of cancer CT images using deep learning techniques. 2021 2nd International Conference on Secure Cyber Computing and Communications (ICSCCC) [Internet]. IEEE; 2021 May 21; Available from: doi:10.1109/ICSCCC51823.2021.9478176

Shindel, P., & Shinde, J. V. (2014, November-December). A survey on multimedia information retrieval systems. Int.J. *Computer Technology and Application, 5.*

.Abdullah, S. K., Akash, K. R. A., Bhubesh, S., & Selvakumar. (2021). Development of a Predictive Model for textual data using Support Vector Machine based on diverse Kernel Functions upon Sentiment Score Analysis. *International Journal of Natural ComputingResearch, 10*(2), 1-20, IGI Global.

Abdullah, A., Parkaya, R., Pudumalar, S., Santhiya, C., & Bhubesh, K. R. A. (2021). Semantic correction system using neural networks. *Proceedings Of The 3rd International Conference Of Green Civil And Environmental Engineering (Gcee 2021*). AIP Publishing. doi:10.1063/5.0072647

Abdullah, A. S. (2022). Assessment of the risk factors of type II diabetes using ACO with self-regulative update function and decision trees by evaluation from Fisher's Z-transformation. *Medical & Biological Engineering & Computing [Internet]*. Springer Science and Business Media LLC.: doi:10.1007/s11517-022-02530-2

Aditi, P. (2014). A Review on Circumscribe Based Video Retrieval. *International Journal of Advanced Research in Computer Science and Software Engineering*, *4*(Nov), 617–620.

Aslam, J. A., & Montague, M. (2013). Models for metasearch. In *Proc. 24th Annu. Int. ACM SIGIR Conf. Res. Develop. Inform. Retrieval*, (pp. 276–284). ACM..

Benavent, X., & Garcia-Serrano, A. (2013). multimedia information retrieval based on late semantic fusion Approaches. *IEEE Transactions on Multimedia*, *13*(dec), 8–14.

Golub, H. & Van Loan. (n.d.). Ssingular value decomposition. *CS theory-info age, 3*, pp 7-10.

Harsha J. K. & Amitkumar, M. (2014). A review paper on multimedia information retrieval based on late semantic fusion approach. *International journal of computer*, 1-4.

Khobragade, V., Patil, L., & Patil, U. (2015). Image Retrieval by Information Fusion of Multimedia Resources [IJARCET]. *International Journal of Advanced Research in Computer Engineering and Technology*, *4*(May), 1721–1727.

Lew, M. S., Sebe, N., Djerba, C., & Jain, R. (2006, February). Content-based multimedia information retrieval: State of the art and challenges. ACM Trans. Multimedia Comp. Commun. *Appl.*, *2*(1), 1–19.

Nuthakki, P., Manju, J., & Geetha, R. S. M & Abdullah, A. S. (2022). A Smart wearable motion sensor and acoustic signal processing based on vocabulary for monitoring children's wellbeing using Big Data. *2022 International Conference on Advanced Computing Technologies and Applications (ICACTA)*, 2022, pp. 1-9. IEEE. 10.1109/ICACTA54488.2022.9752875

Ringer, S. (2009). Multimedia information retrieval. *Synthesis lectures on information concepts, retrieval and services* (pp 6-10). ACM.

Saravanan, D., Sundaram, D., Nalini, N., & Arun, K. (2011). A Study Of Multimedia Information Retrieval Systems. *Research Journal of Science & IT management, .1*(2), 16-21.

Sheik Abdullah, A., Manoj, A., Tarun Kishore, G. T., & Selvakumar, S. (2021). A New Approach to Remote Health Monitoring using Augmented Reality with WebRTC and WebXR. *22nd International Arab Conference on Information Technology (ACIT) [Internet]*. IEEE. 10.1109/ACIT53391.2021.9677324

Sheik Abdullah, A., Parkavi, R., Pudumalar, S., Santhiya, C., & Bhubesh, K. R. A. (2021). Semantic correction system using neural networks. *Proceedings of The 3rd International Conference Of Green Civil And Environmental Engineering (GCEE 2021).* 10.1063/5.0072647

Sheik Abdullah, A., Selvakumar, S., & Venkatesh, M. (2021). Assessment and evaluation of CHD risk factors using weighted ranked correlation and regression with data classification, 25(6), pp. 4979–5001. doi:10.100700500-021-05663-y

Lew, M. (2017). Special issue on deep learning in image and video retrieval. *International Journal of Multimedia Information Retrieval*, 1–3.

Yun Q., Gurong, X., Yang, C., Gao, J., Zhang, A., Chai, P., Zoul, D., & Chen, C. (2021). Effective Steganalysis Based on Statistical Moments of Wavelet Characteristic Function. *Steganalysis, 3,* pp 1-6.

Chapter 12
Preventive Strategies to Reduce Musculoskeletal Disorders of Nursing Personnel; A Systematic Review:
Musculoskeletal Disorders of Nursing Personnel

Narayanage Jayantha Dewasiri
https://orcid.org/0000-0002-5908-8890
Sabaragamuwa University of Sri Lanka, Sri Lanka

W.S.R. Kulasinghe
Base Hospital, Matara, Sri Lanka

Duminda Iresh Kumara Sarambage
Base Hospital, Matara, Sri Lanka

B. Sunil S. De Silva
https://orcid.org/0000-0002-8824-9833
The Open University of Sri Lanka, Sri Lanka

ABSTRACT

The purpose of this study is to investigate the preventive strategies to reduce musculoskeletal disorders of nursing personnel. The findings of this study stated that there are three key themes of strategies to handle the research puzzle. Physical facilities such as lifts, equipment, electric beds, footwear, and other equipment provide physical infrastructure to deal with the issue. Moreover, the findings revealed that the physical facilities alone may not be effective in the long run. The second theme focuses on guidelines, procedures, or principles such as education, staffing, no lift policy, a healthy lifestyle, the culture of safety, training on manual handling, workflow management, need analysis, and stories which provide the supportive structure in addressing the issue. We argue that physical facilities, procedures, guidelines, and principles alone may not work effectively in reducing the musculoskeletal disorders of nurses and there should be a simultaneous implementation of themes one and two. We introduce the Musculoskeletal Prevention Model to deal with the research issue.

DOI: 10.4018/978-1-6684-5925-6.ch012

INTRODUCTION

There are different ways of patient handling, out of which manually handling of patients is a difficult task. The ways and means of patient handling has received a special attention in research since early 1990s in the United States of America. For instance, National Institute for Occupational Safety (NIOS) and Department of Veterans Affairs (DVA) support the researchers to investigate the seriousness of this issue and to find modern solutions for the same. NIOS and DVA are government institutions that focusses on employees' safety as one of their objectives. Hence, they support the researchers to find solutions for this critical issue. Waters et al. (2006) emphasized that unsafe patient handling as the main reason for musculoskeletal injuries among nurses. It is reported that more than 10,000 nurses in the USA face musculoskeletal disorders in each year resulting an inefficient and ineffective work environment (Bureau of Labor Statistics, 2010).

Manual handling is associated with some negative consequences for nursing personal in the long run. For instance, it is generally argued that more than 80% of nursing personal are incapacitated in their career path since there is no safe mechanism to move patients without having a machine assistance. Hence, injuries like musculoskeletal disorders may have a negative impact on the recruiting, retention, and development of nursing personal in the long run. Lagerström et al. (1998), Myers et al. (2002), Hegmann and Garg, (2004), Waters et al. (2006), and Bureau of Labor Statistics (2009) identified that back and shoulder injuries as a major issue for nursing personnel in the long run. Various research studies have focused on preventive strategies to reduce musculoskeletal disorders (MSDs) of nurses across the world. For instance, edification and exercises in physique mechanics and invigorating and transmitting techniques were employed to diminish MSDs in nursing personnel (Videman et al., 1989; Garg & Owen, 1992; Lagerström & Hagberg, 1997). Moreover, Garg and Kapellusch (2012) emphasized that the introduction of patient-handling devices along with a comprehensive program could be effectively used in reducing MSDs amongst nursing personnel. Furthermore, Collins et al. (2004) emphasized four strategies namely, best practices intervention, equipment intervention, training, and written zero-lift policy in reducing MSDs among nursing personnel.

The contrasting views of aforesaid previous studies and lack of comprehensive reviews of effective prevention strategies in patient handling are the main justification for this study. Further, there is a scarcity of research studies conducted in South Asia, investigating the same research issue. Hence, this study will add a definitive value for Sri Lankan nursing personnel and government authorities to implement the most effective preventive strategies in the South Asian context. Accordingly, the research problem of this study has been identified as "what are the most effective preventive strategies in reducing musculoskeletal disorders of nurses?"

Addressing the aforementioned gaps in the literature, the researchers of this study focus on evaluating all available mechanisms or methods to reduce musculoskeletal disorders through a systematic literature review approach. Here, the aim of the study is to identify a possibly most effective method of patient handling, and to develop a new model to deal with this serious issue. The researchers have identified a major question to achieve the research aim; what are the most effective strategies of patient handling in reducing musculoskeletal disorders of nurses? Accordingly, the general research objective of this study has been identified as to identify the most effective strategies of patient handling in reducing musculoskeletal disorders of nursing personnel. The specific research objective has been identified as to develop a Musculoskeletal Prevention Model to deal with the research problem.

LITERATURE REVIEW

Each day nurses assist patients to move, 'position, and mobilize'. However, when this process is done manually, it requires a lot of 'physical effort', and it is more difficult when the patient has tubes and other devices. Thus, 'handling and moving' adult patients must be done safely using special equipment designed for the propose. The following are some ways in which caregivers/nurses provide assistance to patients. It will provide a basic understanding about what is 'patient handling and mobility', the requirement for supporting devices and how these supportive devices would affect the physical care environment (Matz, 2019).

Relocation

There are two general categories: 1) "From one flat space to another" and 2) from "one seated position to another or to a standing position".

Lateral Transfer - Dependent patients should be moved to another flat surface for the treatments. 'Slide' or 'lateral' relocations are usually done, when 'transferring dependent patients for treatments, investigative, and procedure surfaces.' In a situation where there are no rails or armrests the nurses bring the flat surface where the patient should be transferred aligning it to the original surface (where the patient is currently located). In the cace where no supportive equipment is present, the process has to be done manually where one or more nurses can pull or push the sheets along with the patient to the destination surface (Waters, 2007).

Perch to Perch Mechanism

The "Perch" refers any furnishing on which a patient sit. In the case of a long-term illness care instructions and protocols strictly states that the patients must not spend a lot of time on the bed and thus frequent change of positions is required. This could also be keeping in mind that this would require minimum use of bedpans and thus securing the dignity of the patient. More importantly, patients are supposed to be in a right position for a range of treatments, diagnostic, and other procedures. In a manual transfer process from a flat position to a perch position, first of all the caregiver/nurses assist the patient to a seating position and then turn the patient while supporting them in moving their legs and arms to the side of the bed. Then the nurse lifts the patient and lowers the patient to a sitting or a perched position (Marras et al., 2009).

Position / Reposition of a Patient

There are many reasons as to why patients are moved or repositioned. For instance, investigating a patient, performing an activity or procedure such as catheterizing, hygiene tasks on personal level, feeding a patient, in an emergency event it is needed to reposition the patients in an effective manner (Garg and Carlson, 1992; Matz, 2019). It is indeed necessary to change the position of the patient at least by every two hours as it could create bedsore and other allergies. This action can be done by rolling the patient from one side to the other or keeping pillows in different positions so that it would alternate the skin areas which would bear the weight and thus will reduce the pooling of upper-respiratory fluids. This is one of the usual manual move done by nurses. Moreover, it is needed to reposition patients for their convenience and safety. Helping a patient in breathing, process of digesting and comfort by repositioning the patient in the bed, is also a regular annual action done by caretakers/nurses. This also involves taking care of patients who might fall off a chair, wheelchair or something similar. In a conference in 2008, it was revealed that almost half of their time is spent in these types of activities (Waters, 2008).

A patient Is needed to reposition, to address clinical conditions too. For instance, ease breathing, reduce nausea, hypotensive issues, nourishing of incapacitated patients required a reposition to proceed with the respective cause of action. Moreover, it is needed to reposition patients to improve the effectiveness of communication. Aside, keeping eye contact with patients will give them self-respect (Matz, 2019). Ambulation and Mobilization could be considered as another important reasons for repositioning of patients. It is known that a human body does not perform the most vital day to day activity of 'mobilizing/moving' then it 'deteriorate/decline' quickly. It is clearly shown in many studies/researches that if a patient needs quick and better outcomes 'mobilizing' or moving about is paramount. On the other hand, if this process is late then there could be adverse outcomes and also lifelong results (French, 1997).

Another very risky action for both nurses and the patients is lifting up a patient who has fallen. A paramount/vital fact that should be considered is that the caregiver/nurse should make sure that the patient is not injured and seeking whether the patient is stable (Waters, 2008). But at the same time lifting a patient on the floor, who cannot help himself is in no doubt one of the most difficult and a risky task for caregivers/nurses.

Transportation

Long distance transporting and transporting up and down inclinations/slopes can be risky to both the patient and the caregivers/nurses. Many transport devices such as "wheelchairs, gurneys, stretchers, beds, transport chairs, and (less recurrently) mobile bathing trolleys" can be used. Another risk that is faced by both patients and the caregivers/nurses is when the patient might need to be positioned in these devices. Moreover, the caregivers/nurses are faced with an extra risk when they have "to pull, push, thrust, and maneuverer the devices to reach a terminus". However, the greatest challenge is when a caregiver/nurse would decide to utilize the heavy bed with the patient as a transport device in an emergency situation. These have caused long-lasting injuries to the caregivers/nurses (Hegmann and Garg, 2004). Moreover, in the wound care process, the caregiver/nurse will have to lift a patient's body part and then place it in place for a long time.

Toileting

Supporting a patient in his/her toileting process is another challenging task that is rarely discussed. Many institutions and caregivers/nurses make sure that a patients' dignity/self-respect is maintained during the process. However, the following mechanisms of toileting also depends upon the weight, size, and dependency level of the sufferer. Even though, providing toileting facilities to the patient is a vital responsibility of the caregiver/nurse, "misperception, compromised balance, bad lighting, strangeness with environmental barriers, and insufficient room and door clearance" are facts that worsen the situation/task (Randall, 2009).

Showering

Getting a needy patient showered in a safe manner is another responsibility of a nurse, which has a high hazard for both patient and the caregivers. Bathing usually take s place in areas such as patient's bathroom, common bathrooms, bed, and a portable bath location. Hegmann and Garg (2004) argued that there are unique set of challenges in this process; the state of the patient could be fragile, both emotionally and physically; the environment could be wet and slippery and the floor will be inclined; there is a great risk of falling.

Moreover, in surgeries nurses face some challenges when conducting lateral transfers. Patients who are of varying sizes and weights come to care facilitates in various states. Some will arrive in cars and will be able to walk, but there could be many who will not be able to do so. Thus, caregivers will have to lift these patients from different vehicles and the situation get more serious when it is an emergency situation. Another level of caregiving is handling and mobilizing patients who are larger in size and aggressive. The risk of injuries for both the patient and the caregiver/nurse is at a higher level in these situations (Kim, 2012). Thus, special attention should be given to patients in these situations, especially with patients of dementia as they could feel frightened or threatened easily. However, this risk is not only with patients of dementia.

Moreover, manual patient handling is always unsafe as moving of dependent, and larger patients frequently have an added risk of damage for both patients and the caregivers/nurses. In spite of these risks most of the health care facilities are not armed/prepared to handle and over the growing population for high-acuity and increasing number of larger patients. It has also become a fact in the shortage of the global nursing force. There is an effect of manual patient handling on injuries to the aging caregiver workforce, the organizations' difficulty recruiting and retaining qualified nurses, and the number of injured nurses of all ages. Even though the use of "proper" lifting techniques can be shown as a measure to decrease injuries caused by manual patient handling, the injuries caused by handling patients sees to increase. The reason is that it is revealed that "caregivers' biomechanical capabilities" have exceeded. It is identified that no amount of training an assist in minimizing the injuries when it exceeds the tolerance level. Even though we are concerned about "transmitting infections from patent to the caregiver/nurse" we are not aware about the "ergonomic hazards" they face. Exertion of muscles often and over a long time without sufficient time for recovery the "muscle becomes fatigued". A micro-tear can develop into a major- tear when a person continues to exert muscles for a long time period without a rest (Nelson, 2003).

Lifting both heavy and light loads frequently causes excessive spinal loading. "Twisting, reaching, bending, pulling, and similar motions" also contribute to spinal loading. If a person's capacity of the spinal load is surpassed, vertebral endplate micro fractures occur, and scar tissue is formed. According to the Occupational Safety and Health Administration (OSHA), manual patient handling could be considered a significant reason for musculoskeletal injuries, common among health care providers. Researchers have identified that; 'overexertion from manually lifting and moving patients was largely responsible for musculoskeletal injuries found in nurses' (Marras, 2000). A new agenda was released by The National Occupational Research Agenda (NORA) for Healthcare and Social Assistance (HCSA) in 2019. It was developed to recognise 'knowledge and actions' that were vital to enhance job safety and health conditions. In order to develop the agenda, council participant, all experts in their fields, considered the most 'significant issues, gaps in research, and requirements for the HCSA workforce' (Marras, 2000).

STRATEGIES TO PREVENT MUSCULOSKELETAL DISORDERS OF NURSES

The practitioners and researchers across the past few decades focused on developing and implementing strategies to prevent musculoskeletal disorders of nurses. Waters et al. (2006) identified hazardous patient management as a foremost risk factor for nurses which causes musculoskeletal injuries and emphasize on identifying suitable strategies to overcome the same. D'Arcy et al. (2012), Kim et al. (2012), and Pompeii et al. (2009) argued that 31-66% of musculoskeletal injuries are due to the cases on patient handling tasks. Hence, it could be argued that health authorities should provide a universal guideline for the patient handling tasks and develop suitable methods or strategies with the purpose of reducing musculoskeletal injuries. The objective of this section is to critically evaluate the available strategies in order to provide a pathway for a universal model to deal with the issue. Researchers emphasized on different strategies to prevent musculoskeletal pain such as equipment, education, health and safety policy and multi-disciplinary collaboration (Richardson, 2019; Engst et al., 2005; Li et al., 2004; Zhuang et al., 2000; Trinkoff et al., 2003; Lee et al., 2010; Yassi et al., 1995; Vieira, et al., 2006; Videman et al., 2005; Vendittelli et al., 2016; Trinkoff et al., 2002).

The mechanical patient lifting equipment support nurses in reducing the injuries, stress, discomfort of musculoskeletal injuries, and workers' costs. (Engst et al., 2005; Li et al., 2004; Zhuang et al., 2000). Moreover, initiating lift /elevator facilities could be identified as the first step of ensuring a patient's safty and the nurses' well-being which minimizes the patient – nurse physical interactions (American Nurses Association, 2012), but lift facilities are not available in most of the developing countries including Sri Lanka (Trinkoff et al., 2003; Lee et al., 2010). Lee et al. (2013) investigated the impact of patient handling equipment on musculoskeletal pain in the United States and found that lifts tend to reduce work-related pain in shoulders and it is required to reduce the barriers against lift usage of the nursing personal to prevent such injuries. In contrary to aforementioned researches, Richardson (2019) emphasized that there is a lack of education on how to use equipment since there is no such training available in most of the health care centres. Hence, the researchers of this study argue that education on equipment handling and other patient handling mechanisms is important than others strategies.

Education could be considered as an effective strategy to prevent musculoskeletal injuries in the long run. Hence, there are number of training sessions arranged for nursing students and practicing nurses on patient handling mechanisms in preventing from the key issue Richardson (2019). Education plays a vital role even in educating preventive strategies to both the nurses and patients. Hence, there is a need for repeating the information to ensure that the prevention strategies are effectively used. It is revealed that 52.3% of the sample faced injuries due to inadequate training in a Canadian study (Yassi et al., 1995). Moreover, it is revealed that education alone is not adequate to prevent such injuries amongst the nursing category (Harber et al., 1994). Daltroy et al. (1997) stated that it is applicable to other job categories as well.

In addition to the education, it is revealed that there should be an adequate workforce to ensure the patient handling is completed in an effective and efficient manner (Yip, 2004). It allows the management to split the workforce in to shifts rather keeping them worked for hours. Hence, it is reducing the additional burden placed on the nurses where the risk is mitigated amongst the entire staff. There is a limited staff in most of the health institutions in developing countries which may have a negative impact on the number of musculoskeletal injuries in the long run (Vieira, et al., 2006). As a country, Sri Lanka is also facing a similar situation.

Many researchers stated that *no lift policy* is paving way towards the reduction of musculoskeletal injuries in the recent years due to effective utilisation of equipment and education (Videman et al., 2005; Vendittelli et al., 2016; Vieira et al., 2006). The researchers of this study argue that there is a requirement of adequate level of equipment and education in order to implement a *no lift policy* especially in the developing countries. Moreover, it is stated that no lift policy as the most effective method since it provides a clear guidance on how to mobilize the patients in an effective manner (Vendittelli et al., 2016). However, the researchers of this study argue that if there is a deficit of equipment and education in a country, it is better to proceed with a manual lifting policy which will provide a guideline for the same.

Moreover, Trinkoff et al. (2002) revealed that healthy lifestyle including physical fitness as the most effective prevention strategy than other traditional or modern strategies. Richardson (2019) stated that it is all about the physical fitness, being fitter is the key to prevent an injury. However, the researchers of this study argue that it is better to combine physical fitness strategy with other strategies in reducing musculoskeletal injuries rather than focusing on a single strategy.

There are some other strategies including establishing culture of safety, training on manual handling, proper designing and arrangement of the workflow, providing adequate footwear, electric beds, needs analysis, and stories to prevent from musculoskeletal injuries in the long run (Sandelowski, 2000). For instance, management can use previous stories on musculoskeletal injuries in educating its staff members. Storytelling is identified as an effective strategy that elaborates the consequences of lousy patient handling mechanisms or applying no-strategy (Sandelowski, 2000). Further, it is possible to establish a safety culture by undertaking some activities within the healthcare organisation; changes in the leadership style / management approach, timely reporting of an injury, promoting healthy life style and physical fitness, showing the posters and print material to read about the subject, pre-screening before the recruitment of the nurses, regular assessments on the nurses' competencies, and hazard analysis (Ready, 1993). Further, it is vital to provide on the job trainings for the nursing personal rather providing them online trainings. Hence, training within the clinical contexts plas an integral role in educating the staff. Moreover, practical / refresher courses could be arranged in providing manual handling training (North et al., 2013). Further, well-designed workplaces offer a secure place to reduce injuries to nursing personal. Moreover, individual tailoring, proper distribution of resources, and stories provide the right education to prevent musculoskeletal injuries in the long run (Mitchell, 2009). Further, multidisciplinary collaboration such as contact with physio and establishing a health and safety policy may reduce musculoskeletal injuries in the long run.

It is argued that prevention strategies alone are not sufficient to prevent from musculoskeletal injuries if the implementation is at a questionable level. Even though, no-lift policies are available, there is a requirement to highlight and educate on the alternative strategies. Vendittelli et al. (2016) argued that most of the nurses are not aware about the lifting guidelines in the US context. Hence, the situation in developing countries is problematic. Vendittelli et al. (2016) argued on the unavailability of equipment along with insufficient number of staff as the major reasons for the injuries in Michigan. Hence, the researchers of this study argue that there is a requirement to maintain a healthy staff level while educating staff about the lifting guidelines to prevent such issues especially in the developing countries. Moreover, age, selflessness, beliefs, and other personal factors were identified as challenges and issues to implement prevention strategies. Richardson (2019) stated that old nurses do not intend to use methods, and they tend to proceed with the do-it-own approach. Engels et al. (1996) and Vieira et al. (2006) emphasized that workload and time pressures are correlated with musculoskeletal disorders. Hence, this study's researcher argues that the nurses should use a collaborative approach in convincing the management on reducing additional workload and time pressure. Further, they can make a counterargument showing the empirical evidence to the administration.

Challenges / Issues in Implementing Strategies to Overcome the Issue

There are some issues or challenges in implementing strategies to overcome musculoskeletal injuries in the long run. For instance, age of the participants can be considered as a critical factor; older nurses cannot manually handle the patients in an effective manner. If there is no adequate number of workforce to handle the patients, it could be considered as an issue in implementing strategies. Further, equipment availability, time factor, and contextual factors are identified as other crucial challenges in implementing strategies in the work place / healthcare settings (Richardson, 2019). It is imperative to identify such challenges before implementing successful policies to have a better outcome through such initiatives. Then the staff can cope up with such changes.

Age

Previous researchers argued that, it is better to avoid consult ting the older nurses in engaging strategies to overcome musculoskeletal injuries in the long run (Mahmud et al., 2010). Because most of the older nurses are not physically fit and their less involvement in manual handling would cause inverse impact on the successful implementation of the prevention strategies, but the researchers of this study argues that it is better to have their advices/suggestions in implementing such strategies since they have the experience regarding the same.

Equipment Availability

There is a less availability of equipment in most of the healthcare settings especially in developing countries. For instance, there is no lift / elevators available, there is an absence of electrical beds, there is no specialist equipment, and there are no devices to lift or move patients such as trollies (Knibbe, 2007). These barriers would limit the successful implementation of the strategies to overcome musculoskeletal injuries in the long run. Moreover, equipment sharing in diverse wards may cause different issues associated with the strategy (June and Cho, 2011). For instance, if the equipment is shared between diverse wards, it could result in non-availability of the equipment in an emergency and, that could create an issue when implementing the strategy.

Staffing

Inadequate number of staff could be considered as a main challenge to adopt effective strategies in the long run (Hoover, 2011). There are some manual handling activities which required more than one nurse to perform the same. Moreover, insufficient workforce may lead to nurses' involvement faster in every activity. Furthermore, there is an adverse impact when putting people in training in the use of equipment when there is a less workforce (Hunter, 2010). Hence, *on the job training* could be considered as an effective approach in such a situation.

Contextual Barriers

There are some contextual factors which prevent nurses from implementing successful strategies to overcome the issue. For instance, the nurses are assigned for different tasks due to unavailability of medical doctors, their heavy workload, less support to implement strategies to overcome the issue due to bad culture could be considered as different contextual barriers to implement successful strategies in the healthcare settings (Gallagher, 2011). Moreover, in-charge nurses put some control on the implementation of such strategies in the workplace. Further, emergency requirements, hierarchies, and modelling may also prevent nurses to apply prevention strategies in a difficult situation (Choi and Brings, 2016).

Personal Attitudes

There are some nursing personal who believe that prevention strategies may not help them to secure their protection. From the nurses' point of view, it is believed that that use of prevention strategies may have an adverse impact on their personal image of fitness amongst the staff, hence they tend to lift patients in manual modes to showcase their fitness (Brewer et al., 2012). In addition to aforementioned barriers there are other issues such as time which may have an adverse impact on the implementation of prevention strategies. For instance, saving time is considered as one of the major priorities amongst the nursing personnel, because use of equipment may consume time. Moreover, the pressure from the superiors also prevent them in using such strategies to save time (Braun and Clarke 2006).

METHODOLOGY

The purpose of this study is to investigate the most effective strategies of patient handling in reducing musculoskeletal disorders of nursing personnel. The literature review suggested contradictory views on the most effective strategies to prevent musculoskeletal disorders amongst nurses and it has been identified as the general research gap of the current study. Popay et al. (1998) emphasized that there should be a rigour methodology in place in any systematic review to provide a greater contribution to the discipline. Moreover, as emphasized by O'Leary (2013) this study intends to review a sample of articles on musculoskeletal disorders to ensure validity and rigor of the research. Boland et al. (2013) emphasised that the Systematic Literature Review (SLR) approach paves the way towards synthesizing and evaluating the relevant and available literature with special reference to the formulated research question. Hence, SLR focusses on supporting researchers on deeply investigating research questions with the available literature which consists of both published and unpublished records. Accordingly, it enhances the transparency of the findings (Hemingway and Brereton, 2009) through a synergistic approach. Hence, as Melnyk and Fineout-Overholt (2011) emphasised, application of SLR helps to reduce investigator biases while enhancing the validity and reliability of the findings. Therivel and Paridario (2013) emphasised that identification of inconsistencies paves the way towards increasing the accuracy while reducing the inconsistencies of the study design. As emphasised by Cochrane (2014), it can be achieved by utilising the PICO approach. Here, "*P*" stands for Population, "*I*" stands for Intervention, "*C*" applies for comparison, and "O" for the outcome.

Systematic Literature Review Process

The Systematic Literature Review Process presented by Thomas et al. (2004) is used in the current study. The main reason is that it covers a comprehensive process which will support to identify key themes for effective strategies in preventing musculoskeletal injuries. They provided a step by step process to investigate a phenomenon. Creswell (2010) argued that the development of research questions is the building block of any research study. Hence, the nature and type of research questions support in identifying the methodology to investigate the phenomenon (Dewasiri et al., 2018). The research question of this study has been identified as "what are the most effective preventive strategies in reducing musculoskeletal disorders of nurses'. This research question is described under the descriptive, (what) nature, which required a quantitative inquiry. Hence, the researchers of this study have proceeded with a quantitative inquiry in investigating the phenomenon. In applying the PICO approach, the *population* (P) is considered as the nurses, *intervention* is the working environment, *comparison* is conducted on physical facilities, procedures, guidelines, and principles, *outcome* is the most effective preventive strategies to reduce musculoskeletal disorders of nursing personal. The PICO framework provides the possibility to split all the segments of the research study to enable investigators to gather complete access of the available literature as mentioned in the previous section. Accordingly, the researchers have initially proceeded with a generic data base search employing some key words in the data bases such as Science Direct, Sage, PubMed, Emerald, CINAHL, EBSCO host, Google Scholar, Wiley, and Cochrane Library.

The key words used in this investigation were preventive strategies, strategies, prevention, musculoskeletal disorders, musculoskeletal injuries, methods, techniques, nurses, health care centres, and hospitals. The authors were keen on analysing recent studies on the phenomenon, hence, year 2000 is taken as the initial / base year in the data search. Hence, the base year was the first inclusion criteria. The researchers focused on the articles appeared in peer-review academic journals, selected only English as the language as its inclusion criterion, and selected the articles with an abstract, key words, and full text access. The data base search is concluded with a total number of 1297 articles. Then, the researchers removed the unrelated articles in a further modification. Unrelated articles were removed based on the exclusion criterion. The researchers removed articles before year 2000 and then the researchers removed articles with special reference to other stakeholders rather than the nursing population. The data base search is concluded with a total number of 1127 articles. Moreover, 170 articles were identified through other search engines. Accordingly, a total of 1297 articles were identified for the initial screening. Then we removed the irrelevant articles (745) which were not focused on nursing personal. Then, the researchers removed articles which were not focused on musculoskeletal injuries. The final sample was reduced to 67 articles after applying the exclusion criterion. Finally, the articles' abstracts were evaluated in terms of quality of the contents and suitability for the current study. Accordingly, 49 articles were selected as the final sample of the study.

Cochrane (2007) stated that it is important to establish a standard appraisal process to ensure the quality of the articles and to select the most relevant papers to the analysis. Moreover, it may reduce the selection bias while enhancing the validity and the reliability of the sample (Clark and Oxman, 2003). Accordingly, this study employed a critical assessment tool used by Godfrey and Harrison (2010) and developed by the British Sociological Association. It is a vital assessment tool that can be used for both qualitative and quantitative analysis. The researchers can use two various tools to analyse in a comprehensive manner; Critical Appraisal Skills Programme (CASP) tools (2014) and the tool developed by the British Sociological Association. Here, the researchers have not proceeded CASP model due to its

Figure 1. Application of PRISMA Framework for the SLR
(Source: Adapted from Moher et al., 2009)

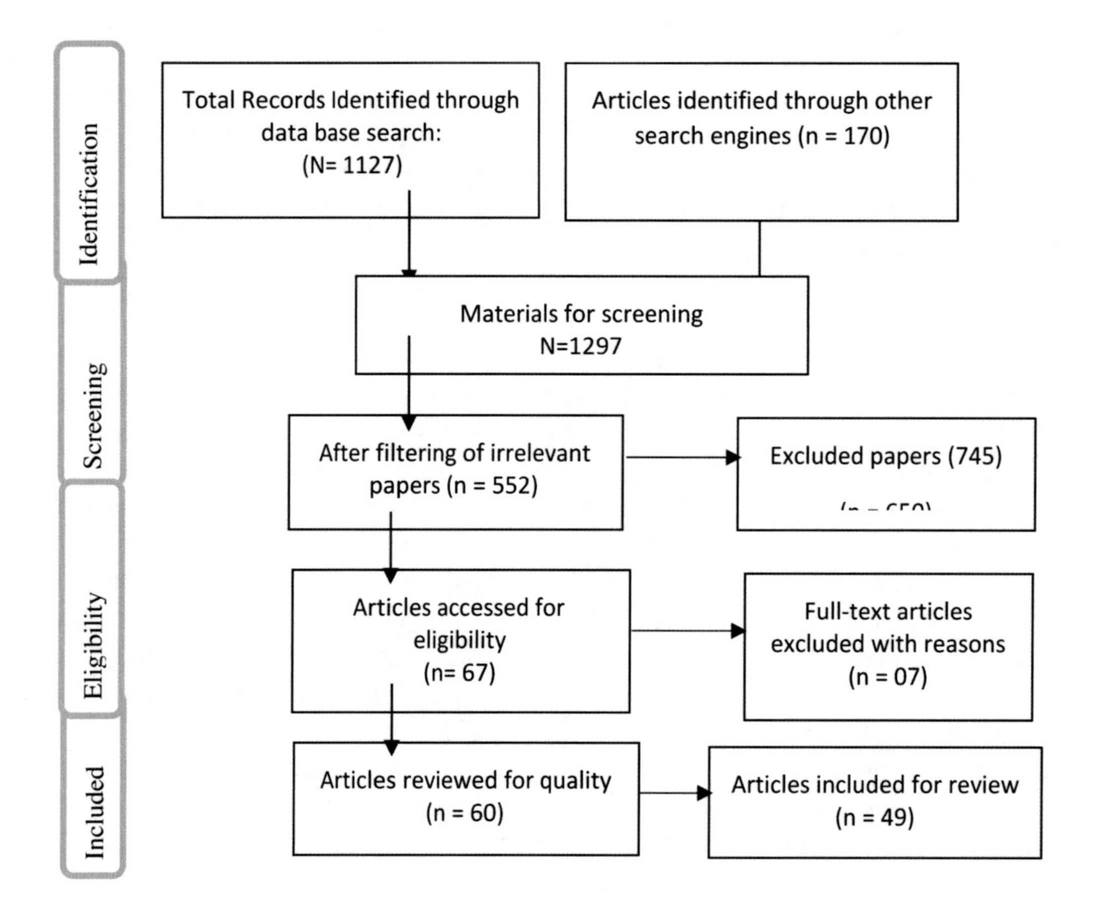

complexity; instead, it proceeded with the model developed by the British Sociological Association, which was later supported by Kmet et al. (2004). Godfrey and Harrison (2010) emphasized that an analysis of a critical review requires generation and conclusion through underlining principles. Accordingly, the researcher of this study has identified several key themes through the systematic literature review and proceeded with a cross over analysis to provide a comprehensive picture about the phenomenon.

RESULTS AND DISCUSSION

The results consist of two major steps. The analysis begins by identifying effective prevention strategies to deal with the research question. Then, the researchers proposed a holistic model to deal with the phenomenon.

Table 1. Summary of Methodologies Used

Methodology	#	%
Quantitative survey data	43	88
Qualitative primary data	05	10.2
Mixed methods approach	1	2
Other triangulation	0	0
Total	49	100

Research Methodologies Used to Study the Puzzle

To extend the analysis, researchers begin by identifying the methodologies used in the sample studies. As Table 2 shows, 88% of the studies rely on quantitative (survey) data, 10% use primary qualitative data, 2% employ mixed methods approach. None use other triangulation approaches, which represents a methodological gap and offers the possibility of reconciling the disparate results of other studies.

This table shows the summary of methodologies used by the 49 sampled studies in explaining the research puzzle.

Prevention Strategies for The Musculoskeletal Disorders of Nurses

Next, researchers identified the prevention strategies examined in the 49 sampled studies. Because some studies explore more than one strategy, the total number of strategies exceeds 19 and the percentages sum to more than 100%. As Table 2 shows, 43 of the 49 sampled studies (88%) examine whether technical equipment could be potentially influencing the prevention of Musculoskeletal Disorders. Other commonly studies strategies are education (38 studies), staffing (29 studies), no lift policy (27 studies), healthy life style (22 studies), culture of safety (5 studies), training on manual handling (4 studies), proper designing and arrangement of the workflow (4 studies), providing adequate footwear (3 studies), electric beds (9 studies), needs analysis (8 studies), and stories (2 studies).

Table 3 reports the percentage of studies that support a specific strategy, from among the 49 sampled studies of the 38 studies investigating education as an effective strategy, 46 (94%) find support for this factor. Preventive strategies showing a high percentage of studies offering support include equipment (71%), staffing and healthy life style (80%), no lift policy (76%), culture of safety (45%), training on manual handling (65%), workflow management (49%), footwear (39%), electric beds (45%), need analysis (43%), and stories (27%).

However, finding that the vast majority of the sampled studies provide support for a specific strategy may reflect "survivorship bias" because journals are unlikely to publish studies that do not provide significant results. Given the contradictions involving the research support for the strategies, developing a new model to deal with the puzzle seems appropriate. The results indicated that education has received the highest acceptance as a single strategy whereas the story telling received the least acceptance. Accordingly, education, equipment, staffing, no-lift policy, healthy life style received the highest acceptance amongst the numerous strategies investigated through this study. It is revealed that 52.3% of the sample faced injuries due to inadequate training in a Canadian study (Yassi et al., 1995). Moreover, it is revealed that education alone is not adequate to prevent such injuries amongst the nursing category (Harber et al., 1994). Daltroy et al. (1997) stated that it is applicable to other job categories as well. Hence, the results show that one strategy alone may not help in reducing musculoskeletal injuries in the long run.

Table 2. Prevention Strategies

Strategy	#	%
Equipment	43	88%
Education	38	78%
Staffing	29	59%
No Lift Policy	27	55%
Healthy Life Style	22	45%
Culture of Safety	5	10%
Training on manual handling	4	8%
Workflow management	4	8%
Footwear	3	6%
Electric Beds	9	18%
Need Analysis	8	16%
Stories	2	4%

Note: For consistency with Table 2 show all percentages carried out to one decimal place.

Table 3. Acceptance of Strategies to prevent musculoskeletal disorders

Strategy	Supported #	%	Not Supported	%
Equipment	35	71%	14	29%
Education	46	94%	3	6%
Staffing	39	80%	10	20%
No Lift Policy	37	76%	12	24%
Healthy Life Style	39	80%	10	20%
Culture of Safety	22	45%	27	55%
Training on manual handling	32	65%	17	35%
Workflow management	24	49%	25	51%
Footwear	19	39%	30	61%
Electric Beds	22	45%	27	55%
Need Analysis	21	43%	28	57%
Stories	13	27%	36	73%

DISCUSSION

This study is conducted employing the critical assessment tool as used by Godfrey and Harrison (2010) and developed by the British Sociological Association. It is an effective critical assessment tool which can be used for crossover analysis. It is imperative to note that all the studies in the sample was published in indexed, peer-reviewed, and refereed journals, hence the overall rigor of the current study is high. It is noted that all the studies conducted the validity and reliability tests ensuring the convergent validity hence, the methodological rigor is high. The articles selected for the analysis are published in world recognized journals such as; American Journal of Industrial Medicine, Critical Care Nursing Clinics, International Journal of Nursing Studies, Ergonomics, AAOHN Journal, Journal of Nursing Management, Research in Nursing and Health, Journal of Nursing Administration, Spine, Journal of Advanced Nursing, Orthopaedic Nursing, and Occupational Medicine. All of the studies have investigated the prevention strategies for musculoskeletal injuries in order to overcome the issue. It is imperative to note that all of the studies investigated more than 5 strategies in a single research. Richardson (2019) investigated 8 of the 12 strategies in a single study. The findings revealed that all of the strategies are equally important and one strategy as a whole cannot perform outstanding results. Out of the sampled studies, Nelson et al. (2006) developed a multidimensional ergonomics platform to prevent injuries due to manual handling activities. Their model comprises of several factors including Patient Handling Assessment Criteria and Decision Algorithms, Peer Leader role, Back Injury Resource Nurses, Patients Ergonomic Assessment Protocol, State-of-the-art Equipment, After Action Reviews, and No Lift Policy. The overall program supported significant reduction in musculoskeletal injuries whereas the total number of worked days reduced by 18%. Moreover, the results presented a job satisfaction of the nursing personal. It is imperative to note that most of the 49 studies focused more than 5 strategies emphasizing their approach as a holistic approach. The researcher of this study believe that one-size-fits-all approach is not suitable in healthcare studies especially in musculoskeletal injuries.

KEY STRATEGIES / THEMES IDENTIFIED IN THE RESEARCH

The results of the systematic literature review provided a set of key strategies to protect nurses from the injuries. These factors could be identified under key three themes; physical facilities, procedures and guidelines, effective and efficient implementation of the strategies. The researcher of this study argues that there should be a holistic approach in addressing the first two key themes while adhering to the effective and efficient implementation of the same. If nurses can work in accordance with these key themes, it is possible to reduce musculoskeletal injuries in the long run. Figure 2 shows the key themes identified in this research in addressing the specific research objective of the study.

Where:

A = Equipment, Footwear, electric beds

B = Education, staffing, no lift policy, Healthy Life Style, culture of safety, trainings on manual handling, workflow management, need analysis, stories

C = Affective Utilization of A and B

A + B + C = Comprehensive picture of the startegies to prevent musculoskeletal injuries

Figure 2. Key themes identified in the research: Musculoskeletal Prevention Model

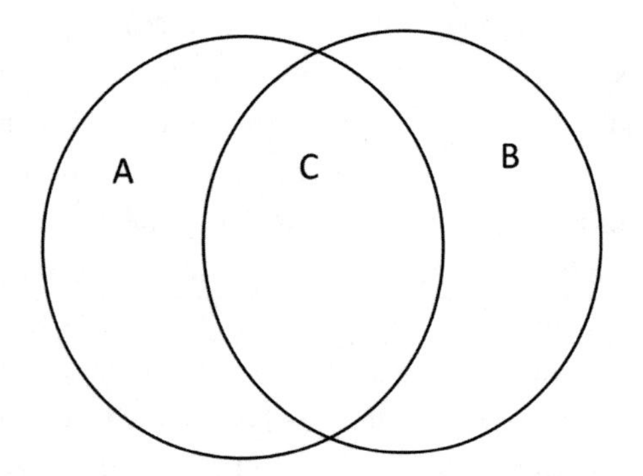

A. Physical facilities

B. Procedures and Guidelines

C. Effective and efficient implementation of both physical facilities and procedures / guidelines.

A + B + C: Comprehensive picture

Theme 1: Physical Facilities (A)

Physical facilities consist of (1) footwear, (2) electric beds, and (3) other equipment. Physical facilities support to replace the manual handling of patients. For instance, use of lifts provides an easy transport within the hospital which reduce the number of occasions on manual handling. It is important to note that there is a requirement for holistic approach rather that focusing on these single dimensions to prevent from musculoskeletal injuries in the long run. Through a qualitative inquiry, Richardson (2019) emphasized on such a holistic model to deal with the puzzle while reducing the barriers to implement the same; age, availability of equipment, adequate staff, contextual barriers, bad attitudes, time availability, and superior pressure.

Theme 2: Procedures and Guidelines (B)

Procedures and guidelines consist of diverse factors such as (1) education, (2) staffing, (3) no lift policy, (4) healthy lifestyle, (5) culture of safety, (6) training on manual handling, (7) workflow management, (8) need analysis, and (9) stories. In addition to the aforementioned procedures and guidelines there are standalone principles in healthcare settings. The procedures and guidelines are important but effective use or adherence to such principles should receive a prominence in the long-run.

Theme 3: Effective Implementation Of Equipment, Procedures, And Guidelines (C)

As stated in the literature review, equipment, rules, procedures, guidelines alone may not have a positive impact on the prevention of the overall musculoskeletal injuries as stated in theme 1. Hence the researcher of this study emphasizes on the holistic model stated in figure 1 and suggest nurses and policy makers to apply the model in preventing such injuries in the long run. Gallagher (2011), Vendittelli et al. (2016) and Richardson (2019) emphasized on a holistic model but they failed to introduce such a collaborative model. Hence, this study adds an original contribution to the existing literature introducing a holistic model to deal with the research puzzle. Further, the barriers stated in the literature review should be minimized while introducing the holistic model. Moreover, it is important to note that all of the barriers such as availability of equipment, adequate staff, contextual barriers, bad attitudes, time availability, and superior pressure could be minimized through the effective implementation of physical equipment and guidelines. For instance, adequacy of staff would turn around when procedures are implemented by enhancing the number of workforce after calculating the workload.

CONCLUSION

This study investigates the prevention strategies in reducing musculoskeletal disorders of nurses in the healthcare settings. Despite of voluminous amount of research conducted there was no single consensus on the prevention strategies across the past few decades. The findings divulge that there are three key themes of strategies to handle the research puzzle. Physical facilities such as lifts, equipment, electric beds, footwear and other equipment provide physical infrastructure to deal with the issue. The findings revealed that physical facilities alone may not be effective in the long run. There should be certain guidelines, procedures, or principles to deal with the research issue. For instance, factors such as (1) education, (2) staffing, (3) no lift policy, (4) healthy life style, (5) culture of safety, (6) trainings on manual handling, (7) workflow management, (8) need analysis, and (9) stories provide the supportive structure in addressing the issue. The researcher of this study argues that physical facilities, procedures, guidelines, and principles alone may not work effectively in reducing musculoskeletal disorders of nurses in the healthcare settings. It is essential to highlight that it is possible to reduce musculoskeletal injuries by implementing such equipment, procedures, or guidelines that are required periodical monitoring. Still, it could not be eliminated from the total healthcare system. Moreover, when a holistic approach is applied, all the barriers mentioned in the discussion would be eliminated in the long run. Hence, the researcher of this study introduces the Musculoskeletal Prevention Model (Figure 2) to deal with the research puzzle.

IMPLICATIONS TO THE PRACTICE

This study has several implications for nurses, policy makers and patients. For nursing personal, it is required to adhere to the model stated in Figure 2 to ensure that musculoskeletal injuries are not taking place when performing day to day activities. It is mandatory to work in accordance with the guidance provided in this research. For policy makers, it is suggested to implement this holistic model while providing infrastructure facilities, rules, regulations, and an effective monitoring mechanism should be on place to deal with this serious research issue. Hence, the researcher suggests to implement such protocol for the betterment of the total healthcare system. Finally, patients can adhere to the holistic model introduced in this study to maintain such practices in the long run. However, they cannot always adhere to the holistic model when they have cognitive impairment. The reduction of musculoskeletal injuries may help nurses to work in an effective and efficient manner.

LIMITATIONS AND FUTURE DIRECTIONS

This research is conducted under different set of limitations. First, the findings of the systematic literature are reliable only when methods and estimations provided in the primary studies are accurate. In other words, the rigor of this study is depending upon the rigor of the sampled studies. The future researchers can focus on testing the level of implementation of the proposed model by developing indicators to test the Musculoskeletal Prevention Model stated in Figure 2.

REFERENCES

American Nurses Association. (2012). *State legislation on safe patient handling*. ANA. http://www.anasafepatienthandling.org/Main-Menu/ANAActions/State-Legislation.aspx .

Boland, A., Cherry, M. G., & Dickson, R. (Eds.). (2013). *Doing a systematic review: a student's guide*. Sage.

Braun, V., & Clarke, V. (2006). Using thematic analysis in psychology. *Qualitative Research in Psychology*, *3*(2), 77–101. doi:10.1191/1478088706qp063oa

Brewer, C. S., Kovner, C. T., Greene, W., Tukov-Shuser, M., & Djukic, M. (2012). Predictors of actual turnover in a national sample of newly licensed registered nurses employed in hospitals. *Journal of Advanced Nursing*, *68*(3), 521–538. doi:10.1111/j.1365-2648.2011.05753.x PMID:22092452

Bureau of Labor Statistics. (2009). *Nonfatal occupational injuries and illnesses requiring days away from work, 2007: News (USDL-08-1716)*. U.S. Department of Labor.

Choi, S. D., & Brings, K. (2016). Work-related musculoskeletal risks associated with nurses and nursing assistants handling overweight and obese patients: A literature review. *Work (Reading, Mass.)*, *53*(2), 439–448. doi:10.3233/WOR-152222 PMID:26835850

Clarke, M., & Oxman, A. D. (2003). Cochrane reviewers' handbook 4.2. 0. *The Cochrane Library*, 2.

Cochrane. (2007). *Systematic Reviews of Health Promotion and Public Health Interventions*. Cochrane. https://ph.cochrane.org/sites/ph.cochrane_PH%20reviews.pdf.

Cochrane Collaboration. (2009) *Cochrane Handbook for Systematic Reviews of Interventions*. Cochrane. www.cochrane-handbooking.org.

D'Arcy, L. P., Sasai, Y., & Stearns, S. C. (2012). Do assistive devices, training, and workload affect injury incidence? Prevention efforts by nursing homes and back injuries among nursing assistants. *Journal of Advanced Nursing*, *68*(4), 836–845. doi:10.1111/j.1365-2648.2011.05785.x PMID:21787370

Daltroy, L. H., Iversen, M. D., Larson, M. G., Lew, R., Wright, E., Ryan, J., & Liang, M. H. (1997). A controlled trial of an educational program to prevent low back injuries. *The New England Journal of Medicine*, *337*(5), 322–328. doi:10.1056/NEJM199707313370507 PMID:9233870

Dewasiri, N. J., Weerakoon, Y. K. B., & Azeez, A. A. (2018). Mixed Methods in Finance Research: The Rationale and Research Designs. *International Journal of Qualitative Methods*, *17*(1), 1–13. doi:10.1177/1609406918801730

Engst, C., Chhokar, R., Miller, A., Tate, R. B., & Yassi, A. (2005). Effectiveness of overhead lifting devices in reducing the risk of injury to care staff in extended care facilities. *Ergonomics*, *48*(2), 187–199. doi:10.1080/00140130412331290826 PMID:15764316

French, P., Flora, L. F. W., Ping, L. S., Bo, L. K., & Rita, W. H. Y. (1997). The prevalence and cause of occupational back pain in Hong Kong registered nurses. *Journal of Advanced Nursing*, *26*(2), 380–388. doi:10.1046/j.1365-2648.1997.1997026380.x PMID:9292374

Gallagher, S. M. (2011). Women's health, size and safe patient handling: What are the ethical issues? *Bariatric Nursing and Surgical Patient Care*, *6*(2), 69–72. doi:10.1089/bar.2011.9973

Garg, A., & Kapellusch, J. M. (2012). Long-Term Efficacy of an Ergonomics Program That Includes Patient-Handling Devices on Reducing Musculoskeletal Injuries to Nursing Personnel. *Human Factors*, *54*(4), 608–625. doi:10.1177/0018720812438614 PMID:22908684

Garg, A., Owen, B. D., & Carlson, B. (1992). An ergonomics evaluation of nursing assistants' job in a nursing home. *Ergonomics*, *35*(9), 979–995. doi:10.1080/00140139208967377 PMID:1387079

Godfrey, C., & Harrison, M. B. (2010). *Systematic Review Resource Package. The Joanna Briggs Institute Method for Systematic Review Research Quick Reference Guide*. Queen's Joanna Briggs Collaboration.

Harber, P., Peña, L., Hsu, P., Billet, E., Greer, D., & Kim, K. (1994). Personal history, training and worksite as predictors of back pain of nurses. *American Journal of Industrial Medicine, 25*(4), 519–526. https://doi. doi:org/10.1002/ajim.4700250406

Hegmann, K. T., & Garg, A. (2004). *Home healthcare: Reducing musculoskeletal hazards.* Final report (NIOSH [CDC] Grant No. U50/CCU 300860). CDC/NIOSH.

Hemingway, P., & Brereton, N. (2009) What is a systematic review? London: Hayward Medical.

Hoover, R. S., & Koerber, A. L. (2011). Using NVivo to answer the challenges of qualitative research in professional communication: Benefits and best practices tutorial. *IEEE Transactions on Professional Communication*, *54*(1), 68–82. doi:10.1109/TPC.2009.2036896

Hunter, B., Branson, M., & Davenport, D. (2010). Saving costs, saving health care providers' backs and creating a safe patient environment. *Nursing Economics*, *28*(2), 130. PMID:20446387

June, K. J., & Cho, S.-H. (2011). Low back pain and work-related factors among nurses in intensive care units. *Journal of Clinical Nursing*, *20*(3-4), 479–487. doi:10.1111/j.1365-2702.2010.03210.x PMID:20673308

Karhula, K., Ronnholm, T., & Sjogren, T. (2006), Development of observation instrument for assessing work load on personnel involved in patient transfer tasks. *Proceedings of NES 38th Annual Congress*, 148-152. NES.

Kim, H., Dropkin, J., Spaeth, K., Smith, F., & Moline, J. (2012). Patient handling and musculoskeletal disorders among hospital workers: Analysis of 7 years of institutional workers' compensation claims data. *American Journal of Industrial Medicine*, *55*(8), 683–690. doi:10.1002/ajim.22006 PMID:22237853

Kim, H., Dropkin, J., Spaeth, K., Smith, F., & Moline, J. (2012). Patient handling and musculoskeletal disorders among hospital workers: Analysis of 7 years of institutional workers' compensation claims data. *American Journal of Industrial Medicine, 55*(8), 683–690. doi:10.1002/ajim.22006 PMID:22237853

Knibbe, H. J., Knibbe, N. E., & Klaassen, A. J. (2007). Safe patient handling program in critical care using peer leaders: Lessons learned in the Netherlands. *Critical Care Nursing Clinics, 19*(2), 205–211. doi:10.1016/j.ccell.2007.02.009 PMID:17512476

Lagerström, M., & Hagberg, M. (1997). Evaluation of a 3-year education and training program for nursing personnel at a Swedish hospital. *AAOHN Journal, 45*(2), 83–92. doi:10.1177/216507999704500207 PMID:9146108

Lagerström, M., Hansson, T., & Hagberg, M. (1998). Work-related low-back problems in nursing. *Scandinavian Journal of Work, Environment & Health, 24*(6), 449–464. doi:10.5271jweh.369 PMID:9988087

Lee, S. J., Faucett, J., Gillen, M., Krause, N., & Landry, L. (2010). Factors associated with safe patient handling behaviors among critical care nurses. *American Journal of Industrial Medicine, 53*(9), 886–897. doi:10.1002/ajim.20843 PMID:20698021

Lee, S. J., Faucett, J., Gillen, M., Krause, N., & Landry, L. (2013). Musculoskeletal pain among critical-care nurses by availability and use of patient lifting equipment: An analysis of cross-sectional survey data. *International Journal of Nursing Studies, 50*(12), 1648–1657. doi:10.1016/j.ijnurstu.2013.03.010 PMID:23648391

Li, J., Wolf, L., & Evanoff, B. (2004). Use of mechanical patient lifts decreased musculoskeletal symptoms and injuries among health care workers. *Injury Prevention, 10*(4), 212–216. doi:10.1136/ip.2003.004978 PMID:15314047

Mahmud, N., Schonstein, E., Schaafsma, F., Lehtola, M. M., Fassier, J.-B., Reneman, M. F., & Verbeek, J. H. (2010). Pre-employment examinations for preventing occupational injury and disease in workers. *Cochrane Database of Systematic Reviews*, (12), CD008881. doi:10.1002/14651858.CD008881 PMID:21154401

Marras, W. S. (2000). Occupational low back disorder causation and control. *Ergonomics, 43*(7), 880–902. doi:10.1080/001401300409080 PMID:10929824

Marras, W. S., Knapik, G. G., & Ferguson, S. (2009). Lumbar spine forces during manoeuvring of ceiling-based and floor-based patient transfer devices. *Ergonomics, 52*(3), 384–397. doi:10.1080/00140130802376075 PMID:19296324

Matz, M. W. (2019). Patient Handling and Mobility Assessments (2nd ed). The Facility Guidelines Institute.

Melnyk, B. M., & Fineout-Overholt, E. (Eds.). (2011). *Evidence-based practice in nursing & healthcare: A guide to best practice*. Lippincott Williams & Wilkins.

Mitchell, T., O'Sullivan, P. B., Smith, A., Burnett, A. F., Straker, L., Thornton, J., & Rudd, C. J. (2009). Biopsychosocial factors are associated with low back pain in female nursing students: A cross-sectional study. *International Journal of Nursing Studies, 46*(5), 678–688. doi:10.1016/j.ijnurstu.2008.11.004 PMID:19118828

Moher, D., Liberati, A., Tetzlaff, J., & Altman, D.PRISMA Group. (2009). Preferred reporting items for systematic reviews and meta-analyses: The PRISMA Statement. *Annals of Internal Medicine*, *151*(4), 264–269. doi:10.7326/0003-4819-151-4-200908180-00135 PMID:19622511

Myers, D., Silverstein, B., & Nelson, N. A. (2002). Predictors of shoulder and back injuries in nursing home workers: A prospective study. *American Journal of Industrial Medicine*, *41*(6), 466–476. doi:10.1002/ajim.10076 PMID:12173371

Nelson, A. L., Lloyd, J. D., Menzel, N., & Gross, C. (2003). Preventing nursing back injuries: Redesigning patient handling tasks. *AAOHN Journal*, *51*(3), 126–134. doi:10.1177/216507990305100306 PMID:12670100

North, N., Leung, W., Ashton, T., Rasmussen, E., Hughes, F., & Finlayson, M. (2013). Nurse turnover in New Zealand: Costs and relationships with staffing practices and patient outcomes. *Journal of Nursing Management*, *21*(3), 419–428. doi:10.1111/j.1365-2834.2012.01371.x PMID:23405958

O'Leary, Z. (2013). *The essential guide to doing your research project. Sage (Atlanta, Ga.).*

Pompeii, L. A., Lipscomb, H. J., Schoenfisch, A. L., & Dement, J. M. (2009). Musculoskeletal injuries resulting from patient handling tasks among hospital workers. *American Journal of Industrial Medicine*, *52*(7), 571–578. doi:10.1002/ajim.20704 PMID:19444808

Popay, J., Rogers, A., & Williams, G. (1998). Rationale and standards for the systematic review of qualitative literature in health services research. *Qualitative Health Research*, *8*(3), 341–351. doi:10.1177/104973239800800305 PMID:10558335

Randall, S. B., Pories, W. J., Pearson, A., & Drake, D. J. (2009). Expanded Occupational Safety and Health Administration 300 log as metric for bariatric patient-handling staff injuries. *Surgery for Obesity and Related Diseases*, *5*(4), 463–468. doi:10.1016/j.soard.2009.01.002 PMID:19359222

Ready, A. E., Boreskie, S. L., Law, S. A., & Russell, R. (1993). Fitness and lifestyle parameters fail to predict back injuries in nurses. *Canadian Journal of Applied Physiology*, *18*(1), 80–90. doi:10.1139/h93-008 PMID:8471996

Sandelowski, M. (2000). Focus on research methods-whatever happened to qualitative description? *Research in Nursing & Health*, *23*(4), 334–340. doi:10.1002/1098-240X(200008)23:4<334::AID-NUR9>3.0.CO;2-G PMID:10940958

Therivel, R., & Paridario, M. R. (2013). *The practice of strategic environmental assessment*. Routledge. doi:10.4324/9781315070865

Thomas, B. H., Ciliska, D., Dobbins, M., & Micucci, S. (2004). A process for systematically reviewing the literature: Providing the research evidence for public health nursing interventions. *Worldviews on Evidence-Based Nursing*, *1*(3), 176–184. doi:10.1111/j.1524-475X.2004.04006.x PMID:17163895

Trinkoff, A. M., Brady, B., & Nielsen, K. (2003). Workplace prevention and musculoskeletal injuries in nurses. *The Journal of Nursing Administration*, *33*(3), 153–158. doi:10.1097/00005110-200303000-00006 PMID:12629302

Trinkoff, A. M., Lipscomb, J. A., Geiger-Brown, J., & Brady, B. (2002). Musculoskeletal problems of the neck, shoulder and back and functional consequences in nurses. *American Journal of Industrial Medicine*, *41*(3), 170–178. doi:10.1002/ajim.10048 PMID:11920961

U.S. Department of Labor, Bureau of Labor Statistics (2018). *Survey of occupational inquiries and illnesses, 2018* [Data set]. Bureau of Labor Statistics.

Vendittelli, D., Penprase, B., & Pittiglio, L. (2016). Musculoskeletal injury prevention for new nurses. *Workplace Health & Safety*, *64*(12), 573–585. doi:10.1177/2165079916654928 PMID:27353509

Videman, T., Ojajärvi, A., Riihimäki, H., & Troup, J. D. (2005). Low back pain among nurses: A follow-up beginning at entry to the nursing school. *Spine*, *30*(20), 2334–2341. doi:10.1097/01.brs.0000182107.14355.ca PMID:16227898

Videman, T., Rauhala, H., Asp, S., Lindström, K., Cedercreutz, G., Kämppi, M., Tola, S., & Troup, J. D. G. (1989). Patient-handling skill, back injuries, and back pain: An intervention study in nursing. *Spine*, *14*(2), 148–156. doi:10.1097/00007632-198902000-00002 PMID:2522242

Vieira, E. R., Kumar, S., Coury, H. J., & Narayan, Y. (2006). Low back problems and possible improvements in nursing jobs. *Journal of Advanced Nursing*, *55*(1), 79–89. doi:10.1111/j.1365-2648.2006.03877.x PMID:16768742

Waters, T.R. (2007). When is it safe to manually lift a patient? *American Journal of Nursing 107, 6*(1), pp. 40–45.

Waters, T. R. (2008). Science to support specific limits on lifting, pushing, and pulling and static postures. Presentation at the *8th Annual Safe Patient Handling Conference*. Lake Buena Vista, Florida, USA.

Waters, T. R., Collins, J., Galinsky, T., & Caruso, C. (2006). NIOSH research efforts to prevent musculoskeletal disorders in the healthcare industry. *Orthopedic Nursing*, *25*(6), 380–389. doi:10.1097/00006416-200611000-00007 PMID:17130760

Yassi, A., Khokhar, J., Tate, R., Cooper, J., Snow, C., & Vallentype, S. (1995). The epidemiology of back injuries in nurses at a large Canadian tertiary care hospital: Implications for prevention. *Occupational Medicine*, *45*(4), 215–220. doi:10.1093/occmed/45.4.215 PMID:7662937

Yip, V. Y. B. (2004). New low back pain in nurses: Work activities, work stress and sedentary lifestyle. *Journal of Advanced Nursing*, *46*(4), 430–440. doi:10.1111/j.1365-2648.2004.03009.x PMID:15117354

Zhuang, Z., Stobbe, T. J., Collins, J. W., Hsiao, H., & Hobbs, G. R. (2000). Psychophysical assessment of assistive devices for transferring patients/ residents. *Applied Ergonomics*, *31*(1), 35–44. doi:10.1016/S0003-6870(99)00023-X PMID:10709750

Chapter 13
Review on Knowledge-Centric Healthcare Data Analysis Case Using Deep Neural Network for Medical Data Warehousing Application

Nilamadhab Mishra
https://orcid.org/0000-0002-1330-4869
Vit Bhopal University, India

Swagat Kumar Samantaray
Vit Bhopal University, India

ABSTRACT

Data in medical data warehouses are often used in data analytics and online analytical processing tools. OLAP techniques do not process enterprise data for hidden or unknown intelligence. The data analytics process takes data from a medical data warehouse as input and identifies the hidden patterns; i.e., data analytics process extracts hidden predictive information from the medical data warehouse through the deep neural networks tools. In this work, the authors attempt to identify the hidden patterns in context to healthcare data analytics case analytics using deep neural networks for medical applications. The authors have experimented with the deep network algorithms for the healthcare data set used through controlled learning that is to be carried out with the medical data set.

INTRODUCTION AND BACKGROUND REVIEW

A traditional medical data warehouse is a central store of data that has been extracted from operational data sources. Data in a medical data warehouse is typically subject-oriented, non-volatile, and of a historic nature, as contrasted with data used in an online transaction processing system. Data in medical

DOI: 10.4018/978-1-6684-5925-6.ch013

data warehouses are often used in data analytics and online analytical processing tools. Online analytical processing techniques do not process enterprise data for hidden or unknown intelligence (Gabrys & Bargiela (2000) (Demuth & Beale, (1993) With the obsolescence of traditional medical data warehouses, new emerging technologies are progressively integrated to gain a better return on investment at the enterprise level. Medical data warehouses offer organizations the ability to gather and store enterprise information in a single conceptual enterprise repository. Basic data modeling techniques are applied to create relationship associations between individual data elements or data element groups. These associations, or "models," often take the form of entity relationship diagrams (ERDs). More advanced techniques include the star schema and snowflake data model concepts. Regardless of the technique chosen, the goal is to build a metadata model that conceptually represents the information usage and relationships within the organization.

Leveraging the metadata model, enterprise users can then apply elementary data analysis techniques to gather business knowledge (Mishra, Lin, & Chang, 2014). For example, ad hoc queries can be run against the medical data warehouse to extract enterprise-level information. These queries would supply information that was impossible to obtain under the legacy system of disparate information silos.

More advanced medical data warehouse toolsets incorporate the concept of multidimensional data or data cubes. This data structure allows information to be multi-indexed, which allows for a rapid drill-down on data attributes. Data cubes are usually used to perform what-if scenarios over-identified data indices. For example, suppose Company X sells jewelry and has offices in Detroit, Pittsburgh, and Atlanta. If the proper attributes were chosen as indices, a user could perform the analysis. This multidimensional analysis of multiple business views is called Online Analytical Processing (OLAP). The primary function of OLAP systems is to provide users the ability to perform manual exploration and analysis of enterprise summaries and detailed information. It is important to understand that OLAP requires the user to know what information he or she is searching for. OLAP techniques do not process enterprise data for hidden or unknown intelligence (Demuth & Beale, 2000.) (Mishra, Lin, & Chang, 2015) (Nørgård, 1997).

Enter the concept of data analytics. During the mid-to-late 1990s, commercial vendors began exploring the feasibility of applying traditional statistical and artificial intelligence analysis techniques to large databases to discover hidden data attributes, trends, and patterns. This exploration evolved into formal data-mining toolsets based on a wide collection of statistical analysis techniques. For a commercial business, the discovery of previously unknown statistical patterns or trends can provide valuable insight into the function and environment of their organization. Data-mining techniques allow businesses to make predictions of future events, whereas OLAP only gives an analysis of past facts. Data-mining techniques can generally be grouped into one of three categories: clustering, classifying, and predictive. Clustering techniques group information based on a set of input patterns using an unsupervised or undirected algorithm. One example of clustering could be the analysis of business consumers for unknown attribute groupings. Input to this example would be well-defined consumer attributes over which the algorithm would search. Classifying techniques group or assign objects to predetermined groupings based on well-defined attributes. The groupings are often clusters discovered using the above techniques. An example would be assigning a consumer to a particular sales cluster based on their income level. Predictive techniques take as input known attributes regarding a particular object or category and apply those attributes to another similar group to identify expected behavior or outcomes. For example, if a group of individuals wearing helmets and shoulder pads is known to be a football team, we can expect another group of individuals with helmets and pads to be a football team as well (Mishra, Lin, & Chang, 2014).

The following list describes many data-mining techniques in use today. Each of these techniques exists in several variations and can be applied to one or more of the categories (Hagan, Demuth, & Beale, 1996.) (Chang, Mishra, & Lin, 2015) (Duin, Juszczak, Paclik, Pekalska, De Ridder, Tax, & Verzakov, 2000).

The regression modeling technique applies standard statistics to data to prove or disprove a hypothesis. One example of this is linear regression, in which variables are measured against a standard or target variable path over time. A second example is a logistic regression, where the probability of an event is predicted based on known values in correlation with the occurrence of prior similar events. The visualization technique builds multi-dimensional graphs to allow a data analyst to decipher trends, patterns, or relationships. The correlation technique identifies relationships between two or more variables in a data group. Variance analysis is a statistical technique to identify differences in mean values between a target or known variable and non-dependent variables or variable groups. The discriminate analysis is a classification technique used to identify or "discriminate" the factors leading to membership within a grouping. Forecasting techniques predict variable outcomes based on the known outcomes of past events. The cluster analysis technique reduces data instances to cluster groupings and then analyzes the attributes displayed by each group. Decision trees separate data based on sets of rules that can be described in the "if-then-else" language. Deep Neural Networks are data models that are meant to stimulate cognitive functions. These techniques "learn" with each iteration through the data, allowing for greater flexibility in the discovery of patterns and trends (Mishra, Chang, & Lin, 2014) (Simpson, 1992).

Extraction is the operation of extracting data from a source system for further use in a medical data warehouse environment. This is the first step of the ETL process. After the extraction, this data can be transformed and loaded into the medical data warehouse. The source systems for a medical data warehouse are typically transaction processing applications. For example, one of the source systems for a sales analysis medical data warehouse might be an order entry system that records all of the current order activities. Designing and creating the extraction process is often one of the most time-consuming tasks in the ETL process and, indeed, in the entire data warehousing process. The source systems might be very complex and poorly documented, and thus determining which data needs to be extracted can be difficult. The data has to be extracted normally not only once, but several times in a periodic manner to supply all changed data to the medical data warehouse and keep it up-to-date. Moreover, the source system typically cannot be modified, nor can its performance or availability be adjusted, to accommodate the needs of the medical data warehouse extraction process. These are important considerations for extraction and ETL in general (Mishra, Chang, & Lin, 2015) (Mishra, 2011) (Hepner, Logan, Ritter, & Bryant, 1990). This chapter, however, focuses on the technical considerations of having different kinds of sources and extraction methods. It assumes that the medical data warehouse team has already identified the data that will be extracted, and discusses common techniques used for extracting data from source databases. Designing this process means making decisions about the following two main aspects:

- Which extraction method do I choose?: This influences the source system, the transportation process, and the time needed for refreshing the warehouse.
- How do I provide the extracted data for further processing?: This influences the transportation method, and the need for cleaning and transforming the data.

The extraction method you should choose is highly dependent on the source system and also on the business needs in the target medical data warehouse environment. Very often, there is no possibility to add additional logic to the source systems to enhance an incremental extraction of data due to the performance or the increased workload of these systems. Sometimes even the customer is not allowed to add anything to an out-of-the-box application system. The estimated amount of the data to be extracted and the stage in the ETL process (initial load or maintenance of data) may also impact the decision of how to extract, it from a logical and a physical perspective. You have to decide how to extract data logically and physically (Mishra, Chang, & Lin, 2018) (Lippmann, 1989) (Mishra, 2017).

LOGICAL EXTRACTION METHODS

Full Extraction: The data is extracted completely from the source system. Because this extraction reflects all the data currently available on the source system, there's no need to keep track of changes to the data source since the last successful extraction. The source data will be provided as-is and no additional logical information (for example, timestamps) is necessary on the source site. An example of a full extraction may be an export file of a distinct table or a remote SQL statement scanning the complete source table. In the case of incremental extraction, At a specific point in time, only the data that has changed since a well-defined event back in history will be extracted. This event may be the last time of extraction or a more complex business event like the last booking day of a fiscal period. To identify this delta change there must be a possibility to identify all the changed information since this specific time event. This information can be either provided by the source data itself such as an application column, reflecting the last-changed timestamp, or a changing table where an appropriate additional mechanism keeps track of the changes besides the originating transactions. In most cases, using the latter method means adding extraction logic to the source system. Many medical data warehouses do not use any change-capture techniques as part of the extraction process. Instead, entire tables from the source systems are extracted to the medical data warehouse or staging area, and these tables are compared with a previous extract from the source system to identify the changed data. This approach may not have a significant impact on the source systems, but it clearly can place a considerable burden on the medical data warehouse processes, particularly if the data volumes are large (Huang, Wang, Tan, & Cui, 2004) (Patnaik & Mishra, 2016).

Physical Extraction Methods

Depending on the chosen logical extraction method and the capabilities and restrictions on the source side, the extracted data can be physically extracted by two mechanisms. In the case of online extraction, the data can either be extracted online from the source system or from an offline structure. Such an offline structure might already exist or it might be generated by an extraction routine. The data is extracted directly from the source system itself. The extraction process can connect directly to the source system to access the source tables themselves or to an intermediate system that stores the data in a preconfigured manner (for example, snapshot logs or change tables). Note that the intermediate system is not necessarily physically different from the source system. With online extractions, you need to consider whether the distributed transactions are using source objects or prepared source objects. In the case of offline extraction, the data is not extracted directly from the source system but is staged explicitly outside the source system. The data already has an existing structure (for example, redo logs, archive logs, or transportable tablespaces) or was created by an extraction routine. A key factor driving the evolution of the modern medical data warehouse is the cloud. So, it is called a cloud-based medical data warehouse (CBDW) or medical data warehouse as a cloud-based service. This CBDW creates access to near-infinite low-cost storage, improved scalability, outsourcing of DW management, and provides security to the cloud vendor. It has the potential to pay for only the storage and computing resources used. The CBDW brings data revolution & provides more people to access data-driven insights. The CBDW enables organizations to focus on what they want to achieve using software rather than on the management of that software and associated hardware (Chavent, 1998) (Hecht-Nielsen, 1992). The main motivation of CBDW is the instant availability of resources with minimal management and without any physical infrastructure at the enterprise level. Through instant availability, the DW application is available for use within hours or even seconds of when a customer purchases it, rather than in weeks or months. Hardware and DW software are also deployed, configured, and managed by the application provider as part of the service. The minimal management tells that users do not spend time worrying about how to patch, upgrade, scale, and optimize the DW software, because the software service does that automatically.

The service is ready to go at any time. There's no setup overhead and no need to spend time doing capacity planning, procuring and installing hardware, installing and configuring software, or any other prep work. Data is entered into the system with minimal worry. There's no time spent transforming data to get it into a form that the DW can handle. The focus is on what questions to ask about data. The service does not require manual tuning and configuration changes to deliver performance and efficiency.

It all just works, without interruptions. There's no need to worry about ongoing management of the system, data protection, security, or other concerns because these are handled by the service. It adapts dynamically and immediately to changes. The service monitors and observes the medical data warehouse and adapts, identifying and making optimizations based on how the service is being used (Heermann & Khazenie, 1992) (Cannas, Fanni, See, & Sias, 2006).

In CBDW, the business users interact with the integrated development environment through the business applications. The data security, backup and recovery, application hosting, and infrastructure scalability can be effectively maintained through the same integrated development environment by the cloud developers (Chang, Li, & Mishra, 2016) (Delen, Walker, & Kadam, 2005) (Chang, Liu, W., & Mishra, 2015).

David floyer in February 2016 analyzed the financial growth between TDW and CBDW across the business enterprises . Net Present Value (NPV) is the difference between the present value of cash inflows and the present value of cash outflows. The NPV in CBDW is three times more than the NPV in CBDW. IRR is the interest rate at which the net present value of all the cash flows. The IRR in CBDW is approximately seven times more than the IRR in TDW. Also, the break-even point (BEP) analysis states that if the enterprise implements a TDW, then after twenty-six months the enterprise starts gaining benefits by recovering the expanses that have been made during TDW setup and tuning, whereas in CBDW, only four months are required to meet the said expenses (Abbass, 2002) (Gabrys & Bargiela, 2000) (Wu, Giger, Doi, Vyborny, Schmidt, & Metz, 1993).

The analysis states that the overall financial growth of CBDW at the enterprise level is much higher than TDW as depicted in figure-1.

Data analytics, the extraction of hidden predictive information from large databases, is a powerful new technology with great potential to help companies focus on the most important information in their medical data warehouses. Data analytics tools predict future trends and behaviors, allowing businesses to make proactive, knowledge-driven decisions. The automated, prospective analyses offered by data analytics move beyond the analyses of past events provided by retrospective tools typical of decision support systems. Data analytics tools can answer business questions that traditionally were too time-consuming to resolve. They scour databases for hidden patterns, finding predictive information that experts may

Figure 1. financial growth rate analysis between TDW and CBDW

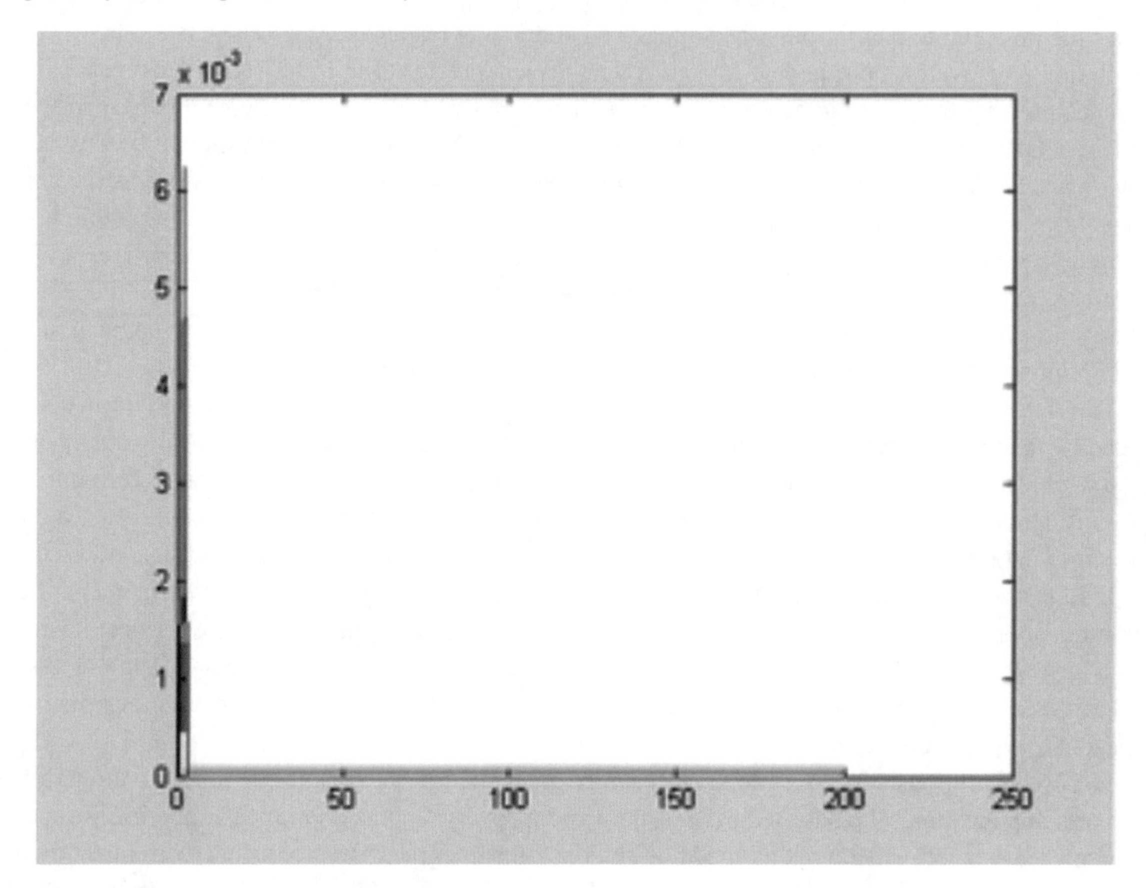

miss because it lies outside their expectations. The most impotent data analytics tool –NN to classify objects by learning nonlinearity. Classification is the process of finding a set of models (or functions) that describe and distinguish data classes or concepts to predict the class of an object whose class label is unknown. The derived model is based on the analysis of a set of training data (i.e. data objects whose class label is known (Gabrys & Bargiela, 2000).

DEEP NEURAL NETWORKS CLASSIFICATION

Artificial deep neural networks are relatively crude electronic networks of "neurons" based on the neural structure of the brain. The process records one at a time, and "learns" by comparing their classification of the record (which, at the outset, is largely arbitrary) with the known actual classification of the record. The errors from the initial classification of the first record are fed back into the network and used to modify the network's algorithm the second time around, and so on for many iterations. The input layer is composed not of full neurons but rather consists simply of the values in a data record, that constitutes inputs to the next layer of neurons. The next layer is called a hidden layer; there may be several hidden layers. The final layer is the output layer, where there is one node for each class. A single sweep forward through the network results in the assignment of a value to each output node, and the record is assigned to whichever class's node had the highest value. In the training phase, the correct class for each record is known (this is termed supervised training), and the output nodes can therefore be assigned "correct" values -- "1" for the node corresponding to the correct class, and "0" for the others. (In practice it has been found better to use values of 0.9 and 0.1, respectively.) It is thus possible to compare the network's calculated values for the output nodes to these "correct" values and calculate an error term for each node (the "Delta" rule). These error terms are then used to adjust the weights in the hidden layers so that, hopefully, the next time around the output values will be closer to the "correct" values. A key feature of deep Neural Networks is an iterative learning process in which data cases (rows) are presented to the network one at a time, and the weights associated with the input values are adjusted each time. After all, cases are presented, the process often starts over again. During this learning phase, the network learns by adjusting the weights to be able to predict the correct class label of input samples. Neural network learning is also referred to as "connectionist learning," due to the connections between the units. Advantages of deep neural networks include their high tolerance to noisy data, as well as their ability to classify patterns on which they have not been trained. The most popular neural network algorithm is the back-propagation algorithm proposed in the 1980s. Once a network has been structured for a particular application, that network is ready to be trained. To start this process, the initial weights (described in the next section) are chosen randomly. Then the training, or learning, begins. The network processes the records in the training data one at a time, using the weights and functions in the hidden layers, then compares the resulting outputs against the desired outputs. Errors are then propagated back through the system, causing the system to adjust the weights for application to the next record to be processed. This process occurs over and over as the weights are continually tweaked. During the training of a network, the same set of data is processed many times as the connection weights are continually refined. Note that some networks never learn. This could be because the input data do not contain the specific information from which the desired output is derived. Networks also don't converge if there is not enough data to enable complete learning. Ideally, there should be enough data so that part of the data can be held back as a validation set (Mishra, Chang, & Lin, 2014) (Hepner, Logan, Ritter, & Bryant, 1990) (Hecht-Nielsen, 1992).

PRACTICAL USAGE OF DEEP NEURAL NETWORKS

Solving the problem of classification is one of the most important implementations of neural networks. The problem of classification is tasks of ranging a pattern in one of several pairwise disjoint sets. Examples of these tasks can be the determination of a bank client's creditworthiness, medical tasks requiring estimation of a disease outcome, tasks of investment management (selling/buying shares or holding them back depending on the market situation), the task of working out viable companies and those susceptible to bankruptcy. Solving problems of classification requires ranging the available static patterns (parameters of the market situation, medical examination data, or information about a client) in certain classes. There can be several methods of data representation. The prevalent one is a method when a pattern is represented by a vector. Components of the vector represent various parameters of the pattern that influence the decision of assigning the pattern to a class. E.g., for medical tasks, the checkup data can serve as the vector components. Thus we have to determine a class where the pattern will be assigned according to the available information about it. The classifier, therefore, ranges the object in a class according to a certain decomposition of an N-dimensional space, which is called input space. The dimensionality of this space is the number of vector components. First of all, it is necessary to determine the complexity level of the system. In real tasks, the situation is very common when the number of patterns is limited and this complicates the evaluation of the task complexity. It is possible to specify three main levels of complexity. The first (the simplest one) is when classes can be separated by straight lines (or hyperplanes if the input space has more than two dimensions). This is so-called linear separability. In the second case, classes cannot be separated by lines (planes), but they can be separated with more complex divisions – nonlinear separability. In the third case, classes intersect and we can only speak of probabilistic separability. In an ideal model after preliminary processing, we must obtain a linearly separable problem, because after that construction of the classifier is significantly simpler. Unfortunately with real problems, we have a limited number of patterns to construct the classifier with. We cannot perform such a preliminary data processing that would result in the linear separability of the patterns (Mishra, Chang, & Lin, 2018) (Mishra, 2017) (Cannas, Fanni, See, & Sias, 2006).

Using deep Neural Networks as a classifier Feed-forward networks are a universal tool of function approximation, therefore they can be used for solving classification tasks. As a rule, deep Neural Networks are the most effective method of classification because they generate several regression models that are used when solving classification tasks by statistical methods. Unfortunately, there are several problems with using deep Neural Networks for real tasks. First, we don't know in advance a network what complexity (size) will be required to realize mapping accurately enough. This complexity may be too high and it will require the complicated architecture of networks. Minsky in his work «Perceptrons» has proved that the simplest single-layer deep Neural Networks can only solve linearly separable problems. This limitation can be overcome by the way of using multi-layer neural networks. Generally, we can say that a network with one hidden layer transforms a vector corresponding to an input pattern into a new space, which can differ in its dimensionality. After that hyperplanes corresponding to neurons of the output layer range it in classes. This way the network recognizes not the initial data characteristics but «the characteristics of characteristics» that are formed by the hidden layer. To construct a classifier it is necessary to determine what parameters influence a decision of ranging a pattern to this or that class. Two problems can arise. First, if the number of parameters is small the situation can develop when the same set of initial data corresponds to examples in different classes. It will be impossible to train the neural network then and the system will not work correctly (it is impossible to find the minimum corresponding to such an initial data set). Initial data must not be contradictive. To solve this problem it is necessary to increase the dimensionality of the attributes space (number of components of the input vector corresponding to the pattern). But after increasing the dimensionality of the attributes space we can face a situation when several attributes would not be enough for training the system and instead of generalization it will simply remember the training samples and will not function correctly. Thus when determining the attributes we have to find a compromise with their number. Further, it is necessary to find a method of representing input data for the neural network, i.e. determine a method of normalization. Normalization is required because deep Neural Networks only work with data represented by numbers in the range between 0 and 1 while input data can have an arbitrary range or can be non-numerical data at all. Various methods can be used, from simple linear transformation to the required range to multivariate analysis of parameters and non-linear normalization, depending on the cross-impact of the parameters (Wu, Giger, Doi, Vyborny, Schmidt, & Metz, 1993) (Salahuddin, Woodruff, Chatterjee, & Lambin, 2022).

Algorithm for Constructing a Classifier Based on the Deep Neural Network

1. Work with the data. Form a database with samples typical for the given task.
2. Decompose the whole set of data into two sets: training and testing sets (decomposition in three sets is also possible: training, testing, and confirmation sets).

Preliminary Processing

1. Select a system of attributes typical for the task and appropriately transform the data for feeding to the network input (normalization, standardization, etc.) It is desirable to obtain linearly separable space of the patterns set.
2. Select a system for coding the output values (classical coding, 2 by 2 coding, etc.)

Constructing, Training, and Evaluating the Network Quality

1. Select the network topology: number of layers, number of neurons in layers, etc.
2. Select a function of neuron activation (e.g., «sigmoid')
3. Select an algorithm for training the system.
4. Evaluate the quality of the network functioning, based on confirmation sets or other criteria. Optimize the architecture (decrease weights, reducing the dimensionality of the attributes space).
5. Settle on the variant of the network that provides the best ability to generalize. Evaluate the quality using the testing set.

Usage and Diagnostics

1. Find out the levels of various factors that influence the decision (heuristic approach).
2. Make sure the network provides the necessary accuracy of classification (the number of incorrectly recognized samples is low).
3. If necessary return to step 2 after changing the method of samples representation or database.
4. Proceed to practical usage of the network for solving the problem.

To construct a high-quality classifier one has to have high-quality data. No method of classifier construction, whether based on deep Neural Networks or a statistical one, will result in a classifier good enough if the given set of examples is not full and representative of the problem that the system would have to work with.

Sometimes we are faced with the problem of delayed reward: rather than being told the correct answer for each input pattern immediately, we may only occasionally get a positive or negative reinforcement signal to tell us whether the entire sequence of actions leading up to this was good or bad. Reinforcement learning provides ways to get a continuous error signal in such situations.

Q-learning associates an expected utility (the Q-value) with each action possible in a particular state. If at time t we are in state s(t) and decide to act a(t), the corresponding Q-value is updated as follows:

where r(t) is the **instantaneous reward** resulting from our action, s(t+1) is the state that it led to, a are all possible actions in that state, and gamma <= 1 is a **discount factor** that leads us to prefer instantaneous over delayed rewards. A common way to implement Q-learning for small problems is to maintain a table of Q-values for all possible state/action pairs. For large problems, however, it is often impossible to keep such a large table in memory, let alone learn its entries in a reasonable time. In such cases, a neural network can provide a compact approximation of the Q-value function. Such a network takes the state s(t) as its input and has an output y_a for each possible action. To learn the Q-value Q(s(t), a(t)), it uses the right-hand side of the above Q-iteration as a target:

$$\delta_{a(t)} = r(t) + \gamma \max_a y_a - y_a(t) \quad (1)$$

Note that since we require the network's outputs at time t+1 to calculate its error signal at time t, we must keep a one-step memory of all input and hidden node activity, as well as the most recent action. The error signal is applied only to the output corresponding to that action; all other output nodes receive no error (they are "don't cares"). Several methods for inductive learning have been developed under the common label *"Machine Learning*". All these methods use a set of samples to generate an approximation of the underlying function that generated the data. The aim is to draw Conclusions from these samples in such a way that when unseen data are presented to a model it is possible to infer the *to-be explained variable* from these data. The methods we discuss here are the Deep Neural Networks Techniques. These methods have been applied to prediction; particularly for Deep Neural Networks are used in pattern recognition and classification. A neural network may be considered as a data processing technique that maps, or relates, some type of input stream of information to an output stream of data deep Neural Networks (NNs) can be used to perform *classification. A*ny function can be approximated to arbitrary accuracy by a neural network [**9**]. NNs consist of *neurons* (or *node*s) distributed across *layer*s. The way these neurons are distributed and the way they are linked with each other define the *structure of the networ*k. Each of the links between the neurons is characterized by a *weight* value. A *neuron* is a processing unit that takes several inputs and gives a distinct output. Apart from the number of its inputs, it is characterized by a function *f* known as the *transfer functio*n. The most commonly used transfer functions are the *hard limi*t, the *pure linea*r, the *sigmoid,* and the *sigmoid* functions (Genzel, Macdonald, & Marz, 2022) (Williamson, Wang, Khandwala, Scheler, & Vagal, 2022).

DATA DESCRIPTION AND CASE SCENARIO ANALYSIS

- Breast Cancer Dataset

Each instance has one of 2 possible classes: benign or malignant

Size of data set: only 699 instances (at that point of time) trained on 420 instances, tested on the other 279.

Number of Attributes: 10 plus the class attribute. Attribute Information: (class attribute has been moved to the last column)

Collected classification results averaged over 10 trials

Best accuracy result: -- 93.7%

Table 1.

# Attribute	Domain
1. Sample code number	id number
2. Clump Thickness	1 - 10
3. Uniformity of Cell Size	1 – 10
4. Uniformity of Cell Shape	1 – 10
5. Marginal Adhesion	1 – 10
6. Single Epithelial Cell Size	1 – 10
7. Bare Nuclei	1 – 10
8. Bland Chromatin	1 – 10
9. Normal Nucleoli	1 – 10
10. Mitoses	1 – 10
11. Class	(2 for benign, 4 for malignant)

- Iris Dataset

This is perhaps the best-known database to be found in the pattern recognition literature. Fisher's paper is a classic in the field and is referenced frequently to this day. (See Duda & Hart, for example.) The data set contains 3 classes of 50 instances each, where each class refers to a type of iris plant. One class is linearly separable from the other 2; the latter are NOT linearly separable from each other. Predicted attribute: class of iris plant. This is an exceedingly simple domain.

Number of Instances: 150 (50 in each of three classes)
Number of Attributes: 4 numeric, predictive attributes and the class

7. Attribute Information:
   1. sepal length in cm
   2. sepal width in cm
   3. petal length in cm
   4. petal width in cm
   5. class:
      -- Iris Setosa
      -- Iris Versicolour
      -- Iris Virginica
   6. Missing Attribute Values: None

Summary Statistics:
   9. Class Distribution: 33.3% for each of the 3 classes.
   Iris-setosa, Iris-versicolor,Iris-virginica.

Table 2.

	Min	Max	Mean	SD	Class Correlation
Sepal length	4.3	7.9	5.84	0.83	0.7826
Sepal width	2.0	4.4	3.05	0.43	0.4194
Petal length	1.0	6.9	3.76	1.76	0.9490 (high!)
Petal width	0.1	2.5	1.20	0.76	0.9565 (high!)

- Diabetes Dataset
    - Each instance has one of 2 possible classes: numeric
    - Size of data set: only 768 instances (at that point of time)
    - trained on 462 instances, tested on the other 306.
    - Number of Attributes: 8 plus the class attribute. Attribute Information: (class attribute has been moved to the last column)

Today's real-world databases are highly susceptible to noisy, missing, and inconsistent data. "How can the data be preprocessed to improve the quality of the data and consequently, of the mining result ". There are several data preprocessing techniques we can use to obtain the cleaned and confirmed dataset. We divide the datasets into subsets. These subsets form two major categories, sets that will be used to define the parameters of the models and sets that will be used to measure their prediction ability. The deep Neural Networks are adjusted(trained) on a part of the available data and tested on another part. Again we will use Set B to adjust the parameters of the models and Set C to measure their prediction ability. This way we will be able to make comparisons of the performance of both types of models on the same dataset. In this study, we will use the term 'Training set' for Set B and 'Test set' for Set C. additionally, due to the nature of the parameters adjustment of the neural network models we need to divide the training set (set B) into three new subset.

MODELS INVESTIGATIONS

All the data used to train and test the NNs were normalized to be in the interval [0.0,1.0] or [-1.0, +1.0]. The training algorithm is Backpropagation. **B**ackpropagation provides computationally efficient methods for changing the weights in a feed-forward network with differentiable activation function units to learn a training set of input-output examples. The total squared error of the o/p computed by the net is minimized by a gradient descent method known as BPR or generalized delta rule. This output is compared with the target value of the sample and the weights of the network are adjusted in a way that a metric that describes the distance between outputs and targets is minimized. There are two major categories of network training *incremental* and *batch* training. During the *incremental* training, the weights of the network are adjusted each time that each one of the input samples is presented to the network, while in *batch* mode training the weights are adjusted only when all the training samples have been presented to the network (Chang, Mishra, & Lin, 2015). The number of times that the training set will be fed to the network is called the *number of epochs*. Issues that arise and are related to the training of a network are: what exactly is the mechanism by which weights are updated when does this iterative procedure cease, and which metric is to be used to calculate the distance between targets and outputs? Answers to these questions are given in the next paragraphs. The *error function* or the *cost function* is used to measure the distance between the targets and the outputs of the network. The weights of the network are updated in the direction that makes the error function minimum. The most common error functions are the *mse* (mean square error) and the *mae* (mean absolute error). In our case study the networks we will be trained and tested using the *mse* function. The mechanism of weight update is known as the *training algorith*m. There are several training algorithms proposed in the literature. We will give a brief description of those that are related to the purposes of our project study. The algorithms described here are related to *feed-forward* networks. A NN is characterized as a *feed-forward* network "if it is possible to attach successive numbers to the inputs and to all of the hidden and output units such that each unit only receives connections from inputs or units having a smaller number" (Tewari, Yousefi, & Webb, 2022) . All these algorithms use the gradient of the *cost function* to determine how to adjust the weights to minimize the *cost functio*n. The gradient is determined using a technique called backpropagation, which involves performing computations backward through the network. Then the weights are adjusted in the direction of the negative gradient.

The power of NN models lies in the way that their *weights* (inter-unit-connection strengths) are adjusted. The procedure of adjusting the weights of a NN based on a specific dataset is referred to as the training of the network on that set *(training se*t). The basic idea behind training is that the network will be adjusted in a way that will be able to learn the patterns that lie in the *training se*t. Using the adjusted network in future situations (unseen data) will be able based on the patterns that learned to generalize giving us the ability to make inferences. In our case, we will train NN models on a part of our time series *(training se*t) and we will measure their ability to generalize on the remaining part *(test se*t). The size of the test set is usually selected to be 40% of the available samples (Chang, Mishra, & Lin, 2015). The way that a network is trained is depicted by the plotted m- figure. Each sample consists of two parts the input and the target part *(supervised learnin*g). Initially, the weights of the network are assigned random values (usually within [-1 1]). Then the input part of the first sample is presented to the network. The network computes an output based on: the values of its weights, the number of its layers, and the type and mass of neurons per layer.

Larger the learning rate the bigger the step. If the learning rate is made too large the algorithm will become unstable and will not converge to the minimum of the error function. If the learning rate is set too small, the algorithm will take a long time to converge. Methods suggested for adopting the learning rate are as follows.

1. start with a high learning rate and steadily decrease it. Changes in the weight vector must be small to reduce oscillations or any divergence.
2. A simple suggestion is to increase the learning rate to improve performance and to decrease the learning rate to worsen the performance.

A significant decision related to the training of a NN is the time at which its weight adjustment will be ceased. As we have explained so far over-trained networks become over-fitted to the training set and they are useless in generalizing and inferring from unseen data. While under-trained networks do not manage to learn all the patterns in the underlying data and due to this reason underperform on unseen data. Therefore there is a tradeoff between over-training and under-training our networks. The methodology that is used to overcome this problem is called *validation* of the trained network. Apart from the *training set* a second set, the *validation se*t, which contains the same number of samples is used. The weights of the network are adjusted using the samples in the *training set* only. Each time that the weights of the network are adjusted its performance (in terms of error function) is measured on the *validation* set. During the initial period of training, both the errors on *training* and *validation* sets are decreased. This is because the network starts to learn the patterns that exist in the data. From several iterations of the training algorithm and beyond the network will start to overfit the training set. If this is the case, the error in the validation set will start to rise. In the case that this divergence continues for several iterations, the training is ceased. The output of this procedure would be a not overfitted network. After describing the way that a NN works and the parameters that are related to its performance we select these parameters in a way that will allow us to achieve optimum performance in the task we are aiming to accomplish. The methodology will follow to define these parameters is described in the next paragraph (Tewari, Yousefi, & Webb, 2022)(Rahman & Subashini, 2022).

One of the major advantages of neural nets is their ability to generalize. This means that a trained net could classify data from the same class as the learning data that it has never seen before. In real-world applications, developers normally have only a small part of all possible patterns for the generation of a neural net. To reach the best generalization, the dataset should be split into three parts:

- The **training set** is used to train a neural net. The error of this dataset is minimized during training.
- The **validation set** is used to determine the performance of a deep neural network on patterns that are not trained during learning.
- A **test set** for finally checking the overall performance of a neural net.

EXPERIMENTS AND VISUAL ANALYSIS

We have proved that IRIS & Breast cancer datasets do not fluctuate randomly. In this chapter, we describe the experiment we undertook to identify the patterns. We also report the result we obtained along with the parameters used to obtain them. We have used different neural network models with variable size hidden units using different activation functions to select the best model and its performance was evaluated on testing data set by giving results in tabular form.

- On iris dataset
  %60 training set
  %40 testing set
  Function: Hyperbolic tangent (tanh)
  Sample: Random

Figures 2-9 depict the numerous scenarios of deep NN implementations on the various medical datasets. The figure-2 identifies the number of pattern clusters in the IRIS dataset. In figure-3, an actual cluster pattern analysis is made based on the breast cancer dataset. IRIS & Breast cancer datasets do not fluctuate randomly. In this work, we discuss the experiment for identifying the patterns. The reports of the results are implemented and analyzed. Different deep neural network models are used with variable size hidden units using different activation functions to select the best model and its performance was evaluated on the testing data set.

Table 3. Classifications accuracy analysis on IRIS based on NN1, NN2, and NN3

Alpha	Model	Epoch	Time	Structure	Accuracy
0.1	NN1	1000	20.485s	4--3	20%
0.06	NN1	1000	21.345s	4--3	30%
0.1	NN2	300	5.81s	4--5--3	40%
0.06	NN2	500	8.251s	4--5--3	80%
0.1	NN3	250	3.900s	4-4-2-3	99.9
0.06	NN3	6000	80.600s	4-6-5-3	99.984

Graph plotting On Iris Dataset f=tanh alpha=0.1 NN:4-2-2-3, e^4
Normalized data: min-max

Figure 2. NN:4-3-3-3, f=tanh, e^4 normalised data by std. dev.

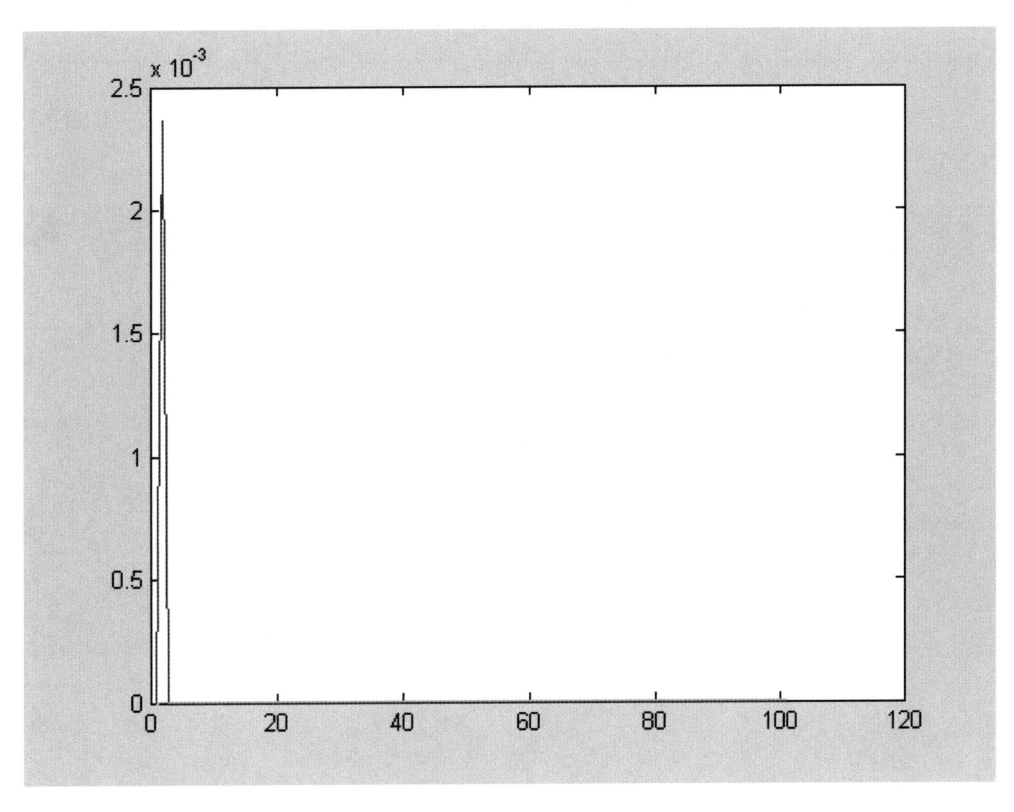

CONCLUSION AND FUTURE WORKS

The success of neural network architecture depends heavily on the availability of effective learning algorithms. The theoretical strength of the "Backpropagation neural network" is yet to be used in hundreds of technologies and the more accurate result may lead if a bigger the database size, if more no. of dimensions involved, if more correct data without noise and out layer, and if the data provided by multiple agencies. The neuro-fuzzy approach has considerable industrial applicability due to its high embedding compatibility with heterogeneous microcontroller devices. The de-fuzzification process provides a method of extracting a crisp value from the fuzzy quantifiers as approximate representative values. Machine learning technics are implemented in many areas of knowledge discovery and semantic knowledge analytics to explore application intelligence. The different frameworks and algorithms are designed and explored for knowledge discovery, representation, semantic analytics, and inferences. The real-world applications are modeled through smart architectures, algorithms, and frameworks to accomplish the knowledge analytics tasks. Having in mind the finding of our study we resulted in the following conclusion & comment: The success of deep neural network architecture depends heavily on the availability of effective learning algorithms. The use of single agency data makes it difficult for the model to recognize trends and patterns that exist in the data. In this research, a discussion is prepared on the overall aspects of traditional and cloud-based data warehousing systems. There is a rapid invocation of cloud-based medical data warehouses across many business enterprises due to high financial growth as compared to the traditional medical data warehouse. In a cloud-based medical data warehouse, many new technologies will be progressively integrated to handle the disparate data sources that consist of sensor data, IoT data, RFID data, business data, social sensing data, smart dust data, and other computing data.

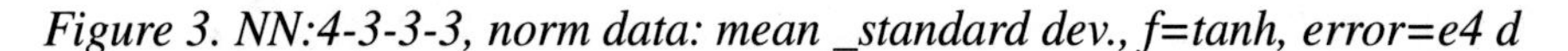

Figure 3. NN:4-3-3-3, norm data: mean _standard dev., f=tanh, error=e4 d

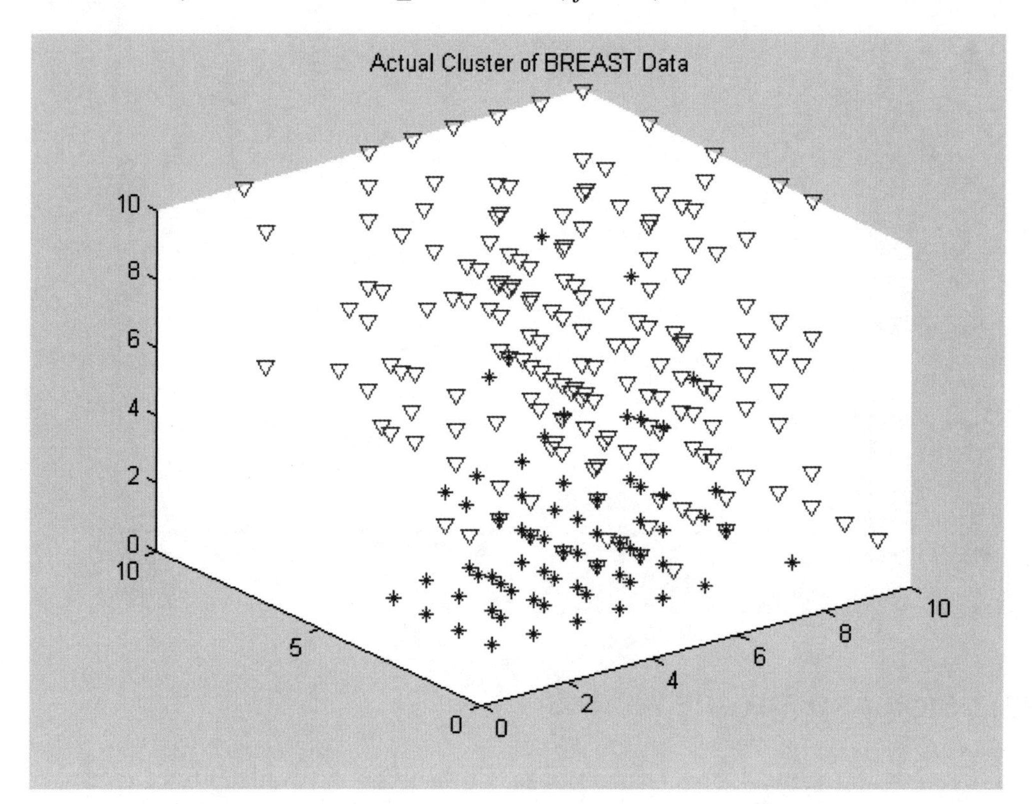

Figure 4. result of sigmoid:(by std and max value) using sigmoid function on normalisediris data, alpha=0.05

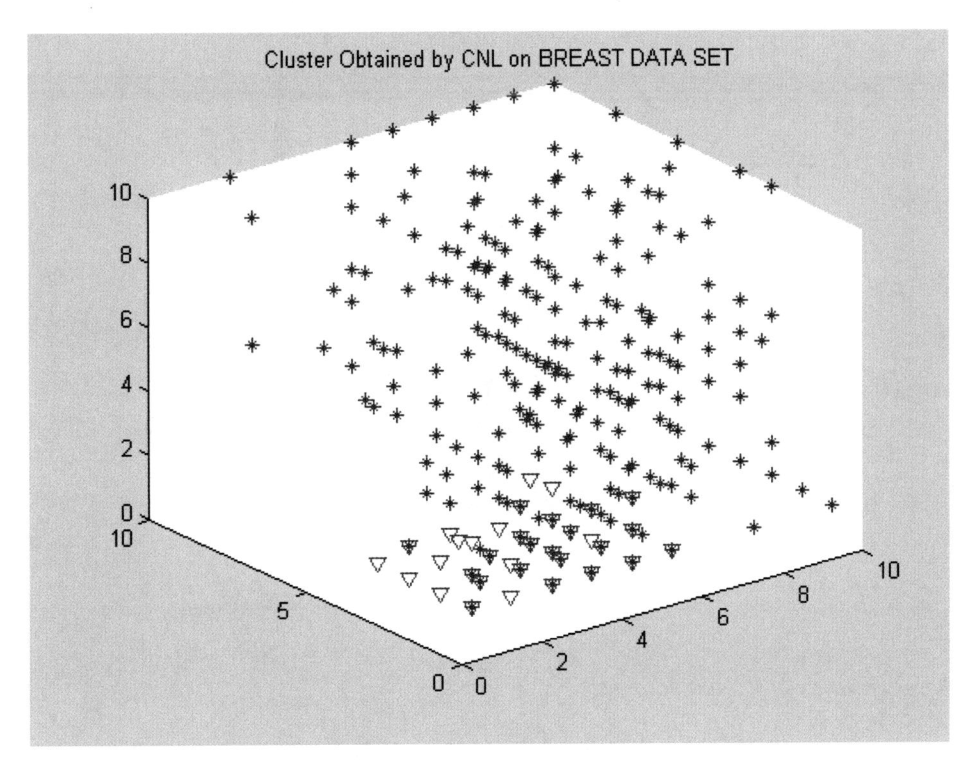

Figure 5. Cluster obtained on IRIS by the convolution NN

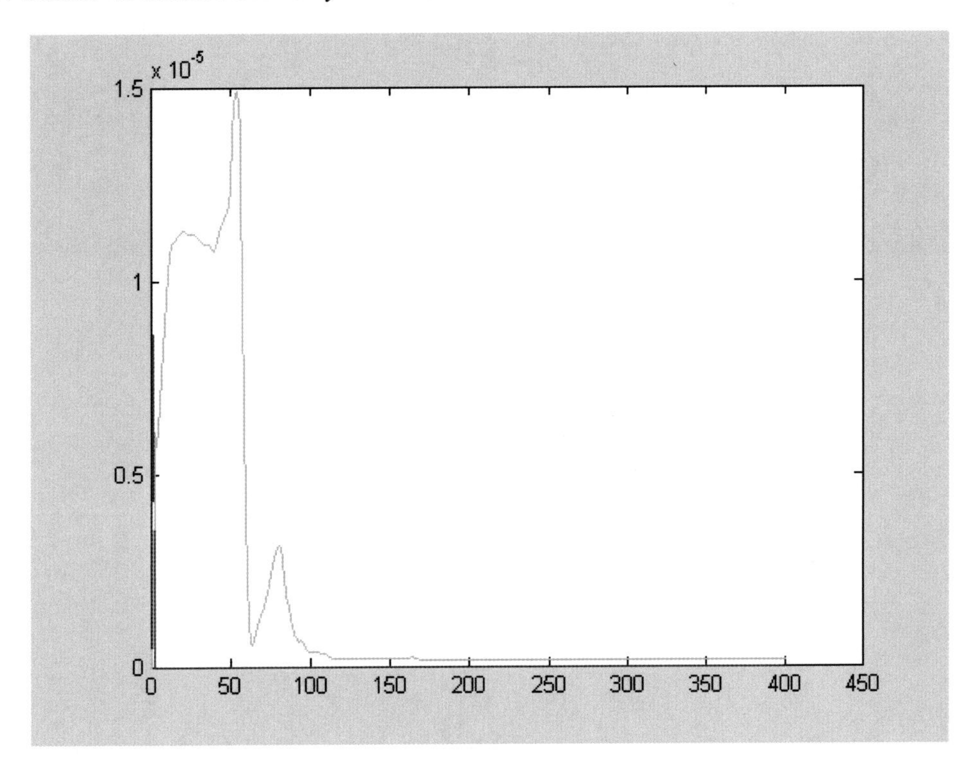

Figure 6. Plots and graph:Norm_breast(frequent data –1) error-e4, hyperbolic tangent func

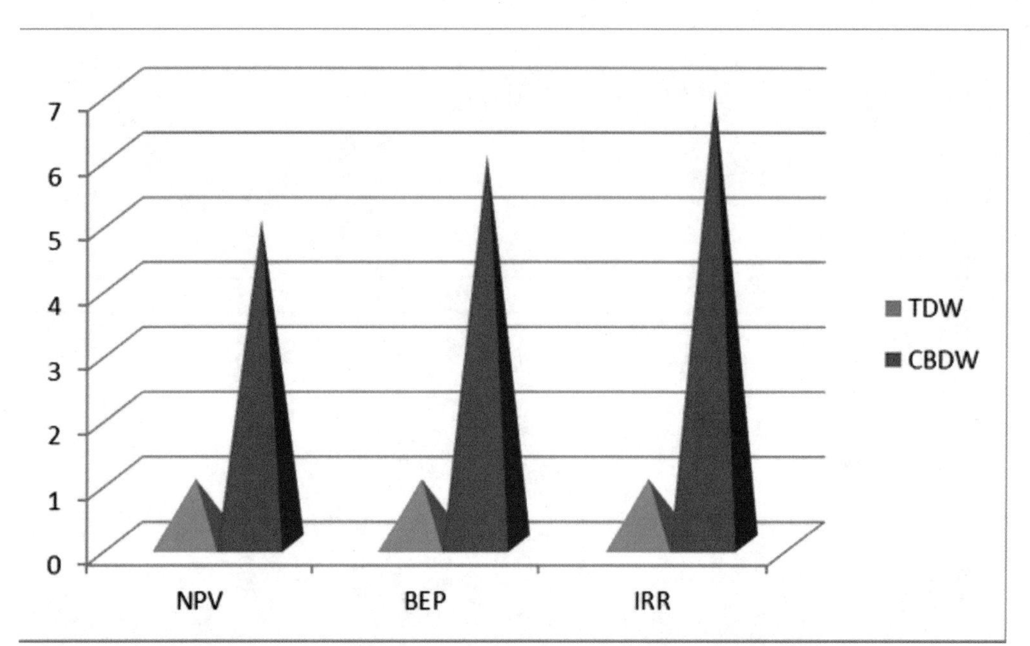

Figure 7. Actual cluster of Breast dataset

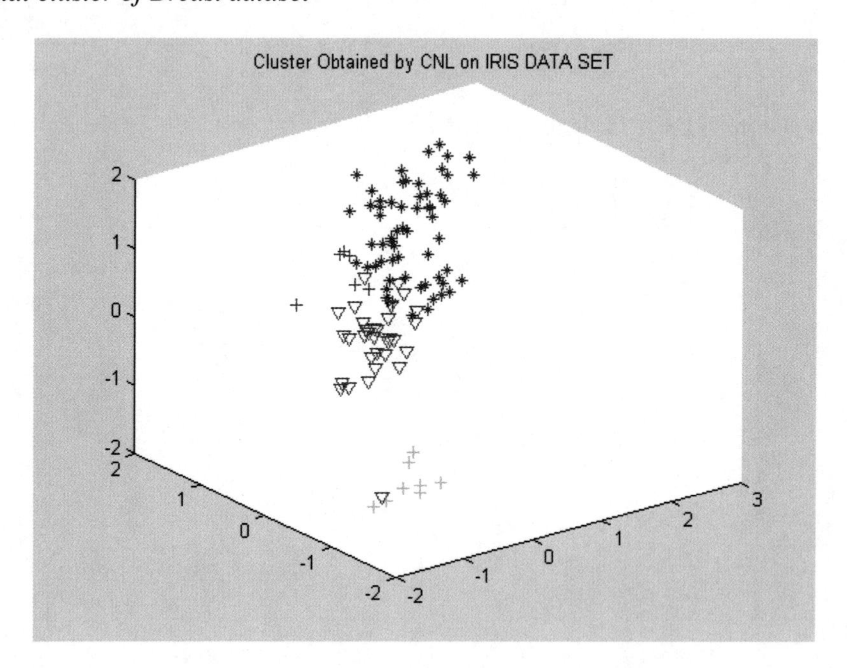

Figure 8. Clusters obtained by deep NN

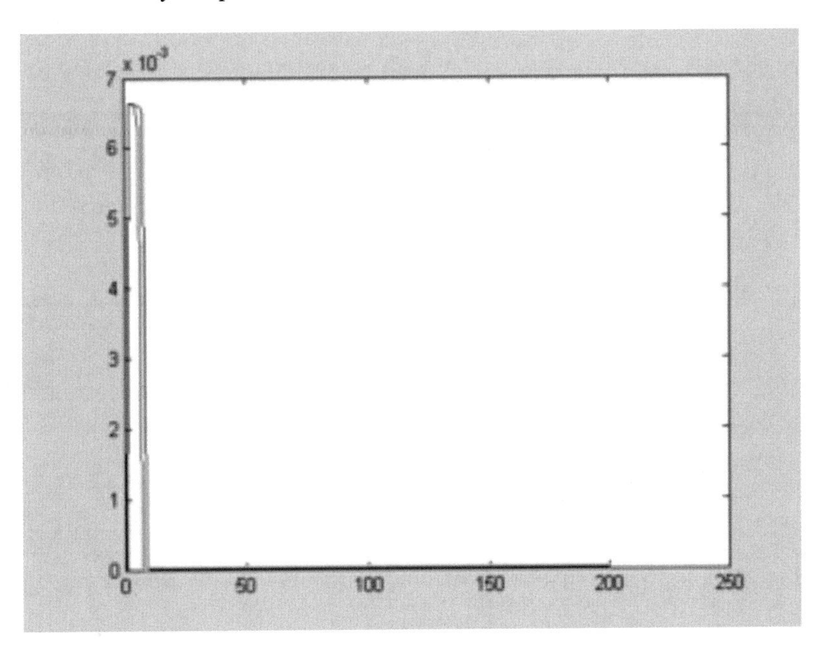

Figure 9. Hyperbolic tangent function, error e2

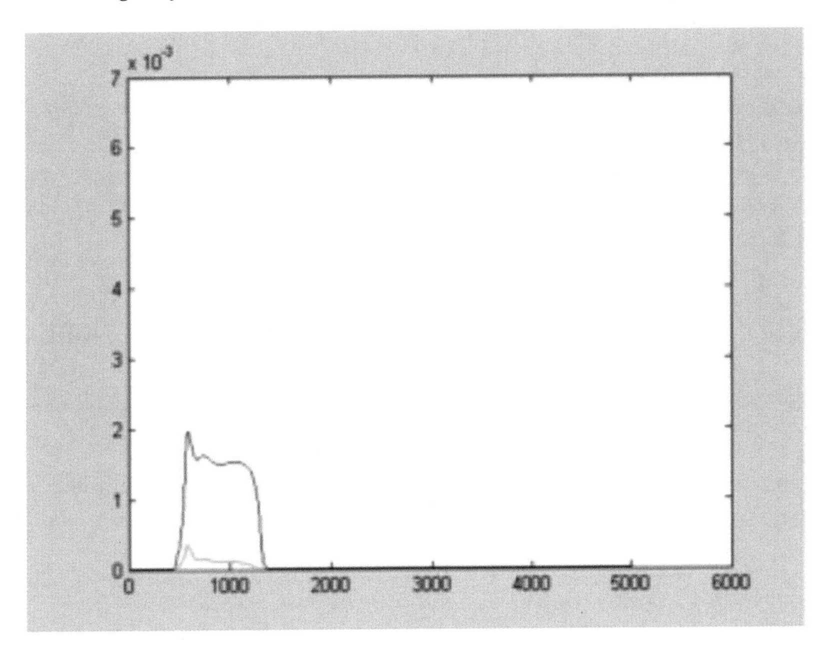

REFERENCES

Abbass, H. A. (2002). An evolutionary artificial deep Neural Networks approach for breast cancer diagnosis. *Artificial Intelligence in Medicine*, *25*(3), 265–281.

Cannas, B., Fanni, A., See, L., & Sias, G. (2006). Data preprocessing for river flow forecasting using neural networks: Wavelet transforms and data partitioning. *Physics and Chemistry of the Earth Parts A/B/C*, *31*(18), 1164–1171.

Chang, H. T., Li, Y. W., & Mishra, N. (2016). mCAF: A multi-dimensional clustering algorithm for friends of social network services. *SpringerPlus*, *5*(1), 757.

Chang, H. T., Liu, S. W., & Mishra, N. (2015). A tracking and summarization system for online Chinese news topics. *Aslib Journal of Information Management*, *67*(6), 687–699.

Chang, H. T., Mishra, N., & Lin, C. C. (2015). IoT Big-Data Centred Knowledge Granule Analytic and Cluster System for BI Applications: A Case Base Analysis. *PLoS One*, *10*(11), e0141980.

Chavent, M. (1998). A monothetic clustering method. *Pattern Recognition Letters*, *19*(11), 989–996.

Delen, D., Walker, G., & Kadam, A. (2005). Predicting breast cancer survivability: A comparison of three data analytics methods. *Artificial Intelligence in Medicine*, *34*(2), 113–127.

Demuth, H., & Beale, M. (1993). Neural Network Toolbox for Use with Matlab--User'S Guide Version 3.0. Matlab.

Demuth, H., & Beale, M. (2000). *Neural network toolbox: for use with Matlab: computation, visualization, programming: User's guide, version 4*. The Mathworks.

Duin, R. P. W., Juszczak, P., Paclik, P., Pekalska, E., De Ridder, D., Tax, D. M. J., & Verzakov, S. (2000). A Matlab toolbox for pattern recognition. *PRTools version, 3*, 109-111.

Gabrys, B., & Bargiela, A. (2000). General fuzzy min-max neural network for clustering and classification. *IEEE Transactions on Neural Networks*, *11*(3), 769–783. doi:10.1109/72.846747 PMID:18249803

Gabrys, B., & Bargiela, A. (2000). General fuzzy min-max neural network for clustering and classification. *IEEE Transactions on Neural Networks*, *11*(3), 769–783.

Genzel, M., Macdonald, J., & Marz, M. (2022). Solving inverse problems with deep neural networks-robustness included. *IEEE Transactions on Pattern Analysis and Machine Intelligence*.

Hagan, M. T., Demuth, H. B., & Beale, M. H. (1996). *Neural network design* (Vol. 20). Pws Pub.

Hecht-Nielsen, R. (1992). Theory of the backpropagation neural network. In Deep Neural Networks for perception (pp. 65-93).

Heermann, P. D., & Khazenie, N. (1992). Classification of multispectral remote sensing data using a back-propagation neural network. *IEEE Transactions on Geoscience and Remote Sensing*, *30*(1), 81–88.

Hepner, G., Logan, T., Ritter, N., & Bryant, N. (1990). Artificial neural network classification using a minimal training set- Comparison to conventional supervised classification. *Photogrammetric Engineering and Remote Sensing*, *56*(4), 469–473.

Huang, J., Wang, Y., Tan, T., & Cui, J. (2004, August). A new iris segmentation method for recognition. In *Proceedings of the 17th International Conference on Pattern Recognition*, (Vol. 3, pp. 554-557). IEEE.

Lippmann, R. P. (1989). Pattern classification using neural networks. *IEEE Communications Magazine*, *27*(11), 47–50.

Mishra, N. (2011). A Framework for associated pattern mining over Microarray database. *International Journal of Global Research in Computer Science*, *2*(2).

Mishra, N. (2017). In-network Distributed Analytics on Data-centric IoT Network for BI-service Applications. *International Journal of Scientific Research in Computer Science, Engineering and Information Technology (IJSRCSEIT), 2*(5), pp.547-552.

Mishra, N., Chang, H. T., & Lin, C. C. (2014). Data-centric knowledge discovery strategy for a safety-critical sensor application. *International Journal of Antennas and Propagation*, 2014.

Mishra, N., Chang, H. T., & Lin, C. C. (2015). An IoT knowledge reengineering framework for semantic knowledge analytics for BI-services. *Mathematical Problems in Engineering*, 2015.

Mishra, N., Chang, H. T., & Lin, C. C. (2018). Sensor data distribution and knowledge inference framework for a cognitive-based distributed storage sink environment. *International Journal of Sensor Networks*, *26*(1), 26–42.

Mishra, N., Lin, C. C., & Chang, H. T. (2014). Cognitive inference device for activity supervision in the elderly. *The Scientific World Journal*, 2014.

Mishra, N., Lin, C. C., & Chang, H. T. (2014, December). A cognitive-oriented framework for IoT big-data management perspective. In *International Conference on Communication Problem-Solving (ICCP),* (pp. 124-127). IEEE.

Mishra, N., Lin, C. C., & Chang, H. T. (2015). A cognitive adopted framework for IoT big-data management and knowledge discovery perspective. *International Journal of Distributed Sensor Networks*, *11*(10), 718390.

Mujeeb Rahman, K. K., & Subashini, M. M. (2022). Identification of Autism in Children Using Static Facial Features and Deep Neural Networks. *Brain Sciences*, *12*(1), 94.

Nørgård, P. M. (1997). *The Neural Network Based System Identification Toolbox: For use with MATLAB.* Matlab.

Patnaik, B. C., & Mishra, N. (2016). A Review on Enhancing the Journaling File System. *Imperial Journal of Interdisciplinary Research, 2*(11).

Salahuddin, Z., Woodruff, H. C., Chatterjee, A., & Lambin, P. (2022). Transparency of deep neural networks for medical image analysis: A review of interpretability methods. *Computers in Biology and Medicine*, *140*, 105111.

Simpson, P. K. (1992). Fuzzy min-max neural networks. I. Classification. *IEEE Transactions on Neural Networks*, *3*(5), 776–786.

Tewari, S., Yousefi, S., & Webb, A. G. (2022). Deep neural network-based optimization for the design of a multi-element surface magnet for MRI applications. *Inverse Problems*.

Williamson, B. J., Wang, D., Khandwala, V., Scheler, J., & Vagal, A. (2022). Improving Deep Neural Network Interpretation for Neuroimaging Using Multivariate Modeling. *SN Computer Science*, *3*(2), 1–8.

Wu, Y., Giger, M. L., Doi, K., Vyborny, C. J., Schmidt, R. A., & Metz, C. E. (1993). Artificial deep Neural Networks in mammography: Application to decision making in the diagnosis of breast cancer. *Radiology*, *187*(1), 81–87.

Chapter 14
Smart System Engineering–Digital Twin

Ambika N.
https://orcid.org/0000-0003-4452-5514
St.Francis College, India

ABSTRACT

The pragmatic model works in an open ecosystem with entrance to GPS knowledge. The proposal has four phases. Tier 1 is the legendary implicit model produced during upfront architecture. It maintains decision-making at the idea conception and preparatory study. Tier 2 is a digital counterpart. It is proficient in including enforcement, wellness, and livelihood data from the mechanical twin. It is an instantiation of the universal arrangement. It introduces group updates and maintains high-level determination. It creates the conceptual scheme, technology blueprint, preceding scheme, and construction. It has the vehicle interface library of the Modelica device. It has a vehicle with a power split. The chassis prototype has a single stage with mass-and speed-dependent resistance features. Tier 3 is the adaptive digital twin. Tier 4 has unsupervised automation ability. The approach improves the system by 7.75% in user experience and 40.6% in performance using the recommendation library compared to the previous contribution.

INTRODUCTION

A computerized twin (Tao, Liu, Hu, & Nee, 2020) (Chaudhary, Khari, & Elhoseny, 2021) is a powerful advanced portrayal of the original framework. The vision of the identical buzzes for joining a corporation, logical, and detector information from original frameworks into the digital framework representative of the advanced matching to work with the investigation, evade issues, and foster informed innovation roadmaps. It incorporates the virtual and actual universes. The computerized alike empowers the ongoing checking of frameworks and cycles. It is an ideal examination of information to head-off issues before they emerge, plan preventive support to diminish/forestall vacations, reveal new business open doors, and plan for future updates. It requires an actual match for information securing and setting-driven collaboration. The computerized alike comprise associated items. The advanced string gives the network all

DOI: 10.4018/978-1-6684-5925-6.ch014

Figure 1. Conceptual view of digital twin (Stojanovic, et al., 2021)

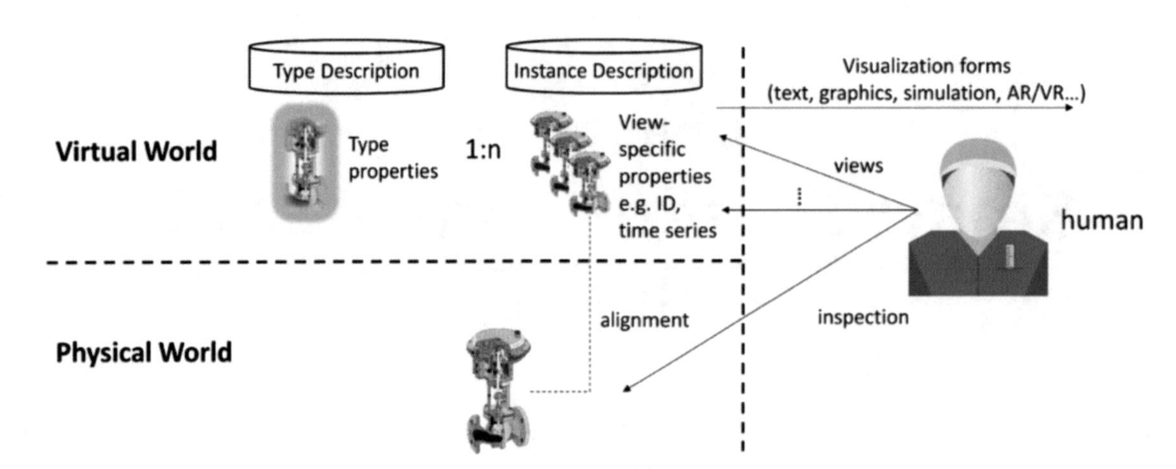

through the framework's lifecycle and gathers information from the actual match to refresh the prototypes in the computerized twin. Figure 1 is the notional view of the digital twin.

Computerized Twin (Farsi, Daneshkhah, Hosseinian-Far, & Jahankhani, 2020) is its capacity to test. It tries different things and thinks of items under various circumstances and utilization conditions. It decreases the need to continuously assemble costly models and mockups, consequently offering massive expense reserve funds during item advancement and testing. The Digital Twin idea is for enormous frameworks like Smart Cities, Aircraft, and huge Buildings, to practically convey virtual frameworks over various handling necessities. These can fill the framework and subpart in a few different registering conditions. The subpart could have sufficient handling ability to identify blunders, gain new data, and even decide how to work on every piece of the framework by anticipating its way of behaving under upsetting circumstances.

In each stage, apparatuses and capacities execute the cycles. The instruments make recordings in different phases. The simulation in the Creation stage may pick some item choices. It recreates some way of behaving of the item. In the Operations stage, it checks and foresees some breaking down. The intelligent entity addresses the digital twin in the design stage. When the item and its advanced partner are out of the Configuration stage, the Production deliberately ease relates models and their product portrayal to test and try different things with the future item. The product parts help in streamlining the actual item. It requires mockups in later stages. The system establishes a connection between the intelligent article and the things in the operation stage.

The pragmatic model (Madni, Madni, & Lucero, 2019) is a vibrant digital description of a physical arrangement. It is a practical occurrence of arrangement updates continuously having representation, preservation, and wellness situation information throughout the physical system's growth sequence. It has the potential to decrease the price of method verifying and experimenting. It provides new penetrations into practice performance. It consists of relevant outcomes utilizing the IoT (Ambika N., 2020) and a digital thread. It provides a connection. The physical situation includes the physical arrangement, visible detectors, and connection interfaces. It works in an open ecosystem with entrance to GPS knowledge. The proposal has four phases. Tier 1 is the legendary implicit model produced in open architecture. It maintains conclusion-making at the idea conception and preparatory study. The pragmatic model is a universal executable arrangement representation of the envisioned method. It is before the mechanical archetype is composed. Tier 2 is a digital counterpart in which the pragmatic composition. It is proficient in including enforcement, wellness, and livelihood data. It is an instantiation of the universal arrangement. It introduces group updates and maintains high-level determination. It creates the conceptual scheme, technology blueprint, preceding scheme, and construction. It has the automobile medium collection of the Modelica device. It has a vehicle with an energy division. The skeleton prototype has a single stage with mass-and speed-dependent resistance features. It uses the brake-lever situation. It emerges from operator performance to measure brake revolution.

The driveline pattern has four engines with a front-wheel approach. The potential separation equipment consists of typical epicyclic tools without impairments. A prototypical battery with a continuous energy reservoir controls the DC machine design with an inductor, resistor, and emf element attached to the shaft core. The motor representation with a flywheel consists of the drive-by-wire accelerator, where the accelerator intakes transform to yield torque. Tier 3 is the Adaptive Digital alike. It proposes an adaptive worker medium to the mechanical and digital counterparts. Tier 4 has the unsupervised automated ability. It has discerned objectives and models engaged in operational circumstances and reinforced knowledge of arrangement and conditions.

The suggestion has two added modules. Previous learning experience analyses the customer experience with the automobile – frequency of using the machine, paths taken by the customer, time duration taken by the customer to reach his destination. It creates a dataset having these parameters. The investigation aims to improve the experience of the user. The recommendation library stores the data over the cloud and suggests it to other users with similar needs. This subcomponent provides suggestions to the customer by collecting the required data. The recommendation improves the system by 7.75% user experience and 40.6% performance using the recommendation library compared to the previous contribution.

The suggestion has six sections. Section two details the background of the technology. The segment three briefs literature survey. Section four details the proposed work. It uses NS2 to simulate, and the same is detailed in segment five. The result concludes in section six.

BACKGROUND

The framework (Batty, 2018) reflects the activity of another. It is an alternate framework typically portrayed as a model. It is deliberation from the construction and cycles that characterize the framework adjusted. The models don't endeavor to reflect everything about a framework. It makes the model naturally not quite the same as the first framework. The possibility of the advanced twin has risen out of the portrayal of the city concerning its resources. Geographic data frameworks are downsizing to the degree of structures, and their augmentation manages the activity. The upkeep utilizing building data models programming gives the setting to broadly advanced portrayals that scale to the level of the multitude of resources in the city.

Computerized twins are virtual duplicates of machines or frameworks reforming the industry. Driven by information gathered from sensors progressively, these refined PC models reflect every feature of an item, cycle, or administration. Each model works without preparation. There are no strategies, principles, or standards.

LITERATURE SURVEY

The multidisciplinary reproduction model (Zhou, Zhang, Li, Ding, & Wang, 2020) uses the Modelica language. This reenactment model comprises four sections- the arranging module, control transport, electric component, and motorized unit. The arranging segment harvests reference movement boundaries for every six tomahawks of the robot as per the ongoing point-to-point area of the automaton seen by location sensing elements. The control transport communicates to the electric module. The electric module could deliver the force, position, and speed. It controls the activities of the mechanical module. The movements are envisioned by a simulated 3D prototype of the machine. The mimicking results foresee the activity status of the robot as per its continuous actual boundaries.

The created virtual portrayal (Polini & Corrado, 2020) depends on a reenactment device and a covering archetypal to address the cycle autograph. The casing typically considers a bunch of focuses for every portion's limit on the surface. The CaUTA programming apparatus produces the collection of mathematical deviations because of the variety of interaction boundaries of the assembling system. The created virtual portrayal frames into two sections. The first imitate a particular actual assembling process. This meta-model produces the different part calculations. It fabricates the process. The CAD model of the part plans uses FEA programming. In the UI of MSC programming, the parts discretize by 3D features. The size of the produced components considers along with the deviations.

The work (Zhang C., Zhou, He, Li, & Cheng, 2019) proposes a knowledge and information-driven structure for the Digital Alike Industrial compartment, where details are answerable for the view of assembling issues, and information gives dependable answers for these issues. It can uphold independent assembling by three empowering advances. The automated twin model adds to the assortment of actual and computerized space. The profound combination of both works with the separate tasks of the cell by the limits of self-performance. This prototype could see and mimic the assembling system created on the constant information distributed by information space. The understanding, anticipating and enhancing the assembling execution with information-based canny abilities. Dynamic information bases go about as the cerebrum of the cell associates actual space, computerized space, information space, and communal space. The association happens through a uniform and interoperable information prototypical. Active information centers outfit cells with the limits of self-intellectual, programmed information route as indicated by assembling issues, and self-improving, in particular, consistent facts collection by separating information from information space. Information-based canny abilities are gained from authentic information in dynamic information bases through artificial Intelligence calculations, which outfit cells with the ability to manage different assembling issues and produce dependable choices.

MBCoT (Zhang, Zhou, Li, & Cao, 2020) is the combination of blockchain innovation and IoT. IT constructs universal associations for actual assembling assets to the digital framework while blockchain interfaces programming characterized by utilitarian hubs of IMS and executes P2P exchanges inside the digital framework in a solid, recognizable, and regionalized manner. The three-layer and five-aspect system of DK-DTMC into tetrad sheets in the designed assessment, including the gadget tier, edge coat, stockpile sheet, and client tier. The gadget associate's gadget twin utilizes IoT. It fills as the exchange listening hub foresees future aggravations. Representatives of KM and figuring units work together with process twin. It fabricates information at the cloud-in view of savvy agreements to acknowledge neighborhood or worldwide ideal state regulator of DK-DTMC. The agent initially buys aggravation of a particular gadget and concludes whether handle it at edge or cloud is contingent upon its time awareness and intricacy. It tackles it by circulating suitable figuring units. The device edge-cloud bundles as gathering administrations in light of the blockchain to attend to higher-level clients in a help situated assembling way.

The model (Park, Woo, & Choi, 2020) depends on the production line plan and the progress of extensible markup language. In the first place, the production line plan and improvement (FDI) formalize movements of every sort, capacity, and data stream applicable to the plant plan and the administration errands executed in SMS. FDI's formalization depends on the multi-facet, industrial facility configuration process for most worldwide assembling undertakings and the reference movement model created by NIST. It comprises four practices. The data relating to the methodology undertakings and exercises are gathered and inspected.

The computerized factory ground has four parts (Tao & Zhang, 2017). The physical plant base incorporates a progression of substances, like people, machines, and materials, existing equitably in actual space. The advances with the physical shop floor give control orders for the physical shop floor and improvement techniques for the shop-floor service system. It is an incorporated assistance stage. It epitomizes the elements of Enterprise Information System, PC helped apparatuses, models, calculations, and so forth into sub-administrations, then, at that point, consolidates them to shape composite administrations for explicit desires from the corporeal workshop base and cybernetic workshop floor. The digital twin data incorporates shop floor information, virtual factory base facts, shop-floor service system details, the intertwined knowledge of the three sections, the current techniques for displaying, upgrading, foreseeing, and so forth. Information in workshop floor virtual identical data is incorporated. It dispenses with the facts confined island. The creation plan is created because of the orders, guidance from different divisions, and history creation information. The finished items are assessed to guarantee whether the pointers like magnitude, form, and execution encounter necessities after production. The qualified items are moved into the storeroom, while the inadequate ones require fixing.

A bike (Tao et al., 2018) is taken as an illustration to outline one of the things to come in application methods of twin-driven item design. The model has three phases, and advanced twin innovation produces results of the whole process. In a reasonable plan, planners can incorporate the actual properties of the bike like tone, substantial, magnitude, motorized possessions, and the different information of its current circumstances like warmth and topographical data by utilizing advanced twin innovation to introduce gathering sensors on the bike. The creators can get the riding propensities for clients and further develop the plan plot by breaking down the data coordinated by advanced twins. In the definite plan stage, planners will refine the plan plot based on clients' criticism, test data, and different issues in buyers' utilization of the past age. In the virtual check stage, the originator can utilize advanced twin innovation to foresee and test item execution straight by recreating configuration conspire and fabricating process variables.

The six-layer twin design (Redelinghuys, Basson, & Kruger, 2020) gives the correspondence between the actual identity and the computerized match, as well as between the indistinguishable and the external biosphere. Engineering focuses on circumstances. The results of different merchants utilize the actual twin. Restrictive and specially created components are kept to a base to decrease advancement and backing costs. The contextual investigation depends on a mechanical gripper that an industry accomplice utilizes in sequential construction systems. The primary subsystem is a gripper intended to work under requesting conditions. Tier 2 of the six-coat engineering is the regulator level of the actual alike. The boundary adjustments and inflated location sensors were associated with computerized intakes on the regulator. The strain and airflow sensing elements associate with simple contributions to the regulator. The control grouping of the gripper was customized utilizing a stepping stool rationale controller in the Siemens TIA entry.

The proposed structure (Zhang, Zhou, Hu, & Li, 2020) empowers using a profound learning approach. The innovation stage initially characterizes a few hypothetical cycles by redoing the recovered knowledge. PKR-Net is figuring out how to comprehend the sketch or 3D CAD model using various information perspectives and produce information for organizers to make decisions. The change stage changes each hypothetical interaction into commonsense activities by examining the attainability and accessibility of engine instruments, cutting apparatuses, and chopping boundaries. The ongoing information and system obtain history data from the actual space of the assessment twin are utilized. The choice stage decides on an ideal cycle intending to finish the machining assignments. The internet of assessment twin uses outwardly reproduce and dissect the activities and produce the interaction plan thinking about assembling time and cost.

The application structure of DT (Zheng, Yang, & Cheng, 2019) comprises three sections. In the application interaction, the DT innovation can understand the full-actual framework planning, the life-cycle dynamic demonstration, and the entire interaction's ongoing streamlining. The admission of bidirectional planning and interoperability of actual and virtual space happens through information connection. The acknowledgment of clever choice happens through iterative improvement and administrative association between two spaces. The original is an intricate, different, and dynamic creation temperature. It comprises individuals, machines, materials, rules, and climate. The assets layer incorporates a range of articles connected with item improvement and assembling. At the execution level, the center of actual space development has components data impression of actual production. The data handling tier is the frequency associating actual area and digital area. The bidirectional planning and interoperation happen using the information cooperation in this layer. There are three primary capacity modules of this layer. The knowledge that should be put away in this layer chiefly comprises two sections, details from actual space and realities from virtual space. The information from the original area includes creation, hardware, material, work, administration, and studio climate details. The facts from virtual space incorporate reproduction information, assessment and forecast points, and choice data. Data planning upholds the simultaneous planning of original information, and virtual studio activity gave the information stockpiling module and information handling module.

The practical model (Madni, Madni, & Lucero, 2019) is an enthusiastic electronic depiction of arrangement. It is a suitable occasion that invigorates diligently having security. It has well-being situation information all through the system's improvement plan. It might potentially lessen the expense of method checking and testing. It gives new doors to preparing an execution. It contains material outcomes utilizing the IoT and an electronic string. The genuine situation consolidates the real strategy, perceptible identifiers, and affiliation interfaces. It works in an open climate with admittance to GPS data. The recommendation has four phases. Level 1 is the mind-boggling undeniable model conveyed using the blunt plan. It stays aware of choice creation at the idea start and primer survey. The practical model is an executable course of action that depicts envisioned technique. It is made before the mechanical model. Level 2 is a high-level accomplice wherein the clearheaded game plan. It is skilled in including approval, healthiness, and work data. It is a send-off of the overall approach. It presents bundle invigorates and stays aware of huge level affirmation. It makes the applied arrangement, advancement chart, going before plan, and improvement. It has the Vehicle Interface bookstore of the Modelica contraption. It has a vehicle with a energy fragment. The case prototype has a single stage with mass-and speed-subordinate resistance features. It uses the brake-switch situation. It ascends out of chairman execution to check brake upset. The driveline configuration includes four engines with a front-wheel approach. The potential separation equipment contains typical epicyclic stuff without preventions. The prototypical battery has a predictable energy store that controls the DC machine plan. It joins an inductor, resistor, and emf to the shaft. The motor depiction with a flywheel involves the drive-by-wire gas pedal, where the gas pedal data sources are changed to yield force. Level 3 is the Adaptive virtual match. It proposes a flexible UI. Level 4 has a solo robotization limit. It has noticed targets and models confronted in the circumstances and upheld data on arrangement and conditions.

It is a 3D model (Sierla et al., 2022) created by LiDAR filtering. The point stockpile is handled to recognize part categories, part boundaries, and 3D areas. The data is computerized to a machine-decipherable format.2D picture acknowledgment recognizes marks, images, and associations from a checked pdf-design P&ID. The knowledge is virtualized to a machine (discernible) configuration. The culmination and rightness of the computerized 2D and 3D data should be approved. These two arrangements convert to a solitary data model and produce the twin. It uses Diagram matching for this purpose. The finished and approved information prototype can be utilized to create a computerized P&ID. This contrasts with the P&ID produced in Step 2. The unique reenactment model is created from the factory information model produced in Step 5.

The review (Shoji, Schudel, Onwude, Shrivastava, & Defraeye, 2022) analyzed the atmosphere warmth on the virus chain of quatern organic products from Spain to Switzerland. The natural products are transported from a homestead to a packhouse, where pre-cooling is performed. In this manner, the organic products are shipped from Spain by a transporter in a refrigerated truck to a circulation place in Switzerland and afterward moved by one more transporter to a neighborhood trade location in Switzerland. Two different datasets undergo assessment. The first dataset comprises a time-temperature report between the packhouse and the DC in 2018 and 2019. The information examines the virus chain at and after the DC and assesses the entire virus chain.

The methodology (Chakraborty & Adhikari, 2021) isolates into two parts. The material science-based ostensible model for information handling and reaction expectations. The information-driven AI model for the time-advancement of the framework boundaries. The physical science-based apparent model is a framework explicit and chosen in light of the possible issue. The information-driven AI model is nonexclusive. Gaussian Process is utilized as the master model.

The work (Zhuang, Miao, Liu, & Xiong, 2021) centers around the demonstrating and utilization of SDT practically speaking for DT applications. It has four levels. The necessities are to utilize SDT to acknowledge ongoing observing and forecast of the actual shop-floor's working status. The demonstrating objects of the actual shop-floor incorporate creation components and creation processes. The creation processes comprise of specialized stream and creation coordinated factors. They are addressed by virtual 3D model liveliness that are framed by the unique difference in spatial positions and working status of actual components. The standard aspect incorporates derivation rules, affiliation rules, and limitation rules. The checking contents incorporate ongoing simultaneous planning of all creation cycles and dynamic presentation of the ongoing status of all creation components. All shop-floor processes are displayed continuously through natural 3D movements, and the ongoing status of all components is shown in the 2D status Kanban. The time arrangements of shop-floor working status are gathered and put away in a data set.

The advanced twin framework (Liu, et al., 2021) gets significant calculation, conduct and setting data and coordinates all the data. The advancement cycle of DTMM remembers. For the copy demonstrating interaction of the computerized twin calculation impersonate model, the converse demonstrating innovation of machining object considering the key machining highlights is taken on. The computerized twin framework gets the assembling highlight trait data, and dissects the machining qualities of the machining object. The mirror improvement of the mathematical model, the conduct model and the setting model. the past mathematical state will be supplanted with the refreshed one. the math model is equipped for mirroring the real morphology and the calculation change of the item object during the machining system. The virtual model and the actual article are converged through the virtual and genuine combination innovation. It shows the geology of the item progressively.

PROPOSED SYSTEM

The pragmatic model (Madni, Madni, & Lucero, 2019) is a vibrant digital description of a physical arrangement. It is a practical occurrence of arrangement updates continuously having representation, preservation, and wellness situation information throughout the physical system's growth sequence. It has the potential to decrease the price of method verifying and experimenting. It provides new penetrations into practice performance. It consists of relevant outcomes utilizing the IoT (Ambika N., 2020) and a digital thread. It provides a connection. The physical situation includes the physical arrangement, visible detectors, and connection interfaces. It works in an open ecosystem, with entrance to GPS knowledge. The proposal has four phases. Tier 1 is the legendary implicit model produced during upfront architecture. It maintains decision-making at the idea conception and preparatory study. The pragmatic model is a universal executable arrangement representation of the envisioned method. It is before the mechanical archetype is composed. Tier 2 is a digital counterpart in which the pragmatic composition. It is proficient in including enforcement, wellness, and livelihood data. It is an instantiation of the universal arrangement. It introduces group updates and maintains high-level determination. It creates the conceptual scheme, technology blueprint, preceding scheme, and construction. It has the Vehicle Interface Library of the Modelica device. It has a vehicle with a power split. The chassis prototype has a single stage with mass-and speed-dependent resistance features. It uses the brake-lever situation. It emerges from operator performance to measure brake revolution. The driveline pattern consists of four engines with a front-wheel approach. The potential separation equipment consists of typical epicyclic gear without impairments. A prototypical battery with a continuous energy reservoir controls the DC machine design with an inductor, resistor, and emf element attached to the shaft core. The motor representation with a flywheel consists of the drive-by-wire accelerator, where the accelerator inputs transform to yield torque. Tier 3 is the Adaptive Digital Twin. It proposes an adaptive user interface. Tier 4 has the unsupervised automated ability. It has discerned objectives and models engaged in operational circumstances and reinforced knowledge of arrangement and conditions.

The proposed model aims to improve the experience with the system.

- Previous learning experience - It analyses the customer experience with the vehicle – frequency of using the automobile, paths taken by the customer, time duration taken by the customer to reach his destination. It creates a dataset having these parameters. The investigation aims to enhance the experience of the user.
- Recommendation library - The same data stored in the engine can be stored over the cloud and suggested to other users with similar needs. This subcomponent provides suggestions to the customer by collecting required data. Figure 2 portrays the same.

Figure 2. Suggested Digital twin model

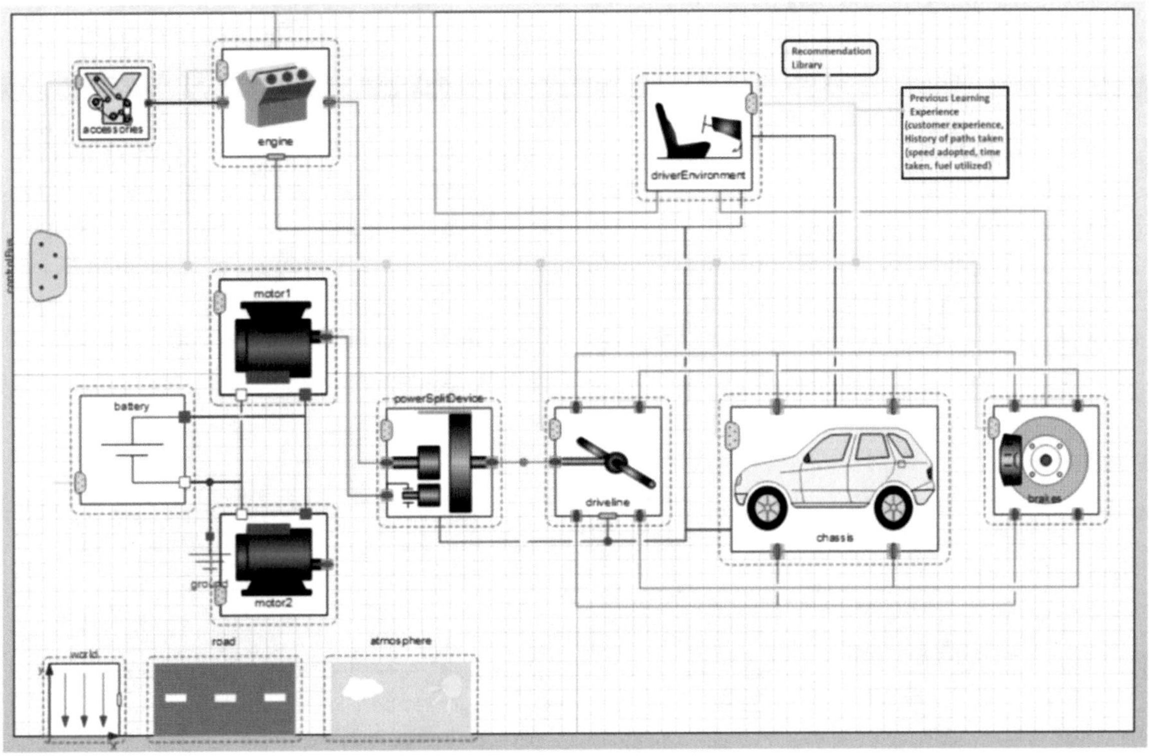

Analysis of the Work

The realistic model (Madni, Madni, & Lucero, 2019) is a lively computerized depiction of an actual plan. It is a reasonable event of course of action refreshes consistently having portrayal, safeguarding, and wellbeing circumstance data all through the framework's development arrangement. It can diminish the cost of strategy checking and testing. It gives new infiltrations into training execution. It comprises (important) results using the IoT and a computerized string. It gives an association. The actual circumstance incorporates the actual plan, noticeable locators, and association interfaces. It works in an open biological system with access to GPS information. The proposition has four stages. Level 1 is a model created during forthright engineering. It keeps up with decision-production at the thought origination and preliminary review. The commonsense model is an executable game plan portrayal of the imagined technique. It is before the mechanical original is formed. Level 2 is a computerized partner where the realistic creation implements health and occupation information from the mechanical twin. It is a launch of the plan. It presents a bunch of refreshes and keeps up with the undeniable level of assurance. It makes the reasonable plan, innovation outline, and development. It has the Vehicle Interface Library of the Modelica gadget. It has a vehicle with a power split. The frame model has a solitary stage with mass-and speed-subordinate obstruction highlights. It utilizes the brake-switch circumstance. It is the outcome of the administrator to quantify brake failure. The driveline design comprises four motors. It follows a front-wheel approach. The potential detachment hardware has epicyclic stuff without impedances. A prototypical battery with a constant energy repository controls the DC machine plan with an inductor, resistor, and emf component connected to the shaft center. The engine is portrayed with a flywheel. It comprises the drive-by-wire gas pedal, where the gas pedal information sources are changed to yield force. Level 3 is the Adaptive Digital Twin. It proposes a versatile UI to the mechanical and advanced partners. Level 4 has solo robotization capacity. It has observed targets and models faced in the functional states and supported information on game plans and conditions.

The suggestion has two added modules. Previous learning experience analyses the customer experience with the automobile – frequency of using the vehicle, paths taken by the customer, time duration taken by the customer to reach his destination. It creates a dataset having these parameters. The investigation aims to improve the experience of the user. The recommendation library accumulates the data over the cloud and suggests it to other users with similar needs. This subcomponent provides suggestions to the customer by collecting the required data. The work is simulated using NS2. Table 1 contains simulation parameters. Figure 3 represents the variation happening during the simulation.

Table 1. Parameters used in the simulation

Restrictions used	Explanation
Zone under investigation	200m * 200m
Number of instances considered	100
Number of destinations considered	4
Number of instances taking the similar destinations	25
Number of instances taking similar paths	12 +13 (for all destinations)
Simulation time	60 ms

Figure 3. Simulation outcome

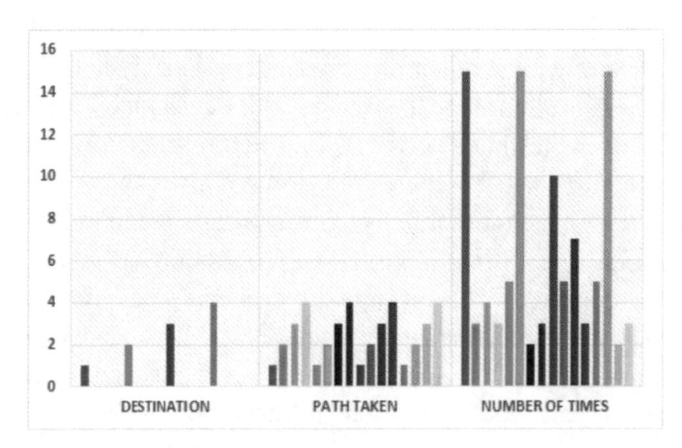

- *User experience* - A client would be willing to use the system if he has a good experience. The suggestion collects the history of the individual driving and recommends appropriately. The system understands the personnel's taste and provides him recommendations. The suggestion improves the system by 7.75% compared to the previous contribution (Madni, Madni, & Lucero, 2019). The same is represented in figure 4.

Figure 4. Comparison of two contribution w.r.t user experience

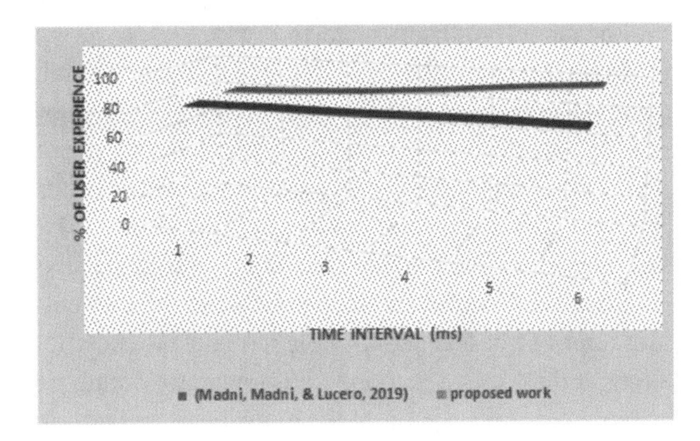

- *Recommendation Library* - The same data stored in the engine imports to the cloud (Nagaraj, 2021) and suggested to other users with similar needs. This subcomponent provides suggestions to the customer by collecting the required data. The work enhances the system performance by 40.6% using the recommendation library. The same is portrayed in Figure 5.

Figure 5. Enhancement of the system performance

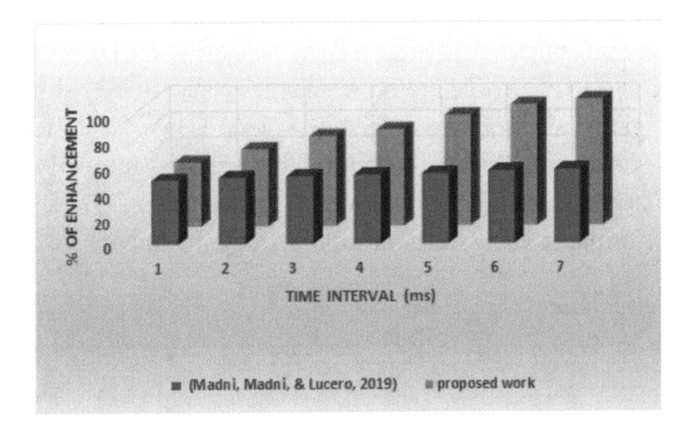

CONCLUSION

A modernized twin is progressed depiction of the first method. The vision of twin calls for joining a business, consistent, and sensor data from unique systems into the virtual structure model of the high-level twin to work with the examination, avoid issues, and cultivate informed development guides. By joining the virtual and real universes, the mechanized twin enables the continuous checking of systems and cycles. It is an optimal assessment of data to head off issues before they arise, plan preventive help to reduce/hinder excursions, uncover new business open entryways, and plan for future updates. It requires a genuine twin for data getting and setting-driven joint effort. The electronic twin includes related things.

The high-level string gives the organization all through the structure's lifecycle and accumulates data from the real twin to revive the models in the mechanized twin.

The pragmatic model (Madni, Madni, & Lucero, 2019) is a vibrant digital description of a physical arrangement. It is a practical occurrence of arrangement updates continuously having representation, preservation, and wellness situation information throughout the physical system's growth sequence. It has the potential to decrease the price of method verifying and experimenting. It provides new penetrations into practice performance. It consists of relevant outcomes utilizing the IoT (Ambika N., 2020) and a digital thread. It provides a connection. The physical situation includes the physical arrangement, visible detectors, and connection interfaces. It works in an open ecosystem, with entrance to GPS knowledge. The proposal has four phases. Tier 1 is the legendary implicit model produced during upfront architecture. It maintains decision-making at the idea conception and preparatory study. The pragmatic model is a universal executable arrangement representation of the envisioned method. It is before the mechanical archetype is composed. Tier 2 is a digital counterpart in which the pragmatic composition. It is proficient in including enforcement, wellness, and livelihood data. It is an instantiation of the universal arrangement. It introduces group updates and maintains high-level determination. It creates the conceptual scheme, technology blueprint, preceding scheme, and construction. It has the Vehicle Interface Library of the Modelica device. It has a vehicle with a power split. The chassis prototype has a single stage with mass-and speed-dependent resistance features. It uses the brake-lever situation. It emerges from operator performance to measure brake revolution. The driveline pattern consists of four engines with a front-wheel approach. The potential separation equipment consists of typical epicyclic gear without impairments. A prototypical battery with a continuous energy reservoir controls the DC machine design with an inductor, resistor, and emf element attached to the shaft core. The motor representation with a flywheel consists of the drive-by-wire accelerator, where the accelerator inputs transform to yield torque. Tier 3 is the Adaptive Digital Twin. It proposes an adaptive user interface. Tier 4 has the unsupervised automated ability. It has discerned objectives and models engaged in operational circumstances and reinforced knowledge of arrangement and conditions. The approach improves the system by 7.75% user experience and 40.6% performance using recommendation library compared to the previous contribution.

REFERENCES

Ambika, N. (2019). Energy-Perceptive Authentication in Virtual Private Networks Using GPS Data. In M. Z. (eds), Security, privacy and trust in the IoT environment (pp. 25-38). Springer. doi:10.1007/978-3-030-18075-1_2

Ambika, N. (2020). Tackling jamming attacks in IoT. In A. M., S. K., & K. S. (eds), Tackling jamming attacks in IoT. (pp. 153-165). Springer. doi:10.1007/978-3-030-37468-6_8

Batty, M. (2018). Digital twins. *Environment and Planning. B, Urban Analytics and City Science*, *45*(5), 817–820. doi:10.1177/2399808318796416

Chakraborty, S., & Adhikari, S. (2021). Machine learning based digital twin for dynamical systems with multiple time-scales. *Computers & Structures*, *243*, 106410. doi:10.1016/j.compstruc.2020.106410

Chaudhary, G., Khari, M., & Elhoseny, M. (2021). *Digital Twin Technology*. CRC Press. doi:10.1201/9781003132868

Devare, M. H. (2019). Convergence of Manufacturing Cloud and Industrial IoT. In G. Kecskemeti (Ed.), *Applying Integration Techniques and Methods in Distributed Systems and Technologies* (pp. 49–78). IGI Global.

Farsi, M., Daneshkhah, A., Hosseinian-Far, A., & Jahankhani, H. (2020). *Digital twin technologies and smart cities*. Springer. doi:10.1007/978-3-030-18732-3

González García, C., Núñez Valdéz, E. R., García Díaz, V., Pelayo García-Bustelo, B. C., & Cueva Lovelle, J. M. (2019). A review of artificial intelligence in the internet of things. International Journal Of Interactive Multimedia And Artificial Intelligence, 5.

Liu, S., Bao, J., Lu, Y., Li, J. L. S., & Sun, X. (2021). Digital twin modeling method based on biomimicry for machining aerospace components. *Journal of Manufacturing Systems*, *58*, 180–195. doi:10.1016/j.jmsy.2020.04.014

Madni, A. M., Madni, C. C., & Lucero, S. D. (2019). Leveraging digital twin technology in model-based systems engineering. *Systems*, *7*(1), 1–13. doi:10.3390ystems7010007

Nagaraj, A. (2022). Adapting Blockchain for Energy Constrained IoT in Healthcare Environment. In Sustainable and Advanced Applications of Blockchain in Smart Computational Technologies (pp. 103-112). Chapman and Hall/CRC.

Nagaraj, A. (2021). Introduction to Sensors in IoT and Cloud Computing Applications. Bentham Science Publishers. doi:10.2174/97898114793591210101

Park, Y., Woo, J., & Choi, S. (2020). A cloud-based digital twin manufacturing system based on an interoperable data schema for smart manufacturing. *International Journal of Computer Integrated Manufacturing*, *33*(12), 1259–1276. doi:10.1080/0951192X.2020.1815850

Polini, W., & Corrado, A. (2020). Digital twin of composite assembly manufacturing process. *International Journal of Production Research*, *58*(17), 5238–5252. doi:10.1080/00207543.2020.1714091

Redelinghuys, A. J., Basson, A. H., & Kruger, K. (2020). A six-layer architecture for the digital twin: A manufacturing case study implementation. *Journal of Intelligent Manufacturing*, *31*(6), 1383–1402. doi:10.100710845-019-01516-6

Shoji, K., Schudel, S., Onwude, D., Shrivastava, C., & Defraeye, T. (2022). Mapping the postharvest life of imported fruits from packhouse to retail stores using physics-based digital twins. *Resources, Conservation and Recycling*, *176*, 105914. doi:10.1016/j.resconrec.2021.105914

Sierla, S., Azangoo, M., Rainio, K., Papakonstantinou, N., Fay, A., Honkamaa, P., & Vyatkin, V. (2022). Roadmap to semi-automatic generation of digital twins for brownfield process plants. *Journal of Industrial Information Integration*, *27*, 100282. doi:10.1016/j.jii.2021.100282

Stojanovic, L., Usländer, T., Volz, F., Weißenbacher, C., Müller, J., Jacoby, M., & Bischoff, T. (2021). Methodology and Tools for Digital Twin Management—The FA3ST Approach. *IoT*, *2*(4), 717–740. doi:10.3390/iot2040036

Tao, F., Cheng, J., Qi, Q., Zhang, M., Zhang, H., & Sui, F. (2018). Digital twin-driven product design, manufacturing and service with big data. *International Journal of Advanced Manufacturing Technology*, *94*(9), 3563–3576. doi:10.100700170-017-0233-1

Tao, F., Liu, A., Hu, T., & Nee, A. Y. (2020). *Digital twin driven smart design*. Academic Press.

Tao, F., & Zhang, M. (2017). Digital twin shop-floor: A new shop-floor paradigm towards smart manufacturing. *IEEE Access: Practical Innovations, Open Solutions*, *5*, 20418–20427. doi:10.1109/ACCESS.2017.2756069

Zhang, C., Zhou, G., Hu, J., & Li, J. (2020). Deep learning-enabled intelligent process planning for digital twin manufacturing cell. *Knowledge-Based Systems*, *191*, 105247. doi:10.1016/j.knosys.2019.105247

Zhang, C., Zhou, G., Li, H., & Cao, Y. (2020). Manufacturing blockchain of things for the configuration of a data-and knowledge-driven digital twin manufacturing cell. *IEEE Internet of Things Journal*, *7*(12), 11884–11894. doi:10.1109/JIOT.2020.3005729

Zhang, C., Zhou, G. H. J., Li, Z., & Cheng, W. (2019). A data-and knowledge-driven framework for digital twin manufacturing cell. *11th CIRP Conference on Industrial Product-Service Systems*. 83, (pp. 345-350). ELSEVIER. 10.1016/j.procir.2019.04.084

Zheng, Y., Yang, S., & Cheng, H. (2019). An application framework of digital twin and its case study. *Journal of Ambient Intelligence and Humanized Computing*, *10*(3), 1141–1153. doi:10.100712652-018-0911-3

Zhou, G., Zhang, C., Li, Z., Ding, K., & Wang, C. (2020). Knowledge-driven digital twin manufacturing cell towards intelligent manufacturing. *International Journal of Production Research*, *58*(4), 1034–1051. doi:10.1080/00207543.2019.1607978

Zhuang, C., Miao, T., Liu, J., & Xiong, H. (2021). The connotation of digital twin, and the construction and application method of shop-floor digital twin. *Robotics and Computer-integrated Manufacturing*, *68*, 102075. doi:10.1016/j.rcim.2020.102075

Chapter 15
Security Implications of IoT Applications with Cryptography and Blockchain Technology in Healthcare Digital Twin Design

Kamalendu Pal
https://orcid.org/0000-0001-7158-6481
University of London, UK

ABSTRACT

Over the last few years, the world has witnessed a fast-paced digital transformation in many aspects of human life in healthcare owing to the coronavirus (COVID-19) pandemic. Business and service providers had to adapt to digital changes quickly to overcome containment challenges and survive in an ever-changing world. Healthcare-related data collection, preservation, and analysis using digital technologies are helping pandemic mitigation strategies. With the rapid development of virtual systems integration methods and data acquisition techniques, digital twin (DT) technology is ushering in a new dawn for modern healthcare services and information systems. However, IoT-based information systems are vulnerable to privacy and security-related issues. This chapter presents an information system framework that consists of IoT with blockchain technology to mitigate vulnerability issues using lightweight cryptography.

INTRODUCTION

Competent healthcare is one of the strategic priorities shared by the primary healthcare service initiatives, such as using the Internet of things (IoT), sensor technologies, and big data analytics. *The digital twin* technology concept is an emerging concept that has become the center of attention for the healthcare industry in recent years. It is at the forefront of the healthcare industry revolution facilitated through advanced data analytics and IoT technology connectivity. This is recognized as a *building block* of the Metaverse, another fast-emerging case representing an immersive digital world that allows real-life

DOI: 10.4018/978-1-6684-5925-6.ch015

experiences and interactions in the healthcare industry. In this way, digital twin technology can tackle the challenge of seamless integration between IoT and data analytics by creating a connected physical and virtual twin (Digital Twin). In addition, a digital twin environment allows for rapid analysis and real-time decisions made through accurate analytics.

The general digitalization process across the healthcare industry and its services, rapidly increasing data processing and analysis capacity enabled by fast-paced technological revolutions, and continuous advancements in cognitive and artificial intelligence (AI) of which have accelerated digital twin technology. It is becoming more evident that Digital Twin runs in parallel with AI and IoT technology resulting in shared challenges. The first step in tackling the challenges is to identify them. Some common challenges are found with data analytics and IoT technology, and the end aim is to identify shared challenges for Digital Twins. The two most important challenges in Digital Twins are: (i) data analytic challenges and (ii) data privacy, security, and trust-related issues.

In data analytics, the most critical challenge is the general Information Technology (IT) infrastructure. The rapid growth of AI needs to be met with high-performance infrastructure in the form of up-to-date hardware and software to help execute machine learning algorithms. The current challenge with the infrastructure is the cost of installing and running these systems. For example, the costs of high-performance graphics processing units (GPUs) that can run machine learning algorithms are heavily costly. As well as this, the infrastructure needs updated software and hardware to run such a system successfully. Overcoming this challenge is seen through GPUs "*as a Service*," providing on-demand GPUs at cost through the cloud. Amazon, Google, Microsoft and NVIDIA, to name a few, are offering unique on-demand services similar to traditional cloud-based applications, breaking the barrier to demand, but the poor infrastructure and high cost are still challenging for data analytics. However, using the cloud for data analytics and Digital Twins still pose challenges in ensuring that the cloud infrastructure offers robust security.

From a data point of view, it is essential to ensure it is not of inferior quality. The data needs to be sorted and cleaned, ensuring the highest data quality is fed into the AI algorithms. In addition, privacy and security are essential topics for the healthcare industry in the context of data analytics performance. Laws and regulations are yet to be fully established because of AI's infancy. The challenge is more security, regulation and measure concerning AI in the future as the technology grows. Future regulation ensures the development of algorithms that take steps to protect user data. For example, the General Data Protection Regulation (GDPR) ensures the privacy and security of personal data worldwide. Despite being an umbrella regulation concerning data and security, this highlights the concerns with handling data when developing AI algorithms.

Regulation is one step to ensure personal data is protected, while another method is federated learning, a decentralized framework for training models. It allows users' data in a learning model to stay localized without data sharing, addressing privacy and security issues when implementing data analytics within a Digital Twin. In addition, with the growth of IoT devices in the healthcare and industry setting comes the challenge of collecting factual data. The challenge is controlling data flow, ensuring it can be organized and used effectively. The challenge becomes a bigger problem with the advent of big data. The use of IoT increases the large volumes of unstructured data. For IoT to manage the amount of data, sorting and organization are necessary and will result in more data being usable and providing value.

One of the supporting technologies of digital twin deployment is the Internet of Things (IoT). The IoT seems crucial in addressing various challenges in healthcare applications (Pal, 2021). These applications are motivated by mobility, mobile communications, web-based services, and the requirements for an operating environment that adapts to how people and healthcare industries want to work. It can provide customized solutions based on the patient's lifestyle and medical background by using IoT in the care-setting environment for successful treatment. IoT technologies support patients, physicians, hospitals, caregivers, and insurance providers. Patients may use wearables like fitness bands and wirelessly connected devices to monitor their physical activity and make health-related decisions. The IoT can unlock existing technologies and contribute to improved healthcare and medical device solutions (Pal, 2022). This technology allows healthcare professionals to apply their skills and training to solve next-generation challenges. It enables them to use data and advanced equipment better, allowing them to take proper and timely steps for patients' medical care. Finally, the available sensors and gateways process data, thereby expanding the possibilities for developing better disease management systems. For example, IoT applications provide software and apps for tracking and managing the hospital's physical properties, such as staff, patients, and equipment.

Collection of healthcare data is essential to provide better treatment, reliable detection of illnesses, storing data in health records for studying and providing appropriate medications and a prevention strategy. In recent years, IoT-based applications have been helping to collect some medical care data. The IoT application's future in healthcare will be game-changing, as it will mobilize demand trends and make data tracking easier. For example, IoT healthcare devices can analyze the collected patient data. In the healthcare industry, IoT monitoring aims to make informed decisions and provide prompt treatment. Real-time alerting and tracking are possible with IoT healthcare applications. In addition, it allows IoT-based applications to provide precise therapies and improved patient care (Pal, 2022).

IoT-based applications also provide automated systems for the tracking of various diseases and better safety for the patient. For security purposes, often this technology is used to monitor the hospital's assets. It is a highly effective technology for tracking objects or individuals. For example, IoT systems are also being used to monitor medicines to ensure correct dosage and monitoring of side effects. In addition, modern IoT-based applications can also remind patients to take their medication on time and in the correct dosage. These applications connect real-world healthcare business objects to wide-area data communication-based service provisions. Based on network architecture, contextual business operational models for healthcare applications, and the world standardization organization, industries are interchangeably using several definitions of IoT. However, IoT systems' two essential components are radio frequency identification (RFID) technology and wireless sensor networks (WSNs).

The WSNs use various resource-constraint sensors or biosensor nodes for healthcare service monitoring applications. The service networks interlink different communication devices (e.g., body sensors, gateways, medical device sensors) using wireless technologies (e.g., fourth generation (4G), fifth generation (5G), Long Term Evolution (LTE) – a standard for wireless broadband, Universal Mobile Telecommunications Service (UMTS) – a third generation broadband, Wi-Fi, satellite communication, and futuristic sixth generation (6G)). Healthcare practitioners require privacy to preserve patients' medical information for diagnostics purposes; user authentication is essential in preserving security-related issues. Based on the gathered pathological information of the concerned patient over the communication network, the practitioner can diagnose a patient's medical condition. At the end of the diagnosis, the practitioner can take the necessary actions. Therefore, deploying IoT-based healthcare information systems without considering privacy and security-related issues would threaten medical practice's effective operation. In other words, IoT-based medical information systems' security is paramount.

In this way, data-driven healthcare systems must seriously consider quality assurance-related issues of medical diagnostics operational data. For example, researchers are using various techniques for healthcare-related data management purposes (Kaswan et al., 2021) (Santosh & Gaur, 2021) (Santosh & Gaur, 2022) (Gaur, 2022).

The medical information system data security must provide adapted mechanisms to mitigate the challenges. Data encryption is crucial before any data is transmitted across a network connection. Blockchain technology is one of the important candidates for the solutions to this challenge (e.g., data confidentiality, integrity, and availability). Blockchain technology and its operations are governed to exchange data, perform actions, and complete transactions in a distributed way. Furthermore, blockchain technology uses public key cryptography and basic techniques (e.g., digital signature, hash functions) to provide security. In addition, through public key infrastructure (PKI), blockchain technology can provide confidentiality of operational data and the system by using encryption methods.

Cryptography methods are instrumental in data encryption and are effective for their appropriateness in ensuring data confidentiality, secrecy, and validity. The communication among IoT devices requires to be encrypted to maintain security, but unfortunately, developing secured solutions based on conventional encryption methods is a challenging task because of the restricted resources available to IoT devices (e.g., limited processing power, storage capacity, battery power) (Luo et al., 2020). For example, an RFID tag cannot use a 1204-bit Rivest, Dhamir, and Adleman (RSA) algorithm because it does not have the appropriate resources to implement it. Hence, a particular type of cryptography technique is emerging in the healthcare IoT ecosystem that manages resource-constraint ubiquitous computing infrastructural devices (Chiadighikaobi & Katuk, 2021). Finally, Alshammari and fellow researchers (Alshammari et al., 2021) have suggested an encryption method that relies on the advanced encryption standard (AES) and a special chaotic substitution box (S-box) technique.

The medical data transmitted in an IoT-based information system is susceptible to affecting the user's privacy, so the information should be communicated to preserve it. Standard information assurance methods (e.g., encryption) are used for this purpose. The encryption technique was used in the prototype system by Sruthi and Rajasekaran (Sruthi & Rajaskaran, 2021). Ayachi and fellow researchers (Ayachi et al., 2021) have highlighted an encryption technique for data on a network-on-chip (NoC) using a light encryption device (LED) algorithm. Lee and Sim (Lee & Sim, 2021) have suggested the privacy-preserving key and a unique mechanism (known as the initialization vector (IV)) of the AES-CBC algorithm every few times, making it more secure. Also, they simplified the directed acyclic graph (DAG) by sending overlap packets to three blocks at a time. In another research, Guan and other researchers (Guan et al., 2021) have presented a ciphertext policy attribute-based encryption (CP-ABE) method to simplify encryption and decryption processes.

Karbasi and Shahpasand (Karbasi & Shahpasand, 2021) presented a lightweight encryption technique to protect IoT systems. A group of researchers presented a simple blockchain model with resource-constrained IoT sensor nodes (Khan et al., 2022). Sowjanya and fellow researchers utilized Elliptic Curve Cryptography (ECC) to make a novel key management system for the CP-ABE framework (Sowjanya et al., 2021). Dwivedi (Dwivedi, 2021) proposed an encryption method which uses dynamism and two separate cipher parts.

Shi and other researchers (Su et al., 2021) presented an access control authorization method for data using blockchain technology. Sleem and Couturier (Sleem & Couturier, 2021) proposed an ultra-lightweight encryption method. Ragab and fellow researchers (Ragab et el., 2021) increased the security of the original corrected block tiny encryption algorithm (CBTEA) block cipher using a unique S-box method. For example, Li and other researchers (Li et al., 2021) used homomorphic encryption to keep people's data safe.

It is also vital that distinct categories of services, which required to protect the enormous amount of healthcare-related data collected and preserve individual privacy. For example, access control may guarantee that data is only accessible by those with the appropriate permissions (Xian & Yuanyuan, 2021) (Gong & Navimipour, 2022). Sensitive personal information about individuals also requires security. Therefore, it is necessary to figure out how and where the WSNs interaction would be crucial to the information system's data safety. For example, researchers use blockchain technology with access control, which they believe can eliminate the requirement for a central middle person while still permitting real-time and trustful data circulation with the system (Villamil et al., 2020). Users of the system may uniquely identify each device by making digital replicas of real things on a blockchain-based network. At the same time, the data they provide is permanently saved and cannot be changed.

Blockchain technology has unique characteristics that can provide transparency, redundancy, reputation, and traceability that create business operational value (Reyna et el., 2018). There are three different types of blockchains: (i) public, (ii) private, and (iii) hybrid. In simple, a public blockchain means that anybody can join and participate. However, private blockchains are the most appropriate form of connecting with IoT and adding value since they are unavailable to the public for use. Nevertheless, hybrid blockchains combine the best features of both private and public blockchains in one system (Auer et al., 2022).

The chapter's main contributions are: (i) provide a hybrid information system framework (i.e., blockchain, IoT); (ii) discuss blockchain technology and its enabling decentralization components, including smart contracts, decentralized storage, advantages of decentralized applications, and recent research works based on blockchain technology for the healthcare industry; (iii) highlight potential and novel opportunities arise from integrating blockchain with 5G network; (iv) briefly discusses the different security issues for IoT applications; (v) provide an overview of lightweight cryptography techniques and its uses for IoT systems security solution; (vi) Finally, the chapter presents the future research direction and conclude with concluding remarks.

BACKGROUND AND RELATED RESEARCH WORK

Healthcare information systems automation has a long history, and it started in the 1960s in the United States of America and congenital Europe. Information technology (IT) plays a vital role from the very beginning in this automation process. In recent decades, the evolution of mobile communication technology has driven the importance of wireless communications usage as one of the ways to connect to the Internet. However, the ability to communicate with people constantly on the go has emerged as one of the essential characteristics of modern healthcare information systems. The research and development activities of the Fifth Generation (5G) and futuristic Sixth Generation (6G) wireless networks are gaining momentum to connect all aspects of healthcare business activities through the network with much higher speed, exceptionally low latency, and ubiquitous connectivity.

The development of IoT technology has led to the universal connection of people, objects, sensors, and services. The central aim of IoT technology deployment is to provide network infrastructure with interconnection ability, interoperable communication methods and software-defined network connectivity, and incorporation of physical/virtual sensors, personal computers, intelligent devices, smart pharmaceutical items, anytime and on any network (Pal, 2022). The development of smartphone technology provides countless objects to be a part of the IoT network through different *mobile phone sensors*. This way, smartphone technologies are used in modern healthcare services. For example, a group of researchers (Hinch et al., 2020) presented an idea of a software-based solution for coronavirus *contact tracing*, highlighting the usability of smartphone devices' proximity sensors.

Architectural Issues for IoT Systems

Regardless of their application or operating environment, IoT devices monitor, control, and enhance medical information systems' connectivity and performance. Many diverse technologies, such as wide-area networks, data analytics, security platforms, and operating systems, are involved in the IoT spectrum for healthcare applications.

There is no standardized architecture for IoT-based information system industrial applications. However, layered architectures are suggested by different vendors and research groups, such as three-layer (Borgia, 2014); five-layer (Bononi et al., 2014); service-oriented edge computing (Gubbi et al., 2013) (Pal & Yasar, 2020). Most of these multi-layered architectures reflect particular industrial applications.

As a result of broad applicability, a plethora of the reported attacks targeting IoT devices is directed to such industrial applications. This chapter discusses security threats for healthcare information systems using Figure 1 layered architecture that consists of three layers: (i) top layer (i.e., application layer), (ii) middle layer (i.e., networking layer), and (iii) bottom layer (i.e., perception layer) for specific operations. In addition, the individual layer must perform specific tasks for the interconnected smart object networks (e.g., operating theatres, hospital intensive care unit, online medical monitoring, and consultation).

In general, an IoT system consists of RFID-based components and sensors. A simple RFID information system consists of an RFID tag, reader, and data storage. A tag reader identifies the object, attached with a unique identity barcode, through radio signals. This system helps to identify, track, and monitor intelligent objects in an IoT network.

Wireless sensors and their network play an essential role in IoT-based information systems by facilitating sensing and communication provisions. For example, a WSN consists of several intelligent sensors used in remote healthcare application environments, and these sensors help to sense and collect business process-related data (e.g., humidity, temperature, airflow). Many IoT devices (e.g., security cameras and intelligent healthcare machinery) provide the foundation of the perception layer. This layer is responsible for collecting regular business operation data. In addition, collected data are sent via one or multiple hops to a gateway station, as shown in the middle layer of Figure 1.

The network layer provides the infrastructural facilities for the collected data from the perception layer and passes it to the application (or service) provision layer. It is the essential layer of the IoT-based information system's architecture, which integrates different communication technologies which help the interconnectivity of smart IoT objects. The top layer gathers the business processes-related industrial data from the middle layer, processes these data, and supports the needed services for IoT-based system users. It also opens up distinct categories of security attacks targeting IoT devices, data, and network infrastructural elements.

Security Analysis

This section presents an IoT system's diverse security attacks based on the above three-layer architecture. Figure 2. presents a security attack analysis diagrammatic representation.

Figure 1. Simple layered architecture for IoT systems

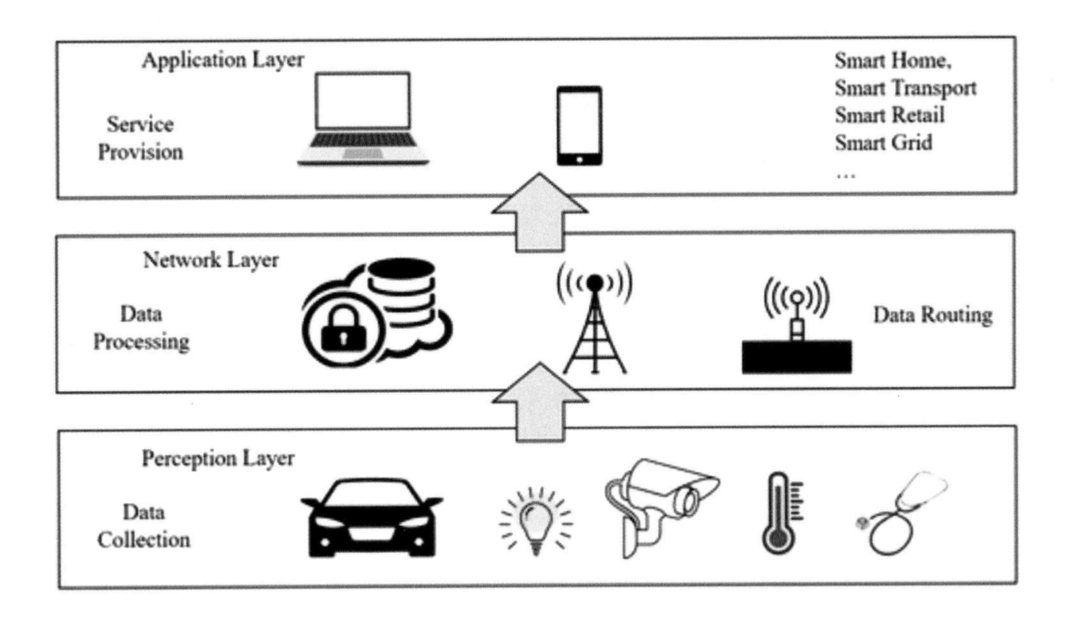

Figure 2. Security attack analysis for IoT-based information systems

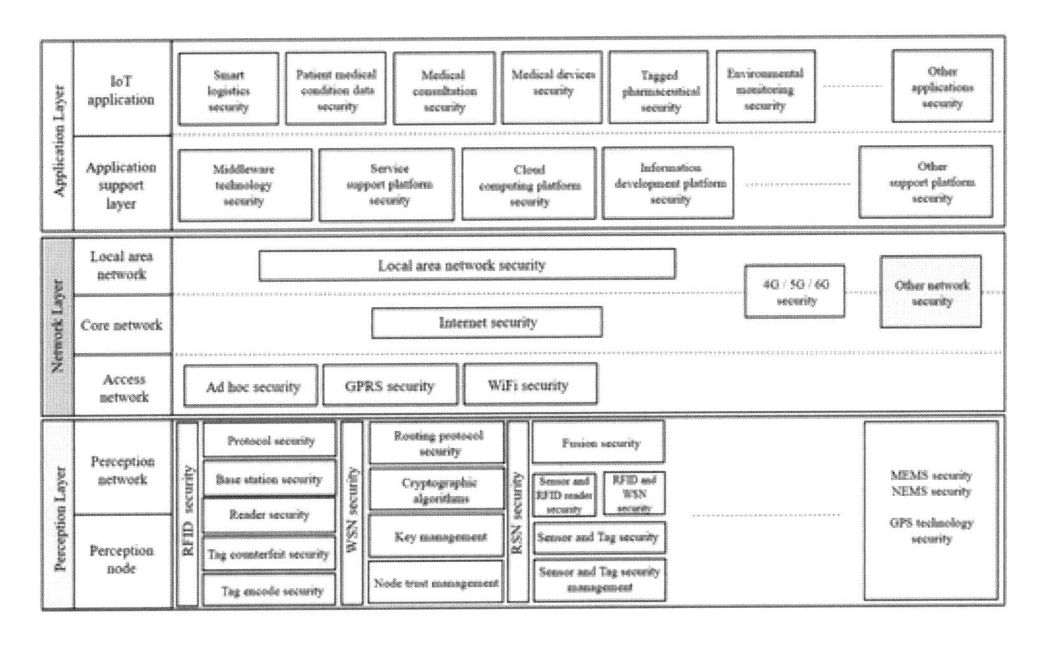

In the above diagrammatic representation, security attacks are classified around the application layer, network layer, and perception layer. Again, the application layer is divided into two parts – the IoT application layer and the application support layer. The network layer is subdivided into the local area, core, and access networks. Each of these subdivisions has its security-related issues. Finally, the perception layer security is analyzed based on the perception network and respective network node.

Figure 3. Various categories of intruder attacks on IoT system

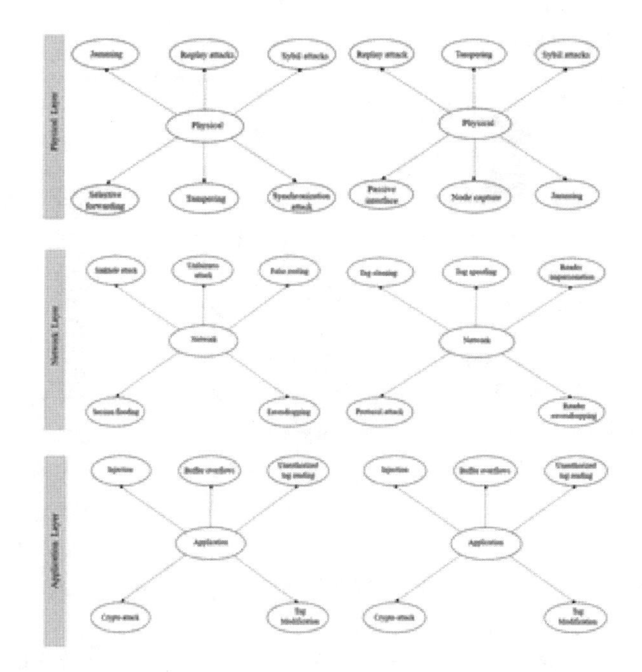

LEGENDS

Jamming – Causing problems by transmitting undesirable radio signals. *Replay attacks* – Capturing a signed packet, and even if it cannot decrypt it, it may gain the trust of the destined entity by re-sending the packet later and creating a problem. *Sybil attack* – Use nodes or devices with multiple identities. These generate traffic that seems many-source, corrupting the fairness of resource usage. *Tampering* – The attacker physically modifies the device or the communication link. *Denial of Service* - Disabling system services by generating repetitive demands. *Eavesdropping* – The attacker can obtain unencrypted information, such as a password supplied in response to a false request.

Different security attack classifications within the IoT landscape exist in the research literature. For example, research shows how to leverage the attack layer (e.g., application, network, perception). Figure 3 represents a diagrammatic representation of attacks and threats on IoT systems from the research literature.

Over time, data security and key transmission have created the idea of cryptography. Cryptography is a strategic way of securing data from unauthorized access by transforming the data into an unrecognizable and unrelatable form. As per IoT requirements, dedicated cryptographic algorithms must be lightweight in terms of area, memory footprint, power, and energy consumption.

This section briefly covers a flow of security measures from Lightweight cryptographic solutions to a comparison among different block ciphers. It includes a comparison between hardware vs software solutions and different recent approaches of the most trusted and researched block cipher, Advanced Encryption Standard (AES), for IoT security.

Lightweight Cryptography

Various cryptographic solutions are available to secure the IoT system's data security. However, not all cryptographic solutions are appropriate for resource-constrained IoT ecosystems. Lightweight cryptographic solutions are being researched thoroughly to have area-efficient and power-efficient solutions. Cryptographic solutions are broadly classified into two categories: (i) asymmetric key cryptography and (ii) symmetric key cryptography. Figure 4 describes the basic functionalities of these two cryptographic methods.

Figure 4. Asymmetric key cryptography and symmetric key cryptography

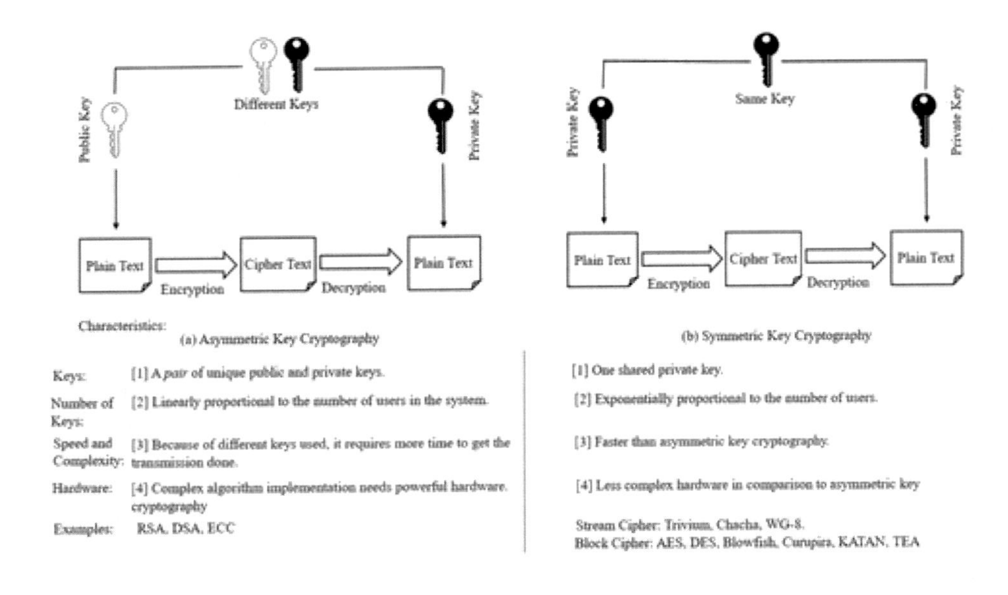

Block chippers have a fixed length of bits and different stages of transformation, which are determined by a symmetric key. Besides, this category of ciphers is very versatile and valuable from an IoT-based information systems perspective. Another advantage is that this process has almost identical encryption and decryption methods; hence, it can be implemented with fewer resources. The following sections describe some of the well-known block chipper designs.

CRYPTOGRAPHY DESIGN OVERVIEW

The advents in computing have changed the meaning of security and the characteristics of modern cryptography. Conventional cryptography refers to modern private vital cyphers, and there are two types of such ciphers: stream ciphers and block ciphers. They differ in the way messages are processed. Messages are transformed into bit-strings, and then encryption/decryption work by bit map operations and manipulations involving a secret key that the sender and receiver share. The transformation of texts into bit-string does not form part of the security of the ciphers. Private key encryption is expected to produce *confusion* and *diffusion* on plaintext.

Stream Ciphers

Historically, stream ciphers came before block ciphers, and the earlier ones were natural successors of the classical ciphers. Stream ciphers are substitution ciphers that process texts one character at a time. Modern stream ciphers are used in applications where the amount of data is large and perhaps unavailable at the outset but needs to be encrypted online such as satellite TV signals and digital mobile phone traffic. In designing such cyphers, cryptographers tried to adhere to Auguste Kerckhoffs's Principles and concentrated on removing the need for statical analysis. Many stream ciphers have been developed, but they differ in how the key is generated.

The one-time Pad: This is a stream cypher that generalizes the Vigenere cypher by taking the keyword to be a random string of characters that is as long as the plaintext, and hence repeated patterns in the ciphertext cannot aid in deducing the key.

Example:

P: GIVEN C EVERY PLAINTEXT IS JUST AS LIKELY ...
Key: SAJRN NFBSS BTYNOLIARH JLBFG YADLS GALB …
C: YIEQE PJWWJ ZIJNW YBEOA RDKZYRAVWAQEWZ …

The one-time pad provides what is termed *'Perfect Security'* by Shannon's Theory of information security: "A cipher has perfect secrecy if and only if there are as many keys as possible plaintexts, and every key is equally likely".

Data Encryption Standard (DES)

In the early 1970s a variety of encipherment devises were available in the market. With the rapid advances in computer and communication technology, the need for secure communication between different organizations started to grow faster. Moreover, encipherment is often introduced within the context of communication protocols. Except for military and governmental purposes, standing encryption systems does make commercial sense and provides good framework for quality control.

In 1973, the American National Bureau of Standards (NBS) initiated a program on standardizing encryption algorithms. It was agreed that the IBM response was the one that fits the published requirements. This was the DES encryption system, which is a development from the earlier scheme *Lucifer*. The DES, also known as the DEA, is a symmetric private key block-cipher. It was designed according to Shannon's Theory of Information security with the aim of achieving confusion and diffusion (Substitution is the mean of confusion, and Transposition as the mean of diffusion).

Figure 5. Description of Feistel Network

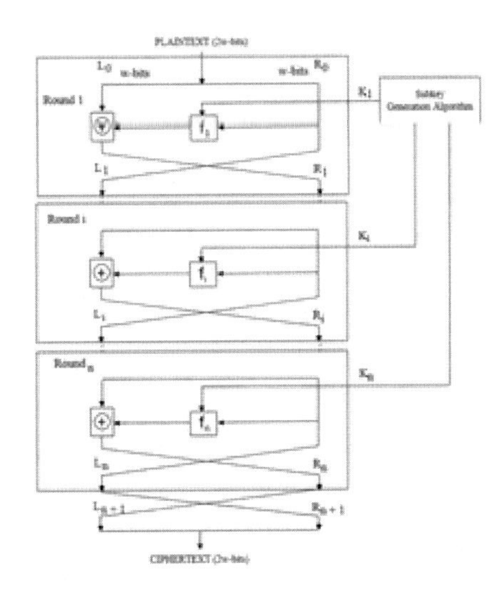

DES is a Feistel 64-bit block cipher, with 16 rounds. The round functions use standard arithmetic and logical operations on up to 64-bit numbers. It is suitable for implementation in software. A DES cipher has a private key of 56-bit length from which 16 48-bit parameters K_1, K_2, …, K_{16} are derived using a complex but otherwise published iterative procedure. The procedure involves certain published permutations, splitting, and a certain bit operation.

The i-th round function of a DES cipher consists of an expansion, followed by addition of K_i subkey, and then passed through a row of 8 S-boxes. Prior to the first Round the input is permuted in a certain way, and after the last round the inverse permutation is applied to get the cipher text.

Figure 6. Description of DES cipher

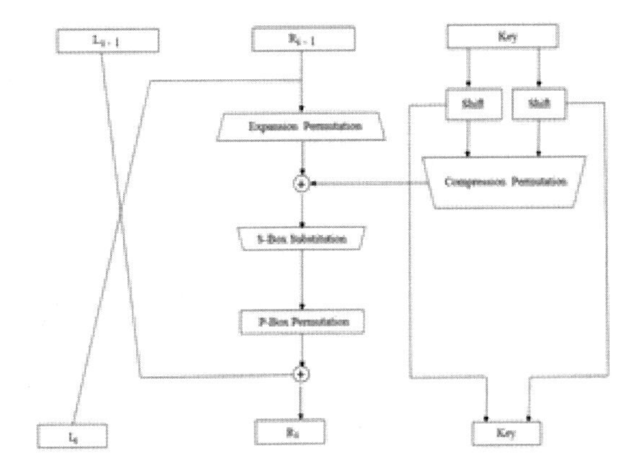

An S-box is table of 4 rows (indexed by 00, 01, 10, 11) and 16 columns (indexed by 0000, 0001, 0010, … , 1111) containing the numbers 0 ... 15. Note that, each these numbers can be expressed as a 4-bit string. An S-box is a substitution that compresses a 48-bit string into a 32-bits as follows: The rows are indexed by 00, 01, 10, and 11. The columns are indexed by 0000, 0001, 0010, …, 1111.

Example: S-Box 1 of the DES cipher

14	4	13	1	2	15	11	8	3	10	6	12	5	9	0	7
0	15	7	4	14	2	13	1	10	6	12	11	9	5	3	8
4	1	14	8	13	6	2	11	15	12	9	7	**3**	10	5	0
15	12	8	2	4	9	1	7	5	11	3	14	10	0	6	13

The j-th 6-bit t block of a 48-bit string is reduced to the 4-bit string in the j-th S-Box which is in the row determined by the numerical value of the first and last position of t, and in the column determined by the numerical value of the other 4 middle bits of t.

Example: If t = 110110 is the input to the S-box above, then it is replaced by the 4-bit in the row indexed by 10 and the column indexed by 1011. Hence, t is replaced by the 4-bit representation of 3, i.e., 0011 (please see the bolded entry in the above table).

As a Feistel cipher, DES decryption is achieved by the same encryption procedure but using the sub-keys K_1, K_2, … , K_{16} in the reverse order (DES, 2022).

Figure 7. Diagrammatic representation of Triple DES (TDES)

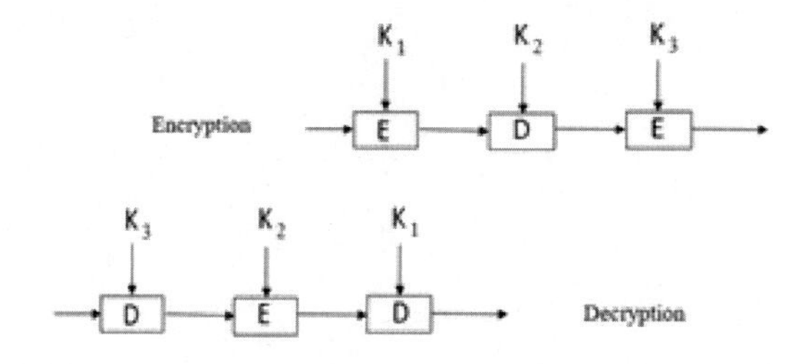

Triple DES There has been two criticisms of the DES at the preliminary stages. The first related to the wisdom of setting a standard for encryption, but it was also criticized for having too short a key. It is now widely accepted that a 56-bit key is not secure and has been broken using "**modest**" computer powers. Other than 56-bit key, have been considered. Longer keys result in more security, but efficiency may become a problem. Other than 16 iterations can be considered as way of improving efficiency, but less than 16 iterations weaken the system.

Triple DES is a block cipher that uses three different 56-bit keys and three executions of DES. Enciphering follows an **encrypt-decrypt-encrypt** (EDE) sequence, and deciphering follows a DED sequence, as shown above. TDEA cipher has the combined effects of taking a 168-bit key and 48 rounds, and yet it is as efficient as a single DES. The efficiency is a result of the fact that after the first two blocks, the three ciphers can work concurrently.

In lightweight block ciphers, design requires very generic bitwise operations (e.g., XOR, AND) and a specific Substitution box (S-box), which promotes an increased number of rounds. In addition, lightweight ciphers need unique cryptographic algorithms to implement information protection strategies.

Design Trends in Lightweight Block Ciphers

Many new generation block ciphers use an additional input alongside the plaintext, and the key called a tweak manages the cypher's operation. This category of ciphers is known as tweakable block ciphers. In recent years, different trends are emerging in designing lightweight block ciphers. The design is often considering hardware and software levels, and different operational efficiency metrics are opening new types of block chippers. The main objectives of these efficiencies measure are to ensure a trade-off between cost, performance, and security. In this way, the best workable solutions that can be achieved are two-fold, and they are (i) a high-cost need to be paid to make a secure and fast chip, and (ii) a slow chip will be less costly and secure.

Lightweight Encryption for IoT Security

In order to get total end-to-end security, the IoT data communication network nodes need to be encrypted. Authentication provides an important method in identification of users and electro-mechanical machineries or devices. This way, authentication can combat attacks to the IoT-based information systems. There are distinct categories of authentication protocols developed for IoT technology: (i) asymmetric-cryptosystem based protocol, symmetric-cryptosystem based protocols (as shown in Figure 8), and hybrid protocols (Ferran et al., 2017).

Since the IoT system users and devices communicate in two-ways, hence it needs authentication mechanisms security purpose. There are diverse types of authentication methods used and some of the recent research is described in the following section.

Blockchain technology

Blockchain technology is simply a database that maintains the history of all the transaction details without requiring a central authority. This database (i.e., global ledger) is secure and distributed. It is used by its many users, without intermediaries, which keeps records of all the transactions created between the nodes on a blockchain network as shown in Figure 6.

Figure 8. Symmetric lightweight cryptography for IoT systems

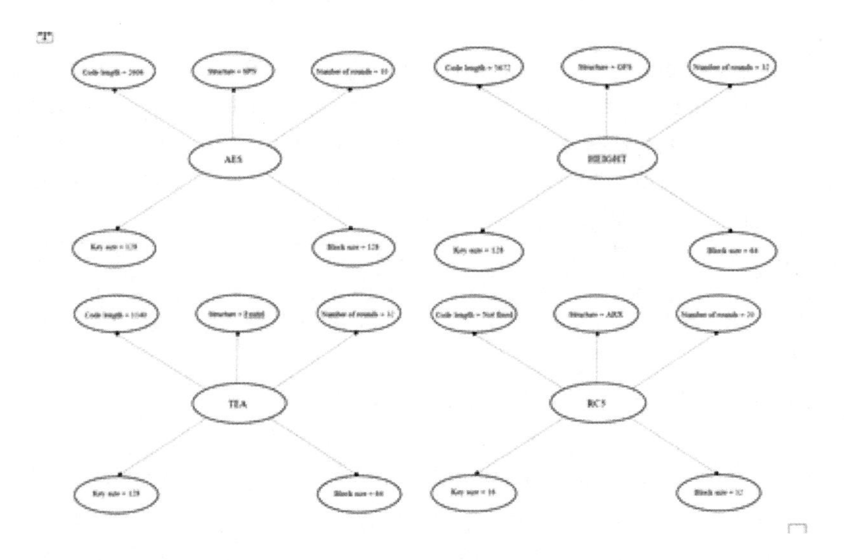

Figure 9. Diagrammatic representation of a blockchain

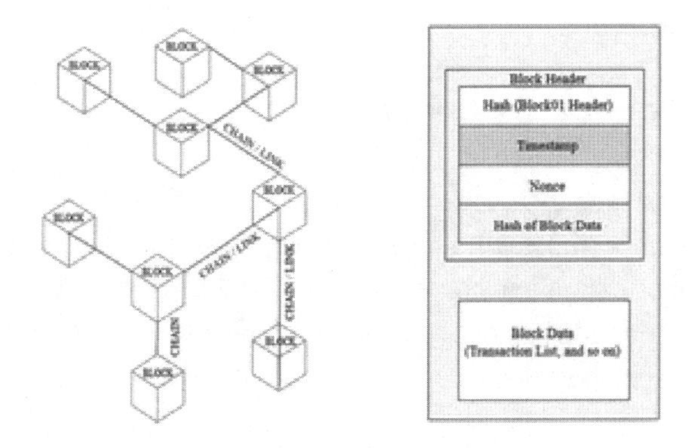

Architecturally a blockchain consists of *nodes*. An individual node is a computational device connected to the network using a program relaying transaction. The registry in which transactions of a system are recorded is known as a *ledger*. Blockchain technology uses a cryptography-based *hash function* for data/information security purposes.

The blockchain working principle allows everyone on the chain (or network) to check the validity of individual transactions through democratic processes of selection (known as *a smart contract*). Smart contracts are programs accessible and auditable by all authorized parties on the blockchain network, whose execution is thus controlled and verifiable.

A smart contract is an automated program capable of running a set of predefined functions when a particular condition(s) occurs. The program is stored on the distributed ledger and is capable of writing the resulting change to the distributed ledger. A diagrammatic representation is shown in Figure x.

Consensus mechanisms are used to ensure that all nodes in the network have the same information and that only valid transactions are recorded in the distributed register. The most common blockchain consensus mechanisms are Proof of Work (PoW), Proof of Stake (PoS), Practical Byzantine Fault Tolerance (PBFT), Hashcash, and Zero Knowledge Proof.

With this brief introduction of blockchain and IoT technology, the following section introduces a hybrid system architecture of these technologies. Integrating the blockchain into the IoT will lead to significant transformations in the healthcare industry. The blockchain can also offer a way of ensuring the security of user data as well as the protection of privacy, thus allowing for a greater adoption of IoT in the healthcare industry.

PROPOSED HEALTHCARE MONITORING FRAMEWORK

The proposed framework is based on a scenario of a remote healthcare system monitoring patients followed remotely by medical staff. In this context, patients are equipped with wearable sensors to measure individual medication conditions (e.g., oxygen saturation, heart rate, pulse, body temperature, blood pressure). The data gathered by these wearable devices are uploaded to a remote blockchain ledger (or database) system. A live monitoring component of this framework analyzes this data to detect a patient's medical condition and raises alarms if required to medical staff, who may take actions based on the health status evaluation of the patient.

Figure 10. Proposed hybrid system framework

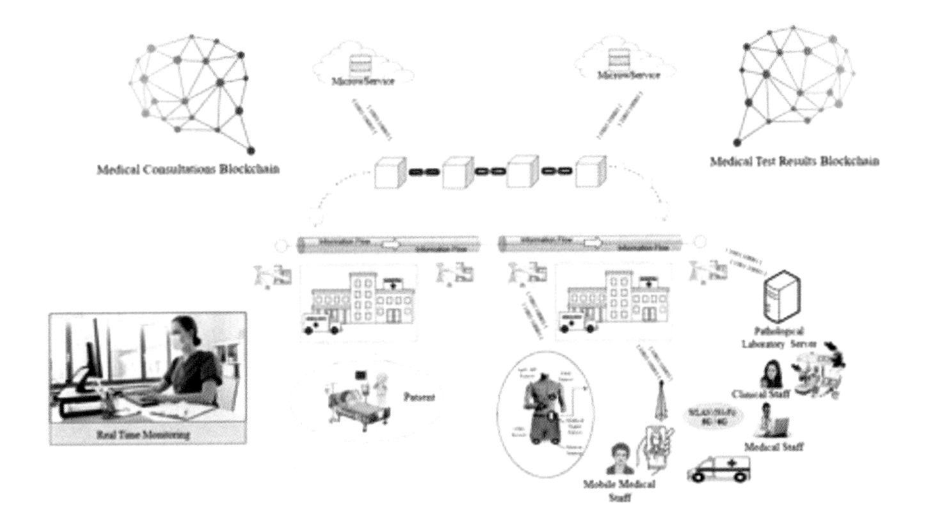

The presented framework illustrated in Figure 10 comprises two blockchain networks (i.e., Medical Consultation Blockchain and Medical Test Results Blockchain).

Research Works for Healthcare Application

With the current pandemic and an increase in population and medical conditions, the workload on global healthcare systems is escalating very rapidly. The application of the fifth generation (5G) wireless networks, IoT-based developments, and blockchain technology is gaining momentum for the healthcare industry's deployment purpose. These new-generation innovative technologies are considered a potential solution to alleviate the pressure on healthcare systems (Kumari et al., 2018) (Gapchup et al., 2016) (Islam et al., 2015). One of the solutions is a remote health monitoring system that uses IoT sensor devices to measure and analyze different health parameters of a patient remotely. For example, Baker and fellow researchers (Baker et al., 2017) highlighted the main components of an end-to-end IoT-based healthcare system for remote monitoring of critically ill patient health conditions.

In another application area, for example, EHR (Hathaliyaa et al., 2019), digitization of patients' health-related information is also necessary to automate healthcare activities. This application shares patients' real-time medical information (e.g., diagnoses and treatment histories) with certain authorized healthcare personnel (HealthIT, 2022). In a different research project, Ekblaw and fellow researchers presented a decentralized patient record management system known as MedRec to manage EHRs using blockchain technology (Ekblaw et al., 2016). The reported system handles security and privacy-related issues, for example, authentication, accountability, confidentiality, and data sharing ability with privacy. Finally, it encourages a different group of users (e.g., public health authorities, medics, and researchers) to use the system, which is designed and developed as a blockchain network.

A diabetes monitoring system named secured mobile-enabled assisting device (SMEAD) was proposed by Saravanan and fellow researchers (Saravanan et al., 2017). SMEAD is designed using blockchain technology, and it performs real-time monitoring of diabetic patients. In addition, the system was designed on the assumption that wearable devices were not appropriate for emergencies and were merely used for monitoring purposes. In addition, the deployed system helps patients who want exceptional care and continuous supervision from specialized medics.

Solanas and other researchers (Solanas et al., 2014) designed and developed an intelligent health (s-health) healthcare system in the context of smart cities. The main goal of intelligent health apps is to consider health within the innovative city application in a sustainable manner. Afterwards, another group of researchers (Capossele et al., 2018) presented a model which fostered the development of such s-health applications. It was intended as an upgraded software edition of the existing e-health solutions (Solanas et al., 2014) (Vora et al., 2018). This system was designed with the help of collected data from different HER and access to the smart cities' data and infrastructure using technologies like IoT and 5G to provide an appropriate real-time feedback mechanism to fellow citizens. In addition, a group of researchers recently highlighted in the importance of IoT technology with blockchain (Solanki et al., 2022).

However, the system designers lacked a few securities-related issues that must be addressed. For example, the trustless property of the software-based platform implied a requirement of secure middleware to get rid of any third-party access. In order to mitigate the issue above, a group of researchers (Capossele et al., 2018) developed a blockchain-based s-health platform to mitigate technical challenges like privacy, security, consistency, interoperability, and trust using 5G capability and IoT technology.

Finally, the proposed system permits the connection of more than one IoT device with high reliability and low latency.

FUTURE WORK

The ubiquitous nature of IoT raises an essential set of issues about users' privacy and how to mitigate the diverseness of individual and commercial system needs regarding privacy services. It needs context-aware, adaptive, and user-centered privacy mitigating options. This way, the diversity of system privacy needs can be tackled using adaptive and context-awareness handling techniques of privacy profiles and governance regulations. It also includes the consideration of privacy in dynamic and heterogeneous operating environments.

The development and importance of edge computing are driving new challenges (e.g., healthcare 5.0, artificial intelligence (AI), machine learning (ML)) for application development. In addition, smart and light technology for lightweight cryptography design and development is essential for future healthcare service deployment. All these research issues will be considered in future work.

CONCLUSION

IoT technologies are used in different healthcare applications. This chapter briefly surveyed some of the industrial applications. In addition, this review briefly presented different architectural issues, attack vectors, and challenges to IoT security. Finally, concepts of block ciphers and architectural components are discussed. Finally, information systems privacy issues (e.g., authentication and encryption techniques) are discussed.

Emerging weaknesses, such as unprotected information exchange channels, unsecured activities in data communication, and unprotected devices, make obvious risks to IoT-based information systems and their networks. It is also true that IoT system devices are attractive points of surface attacks for their irregular system software updates.

Appropriate security measures (e.g., authentication and encryption) and blockchain technology may provide appropriate protection strategies in solving privacy and privacy-related problems in IoT systems. In addition, implementing authentication and encryption mechanisms for resource constraints IoT devices is a daunting task. Lightweight cryptography presents solutions to the problems. This chapter presents IoT-based applications' attack surface and lightweight cryptography solutions, and appropriate IoT threat modelling might help plan adequate system security.

REFERENCES

Abdul-Hussein, R. M., Mohammed, R. S., & Mohammed, A. H. (2021). Review: Security challenges and cyber-attacks for internet of things. In *2021 1st Babylon International Conference on Information Technology and Science (BICITS)*, 81–85. 10.1109/BICITS51482.2021.9509899

Aborujilah, A., Yatim, M. N. M., & Al-Othmani, A. (2021, December). Blockchain-based adoption framework for authentic land registry system in Malaysia [Telecommunication Computing Electronics and Control]. *TELKOMNIKA*, *19*(6), 2038–2049. doi:10.12928/telkomnika.v19i6.19276

Ali, W., Din, I. U., Almogren, A., Guizani, M., & Zuair, M. (2021, September). A lightweight privacy-aware IoT-based metering scheme for smart industrial ecosystems. *IEEE Transactions on Industrial Informatics*, *17*(9), 6134–6143. doi:10.1109/TII.2020.2984366

Alshammari, B. M., Guesmi, R., Guesmi, T., Alsaif, H., & Alzamil, A. (2021, January). Implementing a symmetric lightweight cryptosystem in highly constrained iot devices by using a chaotic s-box. *Symmetry*, *13*(1), 1–20. doi:10.3390ym13010129

Auer, S., Nagler, S., Mazumdar, S., & Mukkamala, R. R. (2022, April). Towards blockchain-IoT based shared mobility: Car-sharing and leasing as a case study. *Journal of Network and Computer Applications*, *200*, 103316. doi:10.1016/j.jnca.2021.103316

Ayachi, R., Mhaouch, A., & Ben Abdelali, A. (2021, May). Lightweight cryptography for network-on-chip data encryption. *Security and Communication Networks*, *2021*, 1–10. doi:10.1155/2021/9943713

Baker, S. B., Xiang, W., & Atkinson, I. (2017). Internet of things for smart healthcare: Technologies, challenges, and opportunities. *IEEE Access: Practical Innovations, Open Solutions*, *5*, 26521–26544.

Berners-Lee, T. (2000). *Weaving the Web: The Original Design and Ultimate Design of the World Wide Web by its inventor*. Harper Business.

Bhatti, S. N., Haywood, G., & Yanagida, R. (2021). End-to-End Privacy for Identity & Location with IP. *29th IEEE International Conference on Network Protocols, Virtual Event*. IEEE. 10.1109/ICNP52444.2021.9651909

Bonomi, F., Milito, R., Natarajan, P., & Zhu, J. (2014). Fog computing: a platform for internet of things and analytics. In *Big Data and Internet of Things: A Road Map for Smart Environments*. Springer. doi:10.1007/978-3-319-05029-4_7

Borgia, E. (2014). The Internet of Things vision: Key features, applications, and open issues. *Computer Communications*, *54*, 1–31. doi:10.1016/j.comcom.2014.09.008

Capossele, A., Conti, M., Gaglione, A., Lazzeretti, R., Missier, P., & Nati, M. (2018). Leveraging blockchain to enable smart-health applications. In *IEEE 4th International Forum on Research and Technology for Society and Industry (RTSI), (pp. 1-6)*. IEEE.

Cenedese, A., Zanella, A., Vangelista, L., & Zorzi, M. (2014). Padova smart city: an urban internet of things experimentation. In *Proceeding of 3rd IEEE World Forum on Internet of Things (WF-IoT)*, (pp. 609-614). IEEE.

Chiadighikaobi, I. R., & Katuk, N. (2021). A scoping study on lightweight cryptography reviews in IoT. *Baghdad Science Journal*, *18*(2), 989–1000. doi:10.21123/bsj.2021.18.2(Suppl.).0989

Crowcroft, J., Gibbens, R., Kelly, F., & Ostring, S. (2003). Modelling incentives for collaboration in Mobile Ad Hoc Networks. *Proceedings of Modeling and Optimization in Mobile, Ad Hoc and Wireless Networks (WiOpt)*.

Crowcroft, J., Gibbens, R., Kelly, F., & Ostring, S. (2004). Modelling Incentives for Collaboration in Mobile Ad Hoc Networks. *International Journal of Performance Evaluation*, *57*(4), 427–439. doi:10.1016/j.peva.2004.03.003

Datta Burton, S., Tanczer, L. M., & Vasudevan, S. Hailes, S., & Carr, M. (2021). The UK Code of Practice for Computer IoT Cybersecurity: where we are and what next. Department for Digital, Culture, Media & Sport.

Deebak, B. D., Al-Turjman, F., Aloqaily, M., & Alfandi, O. (2019). O. (2019). An authentic-based privacy preservation protocol for smart e-Healthcare systems in IoT. *IEEE Access: Practical Innovations, Open Solutions*, *7*, 135632–135649. doi:10.1109/ACCESS.2019.2941575

Dhanda, S. S., Singh, B., & Jindal, P. (2020). Lightweight Cryptography: A Solution to Secure IoT, Wireless Person. *Commun, (2020),* 1–34.

Dwivedi, A. D. (2021, August). Brisk: Dynamic encryption-based cipher for long term security [TELKOMNIKA Telecommun Comput El Control]. *Sensors (Basel)*, *21*(17), 5744. doi:10.339021175744 PMID:34502635

Ferrag, M. A., Maglaras, L. A., Janicke, H., Jiang, J., & Shu, L. (2017). Authentication Protocols for Internet of Things: A Comprehensive Survey. *Security and Communication Networks*, *2017*, 1–41. doi:10.1155/2017/6562953

Gaur, L. (2022). Internet of Things in Healthcare. In Geospatial Data Science in Healthcare for Society 5.0 (pp. 131-140). Springer.

Gong, J., & Navimipour, N. J. (2022). An in-depth and systematic literature review on the blockchain-based approaches for cloud computing. *Cluster Computing*, *25*(1), 383–400. doi:10.100710586-021-03412-2

Guan, Z., Yang, W., Zhu, L., Wu, L., & Wang, R. (2021, June). Achieving adaptively secure data access control with privacy protection for lightweight IoT devices. *Science China. Information Sciences*, *64*(6), 1–14. doi:10.100711432-020-2957-5

Gubbi, J., Buyya, R., Murusic, S., & Palaniswami, M. (2013). Internet of Things (IoT): A vision, architectural elements, and future directions. *Future Generation Computer Systems*, *29*(7), 1645–1660. doi:10.1016/j.future.2013.01.010

Gupta, A., Tripathi, M., Shaikh, T. J., & Sharma, A. (2019, February). A lightweight anonymous user authentication and key establishment scheme for wearable devices. *Computer Networks*, *149*, 29–42. doi:10.1016/j.comnet.2018.11.021

Harbi, Y., Aliouat, Z., Refoufi, A., Harous, S. A., & Bentaleb, A. (2019). Enhanced authentication and key management scheme for securing data transmission in the Internet of Things. *Ad Hoc Networks*, *94*(Nov), 101948. doi:10.1016/j.adhoc.2019.101948

Hinch, R., Probert, W., Nurtay, A., Kendall, M., Wymant, C., Hall, M., Fraser, C., Hall, M., Lythgoe, K., Cruz, A. B., Zhao, L., Stewart, A., Ferretti, L., Parker, M., Meroueh, A., Mathias, B., Stevenson, S., Montero, D., Warren, J., Mather, N. K., Finkelstein, A., Abeler-Domer, L., Bonsall, D., & Fraser, C. (2020). *Effective configurations of a digital contact tracing app: A report to NHSX (NHSX Report).* The Conversation Trust (UK).

Hinch, R., Probert, W., Nurtay, A., Kendall, M., Wymant, C., Hall, M., Fraser, C., Lythgoe, K., Cruz, A. B., Zhao, L., Stewart, A., Ferretti, L., Parker, M., Meroueh, A., Mathias, B., Stevenson, S., Montero, D., Warren, J., Mather, N. K., & Fraser, C. (2020). Effective configurations of a digital contact tracing app: A report to NHSX (NHSX Report). *The Conversation Trust (UK).* https://cdn.theconversation.com/static_files/files/1009/Report_-_Effectiv_App_Configurations.pdf

Hu, Y. C., Perrig, A., & Johnson, D. B. (2003). *Packet leashes: A defense against wormhole attacks in wireless networks.* In *Twenty-Second Annual Joint Conference of the Computer and Communications. INFOCOM, 3,* 1976–1986. IEEE 10.1109/INFCOM.2003.1209219

Islami, S. M. R., Kwak, D., Humaun Kabiri, M .D., Hossain, M., & Kwaki, K. (2015). The Internet of Things for Health Care: A Comprehensive Survey. *IEEE Translations and content mining, 3,* (pp. 678-708). IEEE.

Karbasi, A. H., & Shahpasand, S. (2021). SINGLETON: A lightweight and secure end-to-end encryption protocol for the sensor networks in the Internet of Things based on cryptographic ratchets. *The Journal of Supercomputing, 77*(4), 3516–3554. doi:10.100711227-020-03411-x

Karlof, C., & Wagner, D. (2003). Secure routing in wireless sensor networks: Attacks and countermeasures. *Ad Hoc Networks, 1*(2), 293–315. doi:10.1016/S1570-8705(03)00008-8

Kaswan, K. S., Gaur, L., Dhatterwal, J. S., & Kumar, R. (2021). AI-based natural language processing for the generation of meaningful information electronic health record (EHR) data. In Advanced AI Techniques and Applications in Bioinformatics, 41-86. CRC Press.

Kaushik, K., & Dahiya, S. (2018). Security and Privacy in IoT based EBusiness and Retail, *2018 International Conference on System Modeling & Advancement in Research Trends (SMART),* (pp. 78–81). 10.1109/SYSMART.2018.8746961

Kaushik, K., & Singh, K. (2020). Security and Trust in IoT Communications: Role and Impact. In S. Choudhury, R. Mishra, R. Mishra, & A. Kumar (Eds.), *Intelligent Communication, Control and Devices. Advances in Intelligent Systems and Computing, 989.* Springer. doi:10.1007/978-981-13-8618-3_81

Khan, K. M., Arshad, J., Iqbal, W., Abdullah, S., & Zaib, H. (2022). Blockchain-enabled real-time SLA monitoring for cloud-hosted services. *Cluster Computing, 25*(1), 537–559. doi:10.100710586-021-03416-y

Khan, S., Lee, W. K., & Hwang, S. O. (2022, March). AEchain: A lightweight blockchain for IoT applications. *IEEE Consumer Electronics Magazine, 11*(2), 64–76. doi:10.1109/MCE.2021.3060373

Khubrani, M. M., & Alam, S. (2021, August). A detailed review of blockchain-based applications for protection against pandemic like COVID-19 [Telecommunication Computing Electronics and Control]. *TELKOMNIKA, 19*(4), 1185–1196. doi:10.12928/telkomnika.v19i4.18465

Lee, H., Kang, D., Ryu, J., Won, D., Kim, H., & Lee, Y. (2020, June). A three-factor anonymous user authentication scheme for Internet of Things environments. *Journal of Information Security Application.*, *52*, 102494. doi:10.1016/j.jisa.2020.102494

Lee, S. W., & Sim, K. B. (2021, May). Design and hardware implementation of a simplified dag-based blockchain and new aes-cbc algorithm for iot security. *Electronics (Basel)*, *10*(9), 1127. doi:10.3390/electronics10091127

Li, S., Zhao, S., Min, G., Qi, L., & Liu, G. (2021). Lightweight privacy-preserving scheme using homomorphic encryption in industrial internet of things. *IEEE Internet of Things Journal*, 2021.

Liu, T., Wang, Y., Li, Y., Tong, X., Qi, L., & Jiang, N. (2020, September). Privacy protection based on stream cipher for spatiotemporal data in IoT. *IEEE Internet of Things Journal*, *7*(9), 7928–7940. doi:10.1109/JIOT.2020.2990428

Luo, X., Yin, L., Li, C., Wang, C., Fang, F., Zhu, C., & Tian, Z. (2020). A lightweight privacy-preserving communication protocol for heterogeneous IoT environment. *IEEE Access: Practical Innovations, Open Solutions*, *8*, 67192–67204. doi:10.1109/ACCESS.2020.2978525

Mbed, O. S. (2022). *Mbed OS Features.* armMedbed. https://www.mbed.com/en/platform/mbed-os/ (accessed on July 2022).

Modares, H., Salleh, R., & Moravejosharieh, A. (2011). Overview of security issues in wireless sensor networks. In *Third International Conference on Computational Intelligence, Modelling and Simulation (CIMSiM)*, (pp. 308–311). IEEE. 10.1109/CIMSim.2011.62

Nakamoto, S. (2008). *Bitcoin: A peer-to-peer electronic cash system.* Bitcoin.

Newsome, J., Shi, E., Song, D., & Perrig, A. (2004). The sybil attack in sensor networks: Analysis & defenses. In *Proceedings of the 3rd International Symposium on Information Processing in Sensor Networks*, (pp. 259–268). ACM. 10.1145/984622.984660

Noura, H., Couturier, R., Pham, C., & Chehab, A. (2019). Lightweight stream cipher scheme for resource-constrained IoT devices. In *Proc. Int. Conf. Wireless Mobile Comput., Netw. Commun. (WiMob)*, (pp. 1–8).

Pal, K. (2019). Algorithmic Solutions for RFID Tag Anti-Collision Problem in Supply Chain Management. In *the 9th International Symposium on Frontiers in Ambient and Mobile Systems (FAMS 19)*, 929-934. Procedia Computer Science.

Pal, K. (2021a). *Privacy, Security and Policies: A Review of Problems and Solutions with Blockchain-Based Internet of Things Applications in Industrial Industry.* In the 18th International Conference on Mobile Systems and Pervasive Computing (MobiSPC), Procedia Computer Science, Leuven, Belgium.

Pal, K. (2021b). A Novel Frame-Slotted ALOHA Algorithm for Radio Frequency Identification System in Supply Chain Management. In *11th International Symposium on Frontiers in Ambient and Mobile Systems (FAMS)*, (pp. 871- 876). Procedia Computer Science. 10.1016/j.procs.2021.03.110

Pal, K. (2022a). Application of Game Theory in Blockchain-Based Healthcare Information System. In Malay Dutta Borah, Peng Zhang, and Ganesh Chandra Deka (eds.), Prospects of Blockchain Technology for Accelerating Scientific Advancement in Healthcare, 84-99. IGI Global Publishing.

Pal, K. (2022b). A Decentralized Privacy Preserving Healthcare Blockchain for IoT, Challenges and Solutions. In Malay Dutta Borah, Peng Zhang, Ganesh Chandra Deka (eds.), Prospects of Blockchain Technology for Accelerating Scientific Advancement in Healthcare, 158-188. IGI Global Publishing.

Pal, K. (2022b). Semantic Interoperability in Internet of Things: Architecture, Protocols, and Research Challenges. In M Pejic-Bach and C Dogru (eds), Management Strategies for Sustainability, New Knowledge Innovation, and Personalized Products and Services, 40-171. The IGI Global Publishing.

Pal, K. (2022d). Cryptography and Blockchain Solutions for Security Protection of Internet of Things Applications. In Biswa Mohan Sahoo and Suman Avdhesh Yadav (eds.), Information Security Practices for the Internet of Things, 5G, and Next-Generation Wireless Networks, 152-178. IGI Global.

Pal, K., & Yasar, A. (2020b). Semantic Approach to Data Integration for an Internet of Things Supporting Apparel Supply Chain Management. In *the 17th International Conference on Mobile Systems and Pervasive Computing (MobiSPC),* 197 - 204. Procedia Computer Science.

Pal, K., & Yasar, K. (2020a). Internet of Things and Blockchain Technology in Apparel Manufacturing Supply Chain Data Management. In *the 11th International Conference on Ambient Systems, Networks, and Technologies (ANT 2020),* 450 – 457. Procedia Computer Science.

Ragab, A. A. M., Madani, A., Wahdan, A. M., & Selim, G. M. L. (2021, January). Design, analysis, and implementation of a new lightweight block cipher for protecting IoT smart devices. *Journal of Ambient Intelligence and Humanized Computing*, 1–18. doi:10.100712652-020-02782-6

Reyna, A., Martín, C., Chen, J., Soler, E., & Díaz, M. (2018, November). On blockchain and its integration with IoT. Challenges and opportunities. *Future Generation Computer Systems*, *88*, 173–190. doi:10.1016/j.future.2018.05.046

Sadhukhan, D., Ray, S., Biswas, G. P., Khan, M. K., & Dasgupta, M. (2021). A lightweight remote user authentication scheme for IoT communication using elliptic curve cryptography. *The Journal of Supercomputing*, *77*(2), 1114–1151. doi:10.100711227-020-03318-7

Santosh, K. C., & Gaur, L. (2021). Ai in precision medicine. In Artificial Intelligence and Machine Learning in Public Healthcare, 41-47. Springer.

Santosh, K. C., & Gaur, L. (2021). Introduction to ai in public health. In Artificial Intelligence and Machine Learning in Public Healthcare, 1-10. Springer.

Santosh, K. C., & Gaur, L. (2022). *Artificial Intelligence and Machine Learning in Public Healthcare: Opportunities and Societal Impact.* Springer Nature.

Saravanan, M., Shubha, R., Marks, A. M., & Iyer, V. (2017). SMEAD: A Secured Mobile Enabled Assisting Device for Diabetics Monitoring, *IEEE International Conference on Advanced Networks and Telecommunications Systems (ANTS)*, (pp. 1-6). IEEE.

Shahzadi, R., Anwar, S. M., Qamar, F., Ali, M., & Rodrigues, J. P. C. (2019). Chaos based enhanced RC5 algorithm for security and integrity of clinical images in remote health monitoring. *IEEE Access: Practical Innovations, Open Solutions*, *7*, 52858–52870. doi:10.1109/ACCESS.2019.2909554

Shannon, C. E. (1949). Communication Theory of Secrecy Systems. *The Bell System Technical Journal, 28*(4), 656–715. doi:10.1002/j.1538-7305.1949.tb00928.x

Sharafi, M., Fotouhi-Ghazvini, F., Shirali, M., & Ghassemian, M. (2019). A low power cryptography solution based on chaos theory in wireless sensor nodes. *IEEE Access: Practical Innovations, Open Solutions, 7*, 8737–8753. doi:10.1109/ACCESS.2018.2886384

Shi, E., & Perrig, A. (2004). Designing secure sensor networks. *IEEE Wireless Communications, 11*(6), 38–43. doi:10.1109/MWC.2004.1368895

Shi, N., Tan, L., Yan, C., He, C., Xu, J., Lu, Y., & Xu, H. (2021, September). BacS: A blockchain-based access control scheme in distributed internet of things. *Peer-to-Peer Networking and Applications, 14*(5), 2585–2599. doi:10.100712083-020-00930-5

Singh, K., & Kaushik, K. Ahatsham, & Shahare V. (2020). Role and Impact of Wearables in IoT Healthcare. In: Raju K., Govardhan A., Rani B., Sridevi R., Murty M. (eds) *Proceedings of the Third International Conference on Computational Intelligence and Informatics. Advances in Intelligent Systems and Computing, (vol 1090).* Springer.

Sleem, L., & Couturier, R. (2021, May). Speck-R: An ultra-light-weight cryptographic scheme for internet of things. *Multimedia Tools and Applications, 80*(11), 17067–17102. doi:10.100711042-020-09625-8

Solanas, A., Patsakis, C., Conti, M., Vlachos, I. S., Ramos, V., Falcone, F., Postolache, O., Perez-Martinez, P. A., Pietro, R. D., Perrea, D. N., & Martinez-Balleste, A. (2014). Smart health: A context-aware health paradigm within smart cities. *IEEE Communications Magazine, 52*(8), 74–81.

Solanki, A., Jain, V., & Gaur, L. (Eds.). (2022). *Applications of Blockchain and Big IoT Systems: Digital Solutions for Diverse Industries*. CRC Press.

Sowjanya, K., Dasgupta, M., & Ray, S. (2021, August). A lightweight key management scheme for key-escrow-free ECC-based CP-ABE for IoT healthcare systems. *Journal of Systems Architecture, 117*, 102108. doi:10.1016/j.sysarc.2021.102108

Sruthi, M., & Rajasekaran, R. (2021). Hybrid lightweight signcryption scheme for IoT. *Open Computer Science, 11*(1), 391–398. doi:10.1515/comp-2020-0105

Sun, Y. F., Lo, F. P. W., & Lo, B. (2021). Light-weight internet-of-things device authentication, encryption and key distribution using end-to-end neural cryptosystems. *IEEE Internet of Things Journal, 14*(8), 1–10. doi:10.1109/JIOT.2021.3123822

Usman, M., Ahmed, I., Aslam, M. I., Khan, S., & U. A. Shah U. A. (2017*). SIT: A lightweight encryption algorithm for secure Internet of Things.* arXiv:1704.08688. https://arxiv.org/abs/1704.08688

Villamil, S., Hernández, C., & Tarazona, G. (2020, October). An overview of internet of things [Telecommunication Computing Electronics and Control]. *TELKOMNIKA, 18*(5), 2320–2327. doi:10.12928/telkomnika.v18i5.15911

Wazid, M., Das, A. K., Odelu, V., Kumar, N., Conti, M., & Jo, M. (2017, February). Design of secure user authenticated key management protocol for generic IoT networks. *IEEE Internet of Things Journal, 5*(1), 269–282. doi:10.1109/JIOT.2017.2780232

Whaiduzzaman, M., Hossain, M. R., Shovon, A. R., Roy, S., Laszka, A., Buyya, R., & Barros, A. (2020). A Privacy-Preserving Mobile and Fog Computing Framework to Trace and Prevent COVID-19 Community Transmission. *IEEE Journal of Biomedical and Health Informatics, 24*(12), 3564–3575. doi:10.1109/JBHI.2020.3026060 PMID:32966223

Wu, F., Li, X., Sangaiah, A. K., Xu, L., Kumari, S., Wu, L., & Shen, J. (2018, May). A lightweight and robust two-factor authentication scheme for personalized healthcare systems using wireless medical sensor networks. *Future Generation Computer Systems*, *82*, 727–737. doi:10.1016/j.future.2017.08.042

Xiang, W., & Yuanyuan, Z. (2022). Scalable access control scheme of internet of things based on blockchain based on blockchain. *Procedia Computer Science*, *198*, 448–453. doi:10.1016/j.procs.2021.12.268

Xie, X., & Chen, Y. C. (2021, April). Decentralized data aggregation: A new secure framework based on lightweight cryptographic algorithms. *Wireless Communications and Mobile Computing*, *2021*(3), 1–12.

Yu, B., Yang, M., Wang, Z., & Gao, C. S. (2006). Identify Abnormal Packet Loss in Selective Forwarding Attacks. *Chinese Journal of Computers*, *9*, 1540–1550.

Zia, T., & Zomaya, A. (2006). Security issues in wireless sensor networks. In *International Conference on Systems and Networks Communications, ICSNC'06*, (p. 40). IEEE.

Compilation of References

Abbass, H. A. (2002). An evolutionary artificial deep Neural Networks approach for breast cancer diagnosis. *Artificial Intelligence in Medicine*, *25*(3), 265–281.

Abdul-Hussein, R. M., Mohammed, R. S., & Mohammed, A. H. (2021). Review: Security challenges and cyber-attacks for internet of things. In *2021 1st Babylon International Conference on Information Technology and Science (BICITS)*, 81–85. 10.1109/BICITS51482.2021.9509899

Aborujilah, A., Yatim, M. N. M., & Al-Othmani, A. (2021, December). Blockchain-based adoption framework for authentic land registry system in Malaysia [Telecommunication Computing Electronics and Control]. *TELKOMNIKA*, *19*(6), 2038–2049. doi:10.12928/telkomnika.v19i6.19276

Afaq, A., Gaur, L., Singh, G., & Dhir, A. (2021). COVID-19: transforming air passengers' behaviour and reshaping their expectations towards the airline industry. Tourism Recreation Research., https://doi.org/10.1080/02508281.2021.2008211.

Ahmadi, H., Nag, A., Khar, Z., Sayrafian, K., & Rahardja, S. (2021). Networked Twins and Twins of Networks: An Overview on the Relationship between Digital Twins and 6G. *IEEE Communications Standards Magazine, 5* (4), pp. 154-160. doi:10.1109/MCOMSTD.0001.2000041

Aich, S., Sinai, N. K., Kumar, S., Ali, M., Choi, Y. R., Joo, M. I., & Kim, H. C. (2021, February). Protecting Personal Healthcare Record Using Blockchain & Federated Learning Technologies. In 2021 23rd International Conference on Advanced Communication Technology (ICACT) (pp. 109-112). IEEE. 10.23919/ICACT51234.2021.9370566

Aidan Fuller, Z. F. (28 May 2020). Digital Twin: Enabling Technologies, Challenges and Open Research. *IEEE.*

Ali, W., Din, I. U., Almogren, A., Guizani, M., & Zuair, M. (2021, September). A lightweight privacy-aware IoT-based metering scheme for smart industrial ecosystems. *IEEE Transactions on Industrial Informatics*, *17*(9), 6134–6143. doi:10.1109/TII.2020.2984366

Alrashed, S., Min-Allah, N., Ali, I., & Mehmood, R. (2022). COVID-19 outbreak and the role of digital twin. *Multimedia Tools and Applications*. doi:10.100711042-021-11664-8

Alshammari, B. M., Guesmi, R., Guesmi, T., Alsaif, H., & Alzamil, A. (2021, January). Implementing a symmetric lightweight cryptosystem in highly constrained iot devices by using a chaotic s-box. *Symmetry*, *13*(1), 1–20. doi:10.3390ym13010129

Amann, J., Blasimme, A., Vayena, E., Frey, D., & Madai, V. I. (2020). Explainability for artificial intelligence in health-care: A multidisciplinary perspective. *BMC Medical Informatics and Decision Making*, *20*(1), 1–9. doi:10.118612911-020-01332-6 PMID:33256715

Ambika, N. (2019). Energy-Perceptive Authentication in Virtual Private Networks Using GPS Data. In M. Z. (eds), Security, privacy and trust in the IoT environment (pp. 25-38). Springer. doi:10.1007/978-3-030-18075-1_2

Ambika, N. (2020). Tackling jamming attacks in IoT. In A. M., S. K., & K. S. (eds), Tackling jamming attacks in IoT. (pp. 153-165). Springer. doi:10.1007/978-3-030-37468-6_8

American Nurses Association. (2012). *State legislation on safe patient handling*. ANA. http://www.anasafepatienthandling.org/Main-Menu/ANAActions/State-Legislation.aspx .

Amir Latif, R. M., Hussain, K., Jhanjhi, N. Z., Nayyar, A., & Rizwan, O. (2020). A remix IDE: Smart contract-based framework for the healthcare sector by using Blockchain technology. *Multimedia Tools and Applications*, 1–24. https://ieeexplore.ieee.org/abstract/document/9214512

Annangi, P., Ravishankar, H., Patil, R., Tore, B., Aase, S. A., & Steen, E. (2020, September). AI assisted feedback system for transmit parameter optimization in Cardiac Ultrasound. In *2020 IEEE International Ultrasonics Symposium (IUS)* (pp. 1-4). IEEE. 10.1109/IUS46767.2020.9251501

Antarsih, N. R., Setyawati, S. P., Ningsih, S., Sulaiman, E., & Pujiastuti, N. (2022, January). *Telehealth Business Potential in Indonesia*. In *International Conference on Social, Economics, Business, and Education (ICSE 2021)* (pp. 73-78). Atlantis Press.

Ao, F., Zhang, M., Liu, Y., & Nee, A. Y. (2018). Digital twin driven prognostics and health management for complex equipment. *CIRP Annals*, *67*(1), 169–172. doi:10.1016/j.cirp.2018.04.055

Arun, S. (2017), Digital Twin - An Emerging Technology for Geospatial World. *Satpalda Geospatial Services*. https://www.satpalda.com/blogs/digital-twin-an-emerging-technology-for-geospatial-world

Auer, S., Nagler, S., Mazumdar, S., & Mukkamala, R. R. (2022, April). Towards blockchain-IoT based shared mobility: Car-sharing and leasing as a case study. *Journal of Network and Computer Applications*, *200*, 103316. doi:10.1016/j.jnca.2021.103316

Augusto, C., & … . "Test-Driven Anonymization in Health Data: A Case Study on Assistive Reproduction," *2020 IEEE International Conference On Artificial Intelligence Testing (AITest)*, 2020, pp. 81-82, 10.1109/AITEST49225.2020.00019

Autiosalo, J., Vepsalainen, J., Viitala, R., & Tammi, K. (2019). A Feature-Based Framework for Structuring Industrial Digital Twins. *IEEE Access, 8*, 1193–1208. [CrossRef]

Autiosalo, J.; Vepsalainen, J.; Viitala, R.; Tammi, K. A (2019). Feature-Based Framework for Structuring Industrial Digital Twins. *IEEE Access 8,* 1193–1208.

Ayachi, R., Mhaouch, A., & Ben Abdelali, A. (2021, May). Lightweight cryptography for network-on-chip data encryption. *Security and Communication Networks*, *2021*, 1–10. doi:10.1155/2021/9943713

Baker, S. B., Xiang, W., & Atkinson, I. (2017). Internet of things for smart healthcare: Technologies, challenges, and opportunities. *IEEE Access: Practical Innovations, Open Solutions*, *5*, 26521–26544.

Barnard, Y., Bradley, M. D., Hodgson, F., & Lloyd, A. D. (2013). Older adults' learning to use new technologies: Perceived difficulties, experimentation behavior, and usability. *Computers in Human Behavior*, *29*(4), 1715–1724. doi:10.1016/j.chb.2013.02.006

Barricelli, B.; Casiraghi, E.; Gliozzo, J.; Petrini, A.; Valtolina, S. (n.d.). Human Digital Twin for Fitness Management. *IEEE* doi:. doi:10.1109/ACCESS.2020.2971576

Bartoletti, I. "AI in healthcare: Ethical and privacy challenges." *Conference on Artificial Intelligence in Medicine in Europe*. Springer, Cham, 2019. 10.1007/978-3-030-21642-9_2

Batty, M. (2018). Digital twins. *Environment and Planning. B, Urban Analytics and City Science*, *45*(5), 817–820. doi:10.1177/2399808318796416

Bayer, S., Kuzmickas, P., Boissy, A., Rose, S. L., & Mercer, M. B. (2021). Categorizing and rating patient complaints: An innovative approach to improve patient experience. *Journal of Patient Experience*, *8*, 2374373521998624. doi:10.1177/2374373521998624 PMID:34179397

Beard, J. R.,, Officer, A.,, de Carvalho, I. A.,, Sadana, R.,, Pot, A.M.,, Michel, J.-P.,, Lloyd-Sherlock, P.,, & Epping-Jordan, J. E., Peeters, G. M. E. E., & Mahanani, W. R. (2016). The world report on ageing and health:A policy framework for healthy ageing. *Lancet*, *387*, 2145–2154.

Beil, C., & Kolbe, T. H. (2020). Combined Modelling of Multiple Transportation Infrastructure Within 3D City Models and its Implementation in CityGML 3.0. [CrossRef]. *ISPRS Ann. Photogramm. Remote Sens. Spatial Inf. Sci.*, *6*, 29–36. doi:10.5194/isprs-annals-VI-4-W1-2020-29-2020

Beneito-Montagut, R., Cassián-Yde, N., & Begueria, A. (2018). *What do we know about the relationship between internet-mediated interaction and social isolation and loneliness in later life?* Quality in Aging and Older Adults. doi:10.1108/QAOA-03-2017-0008

Bentley Systems Incorporated. (2021). Discover OpenCities Planner–Connect The Data, People, Workflows, and Ideas Necessary to Support Today's Infrastructure Projects. *Report P-18.* https://www.bentley.com/es/products/brands/opencities-planner .

Bentley Systems Incorporated. (2021). Discover OpenCities Planner–Connect The Data, People, Workflows, and Ideas Necessary to Support Today's Infrastructure Projects. *Report P-18.* https://www.bentley.com/es/products/brands/opencities-planner.

BergthorBjornsson, C. B. (2019). Digital twins to personalize medicine. *Biomedical Central-. Genome Medicine.*

Berners-Lee, T. (2000). *Weaving the Web: The Original Design and Ultimate Design of the World Wide Web by its inventor*. Harper Business.

Bhandari, M., Parajuli, P., Chapagain, P., & Gaur, L. (2022). Evaluating Performance of Adam Optimization by Proposing Energy Index. In K. Santosh, R. Hegadi, & U. Pal (Eds.), Recent Trends in Image Processing and Pattern Recognition. RTIP2R 2021. Communications in Computer and Information Science (Vol. 1576). Springer. https://doi.org/10.1007/978-3-031-07005-1_15.

Bhatti, S. N., Haywood, G., & Yanagida, R. (2021). End-to-End Privacy for Identity & Location with IP. *29th IEEE International Conference on Network Protocols, Virtual Event*. IEEE. 10.1109/ICNP52444.2021.9651909

Biesinger, F., & Weyrich, M. (2019). The Facets of Digital Twins in Production and the Automotive Industry. In *23rd International Conference on Mechatronics Technology (ICMT)*, Salerno, Italy. 10.1109/ICMECT.2019.8932101

Biswas, M., Chaki, S., Ahammed, F., Anis, A., Ferdous, J., Siddika, A. M., & Gaur, L. (2022). Prototype development of an assistive smart-stick for the visually challenged persons. *Proceedings of 2nd International Conference on Innovative Practices in Technology and Management*, (pp. 477-482). Science Open. doi:10.1109/ICIPTM54933.2022.9754183

Biswas, M., Kaiser, M. S., Mahmud, M., Al Mamun, S., Hossain, M. S., & Rahman, M. A. (2021). An XAI Based Autism Detection: The Context Behind the Detection. In M. Mahmud, M. S. Kaiser, S. Vassanelli, Q. Dai, & N. Zhong (Eds.), Lecture Notes in Computer Science: Vol. 12960. Brain Informatics. BI 2021. Springer. https://doi.org/10.1007/978-3-030-86993-9_40.

Biswas, M., Tania, M. H., Kaiser, M. S., Kabir, R., Mahmud, M., & Kemal, A. A. (2021). ACCU3RATE: A mobile health application rating scale based on user reviews. *PLoS One*, *16*(12), e0258050.

Boată, A., Angelescu, R., & Dobrescu, R. (2021). Using digital twins in health care. UPB Scientific Bulletin, Series C, *Electrical Engineering and Computer Science*, *83*(4), 53–62.

Boland, A., Cherry, M. G., & Dickson, R. (Eds.). (2013). *Doing a systematic review: a student's guide*. Sage.

Bonomi, F., Milito, R., Natarajan, P., & Zhu, J. (2014). Fog computing: a platform for internet of things and analytics. In *Big Data and Internet of Things: A Road Map for Smart Environments*. Springer. doi:10.1007/978-3-319-05029-4_7

Boockvar, K. S., Judon, K. M., Eimicke, J. P., Teresi, J. A., & Inouye, S. K. (2020). Hospital Elder Life Program in Long-Term Care (HELP-LTC): A Cluster Randomized Controlled Trial. *Journal of the American Geriatrics Society*, *68*(10), 2329–2335. doi:10.1111/jgs.16695 PMID:32710658

Bora, G. (2020). https://economictimes.indiatimes.com/small-biz/startups/features/covid-19-in-the-times-of-touch-me-not-environment-drones-are-the-new-best-friends/articleshow/74924233.cms?utm_source=contentofinterest&utm_medium=text&utm_campaign=cppst

Borgia, E. (2014). The Internet of Things vision: Key features, applications, and open issues. *Computer Communications*, *54*, 1–31. doi:10.1016/j.comcom.2014.09.008

Botín-Sanabria, D. M., Mihaita, A. S., Peimbert-García, R. E., Ramírez-Moreno, M. A., Ramírez-Mendoza, R. A., & Lozoya-Santos, J. D. J. (2022). Digital twin technology challenges and applications: A comprehensive review. *Remote Sensing*, *14*(6), 1335. doi:10.3390/rs14061335

Boulos, M. N. (2021). *Digital Twins: From Personalised Medicine to Precision Public Health*. Researchgate.

Braun, V., & Clarke, V. (2006). Using thematic analysis in psychology. *Qualitative Research in Psychology*, *3*(2), 77–101. doi:10.1191/1478088706qp063oa

Brewer, C. S., Kovner, C. T., Greene, W., Tukov-Shuser, M., & Djukic, M. (2012). Predictors of actual turnover in a national sample of newly licensed registered nurses employed in hospitals. *Journal of Advanced Nursing*, *68*(3), 521–538. doi:10.1111/j.1365-2648.2011.05753.x PMID:22092452

Briggs, B., & Buchholz, S. (2020). Deloitte Tech Trends 2020. *Insights*, *2020*, 1–130.

Broadbent, E., Stafford, R., & MacDonald, B. (2009). Acceptance of healthcare robots for the older population: Review and future directions. *International Journal of Social Robotics*, *1*(4), 319–330. doi:10.100712369-009-0030-6

Bruynseels, K., Santoni de Sio, F., & Van den Hoven, J. (2018). Digital twins in health care: Ethical implications of an emerging engineering paradigm. *Frontiers in Genetics*, 31.

Bureau of Labor Statistics. (2009). *Nonfatal occupational injuries and illnesses requiring days away from work, 2007: News (USDL-08-1716)*. U.S. Department of Labor.

Campos-Ferreira, A., Lozoya-Santos, J. J., Vargas-Martínez, A., Mendoza, R., & Morales-Menéndez, R. (2019). Digital Twin Applications: A review. In *Memorias del Congreso Nacional de Control Automático*, (pp. 606–611). Asociación de México de Control Automático.

Campos-Ferreira, A., Lozoya-Santos, J. J., Vargas-Martínez, A., Mendoza, R., & Morales-Menéndez, R. Digital Twin Applications: A review. In *Memorias del Congreso Nacional de Control Automático*, (pp. 606–611). Asociación de México de Control Automático.

Cannas, B., Fanni, A., See, L., & Sias, G. (2006). Data preprocessing for river flow forecasting using neural networks: Wavelet transforms and data partitioning. *Physics and Chemistry of the Earth Parts A/B/C, 31*(18), 1164–1171.

Canzoneri, M., De Luca, A., & Harttung, J. (2021). Digital Twins: A General Overview of the Biopharma Industry. *Advances in biochemical engineering/biotechnology, 177*, pp. 167-184. doi:10.1007/10_2020_157

Capossele, A., Conti, M., Gaglione, A., Lazzeretti, R., Missier, P., & Nati, M. (2018). Leveraging blockchain to enable smart-health applications. In *IEEE 4th International Forum on Research and Technology for Society and Industry (RTSI), (pp. 1-6).* IEEE.

Carvalho, A., Melo, P., Oliveira, M., & Barros, R. The 4-corner model as a synchromodal and digital twin enabler in the transportation sector. In Proceedings of the 2020 IEEE International Conference on Engineering, Technology and Innovation (ICE/ITMC), (pp. 15–17). IEEE. [CrossRef] 10.1109/ICE/ITMC49519.2020.9198592

Cenedese, A., Zanella, A., Vangelista, L., & Zorzi, M. (2014). Padova smart city: an urban internet of things experimentation. In *Proceeding of 3rd IEEE World Forum on Internet of Things (WF-IoT)*, (pp. 609-614). IEEE.

Chakraborty, S., & Adhikari, S. (2021). Machine learning based digital twin for dynamical systems with multiple timescales. *Computers & Structures, 243*, 106410. doi:10.1016/j.compstruc.2020.106410

Chang, H. T., Liu, S. W., & Mishra, N. (2015). A tracking and summarization system for online Chinese news topics. *Aslib Journal of Information Management, 67*(6), 687–699.

Chang, H. T., Li, Y. W., & Mishra, N. (2016). mCAF: A multi-dimensional clustering algorithm for friends of social network services. *SpringerPlus, 5*(1), 757.

Chang, H. T., Mishra, N., & Lin, C. C. (2015). IoT Big-Data Centred Knowledge Granule Analytic and Cluster System for BI Applications: A Case Base Analysis. *PLoS One, 10*(11), e0141980.

Chang, W. Z. D., & Bourgeois, M. (2012). Effects of memory aids on the conversations of elderly Chinese persons. *Asia Pacific Journal of Speech, Language and Hearing, 15*(4), 245–263. doi:10.1179/136132812804731767

Chaudhary, G., Khari, M., & Elhoseny, M. (2021). *Digital Twin Technology*. CRC Press. doi:10.1201/9781003132868

Chavent, M. (1998). A monothetic clustering method. *Pattern Recognition Letters, 19*(11), 989–996.

Cheng, Y. "A Development Architecture for the Intelligent Animal Care and Management System Based on the Internet of Things and Artificial Intelligence," 2019 International Conference on Artificial Intelligence in Information and Communication (ICAIIC), 2019, pp. 078-081, 10.1109/ICAIIC.2019.8669015

Chiadighikaobi, I. R., & Katuk, N. (2021). A scoping study on lightweight cryptography reviews in IoT. *Baghdad Science Journal, 18*(2), 989–1000. doi:10.21123/bsj.2021.18.2(Suppl.).0989

Choi, S. D., & Brings, K. (2016). Work-related musculoskeletal risks associated with nurses and nursing assistants handling overweight and obese patients: A literature review. *Work (Reading, Mass.), 53*(2), 439–448. doi:10.3233/WOR-152222 PMID:26835850

Choudhary, M. (2020), What are use cases of Digital Twin? *Geospatial World.* https://www.geospatialworld.net/blogs/what-are-use-cases-of-digital-twin/

Christodoulidis, S., Anthimopoulos, M., Ebner, L., Christe, A., & Mougiakakou, S. (2016). Multisource transfer learning with convolutional neural networks for lung pattern analysis. *IEEE Journal of Biomedical and Health Informatics, 21*(1), 76–84.

Clarke, M., & Oxman, A. D. (2003). Cochrane reviewers' handbook 4.2. 0. *The Cochrane Library*, 2.

Cochrane Collaboration. (2009) *Cochrane Handbook for Systematic Reviews of Interventions*. Cochrane. www.cochrane-handbooking.org.

Cochrane. (2007). *Systematic Reviews of Health Promotion and Public Health Interventions*. Cochrane. https://ph.cochrane.org/sites/ph.cochrane_PH%20reviews.pdf.

Collard, H. R., Tino, G., Noble, P. W., Shreve, M. A., Michaels, M., Carlson, B., & Schwarz, M. I. (2007). Patient experiences with pulmonary fibrosis. *Respiratory Medicine*, *101*(6), 1350–1354.

Conejos, P., Martínez, F., Hervas, M., & Alonso, J. C. (2020). Building and Exploiting a Digital Twin for the Managmenet of Drinking Water Distribution Networks. [CrossRef]. *Urban Water Journal*, *17*(8), 704–713. doi:10.1080/1573062X.2020.1771382

Costabel, U., Du Bois, R. M., & Egan, J. J. (Eds.). (2007). *Diffuse parenchymal lung disease* (Vol. 36). Karger Medical and Scientific Publishers.

Cottin, V., Nunes, H., Mouthon, L., Gamondes, D., Lazor, R., & Hachulla, E., & Groupe d'Etudes et de Recherche sur les Maladies "Orphelines" Pulmonaires. (2011). Combined pulmonary fibrosis and emphysema syndrome in connective tissue disease. *Arthritis and Rheumatism*, *63*(1), 295–304.

Crowcroft, J., Gibbens, R., Kelly, F., & Ostring, S. (2003). Modelling incentives for collaboration in Mobile Ad Hoc Networks. *Proceedings of Modeling and Optimization in Mobile, Ad Hoc and Wireless Networks (WiOpt).*

Crowcroft, J., Gibbens, R., Kelly, F., & Ostring, S. (2004). Modelling Incentives for Collaboration in Mobile Ad Hoc Networks. *International Journal of Performance Evaluation*, *57*(4), 427–439. doi:10.1016/j.peva.2004.03.003

Cutler, N. E. (2015). Will the Internet Help Your Parents to Live Longer? Isolation, Longevity, Health, Death, and Skype™. *Journal of Financial Service Professionals*, *69*(2).

D'Arcy, L. P., Sasai, Y., & Stearns, S. C. (2012). Do assistive devices, training, and workload affect injury incidence? Prevention efforts by nursing homes and back injuries among nursing assistants. *Journal of Advanced Nursing*, *68*(4), 836–845. doi:10.1111/j.1365-2648.2011.05785.x PMID:21787370

Da Nóbrega, R. V. M., Peixoto, S. A., da Silva, S. P. P., & Rebouças Filho, P. P. (2018, June). Lung nodule classification via deep transfer learning in CT lung images. In *IEEE 31st international symposium on computer-based medical systems (CBMS)* (pp. 244-249). IEEE.

Dahmen, U., & Rossmann, J. (2018). Experimentable Digital Twins for a Modeling and Simulation-based Engineering Approach. In *Proceedings International Systems Engineering Symposium (ISSE)*. IEEE. 10.1109/SysEng.2018.8544383

Daltroy, L. H., Iversen, M. D., Larson, M. G., Lew, R., Wright, E., Ryan, J., & Liang, M. H. (1997). A controlled trial of an educational program to prevent low back injuries. *The New England Journal of Medicine*, *337*(5), 322–328. doi:10.1056/NEJM199707313370507 PMID:9233870

Datta Burton, S., Tanczer, L. M., & Vasudevan, S. Hailes, S., & Carr, M. (2021). The UK Code of Practice for Computer IoT Cybersecurity: where we are and what next. Department for Digital, Culture, Media & Sport.

David Jones, C. S. (May 2020). Characterising the Digital Twin: A systematic literature review. *Science Direct*, 36-52.

Day, R., & Hitchings, R. (2011). 'Only old ladies would do that': Age stigma and older people's strategies for dealing with winter cold. *Health & Place*, *17*(4), 885–894. doi:10.1016/j.healthplace.2011.04.011 PMID:21606000

De Maeyer, C., & Markopoulos, P. (2021). Future outlook on the materialisation, expectations and implementation of Digital Twins in healthcare. *34th British Human Computer Interaction Conference Interaction Conference,* (pp. 180-191). Science Open. doi:10.14236/ewic/HCI2021.18

Deebak, B. D., Al-Turjman, F., Aloqaily, M., & Alfandi, O. (2019). O. (2019). An authentic-based privacy preservation protocol for smart e-Healthcare systems in IoT. *IEEE Access: Practical Innovations, Open Solutions*, *7*, 135632–135649. doi:10.1109/ACCESS.2019.2941575

Delen, D., Walker, G., & Kadam, A. (2005). Predicting breast cancer survivability: A comparison of three data analytics methods. *Artificial Intelligence in Medicine*, *34*(2), 113–127.

Delgoshaei, B., Mobinizadeh, M., Mojdenar, R., Afzal, E., Arabloo, J., & Mohamadi, E. (2017). Telemedicine: A systematic review of economic evaluations. *Medical Journal of the Islamic Republic of Iran*, *31*(1), 113. doi:10.14196/mjiri.31.113 PMID:29951414

Dembski, F., Wossner, U., Letzgus, M., Ruddat, M., & Yamu, C. (2020). Urban Digital Twins for Smart Cities and Citizens: The Case Study of Herrenberg, Germany. [CrossRef]. *Sustainability*, *12*(6), 2307. doi:10.3390u12062307

Demuth, H., & Beale, M. (1993). Neural Network Toolbox for Use with Matlab--User'S Guide Version 3.0. Matlab.

Demuth, H., & Beale, M. (2000). *Neural network toolbox: for use with Matlab: computation, visualization, programming: User's guide, version 4*. The Mathworks.

Depeursinge, A., Iavindrasana, J., Hidki, A., Cohen, G., Geissbuhler, A., Platon, A., ... Müller, H. (2010). Comparative performance analysis of state-of-the-art classification algorithms applied to lung tissue categorization. *Journal of Digital Imaging*, *23*(1), 18–30.

Devare, M. H. (2019). Convergence of Manufacturing Cloud and Industrial IoT. In G. Kecskemeti (Ed.), *Applying Integration Techniques and Methods in Distributed Systems and Technologies* (pp. 49–78). IGI Global.

Dewasiri, N. J., Weerakoon, Y. K. B., & Azeez, A. A. (2018). Mixed Methods in Finance Research: The Rationale and Research Designs. *International Journal of Qualitative Methods*, *17*(1), 1–13. doi:10.1177/1609406918801730

Dey, R., Lu, Z., & Hong, Y. (2018, April). Diagnostic classification of lung nodules using 3D neural networks. In *2018 IEEE 15th international symposium on biomedical imaging (ISBI 2018)* (pp. 774-778). IEEE.

Dhanda, S. S., Singh, B., & Jindal, P. (2020). Lightweight Cryptography: A Solution to Secure IoT, Wireless Person. *Commun, (2020),* 1–34.

Dillenseger, A., Weidemann, M. L., Trentzsch, K., Inojosa, H., Haase, R., Schriefer, D., Voigt, I., Scholz, M., Akgün, K., & Ziemssen, T. (2021). Digital biomarkers in multiple sclerosis. *Brain Sciences*, *11*(11), 1519. doi:10.3390/brainsci11111519

Duan, Y., Coatrieux, G., & Shu, H. Z. (2015, August). Computed tomography image source identification by discriminating CT-scanner image reconstruction process. In *37th Annual International Conference of the IEEE Engineering in Medicine and Biology Society (EMBC)* (pp. 5622-5625). IEEE.

Duin, R. P. W., Juszczak, P., Paclik, P., Pekalska, E., De Ridder, D., Tax, D. M. J., & Verzakov, S. (2000). A Matlab toolbox for pattern recognition. *PRTools version, 3*, 109-111.

Durrani, H., & Khoja, S. (2009). A systematic review of the use of telehealth in Asian countries. *Journal of Telemedicine and Telecare*, *15*(4), 175–181. doi:10.1258/jtt.2009.080605 PMID:19471028

Dwivedi, A. D. (2021, August). Brisk: Dynamic encryption-based cipher for long term security [TELKOMNIKA Telecommun Comput El Control]. *Sensors (Basel)*, *21*(17), 5744. doi:10.339021175744 PMID:34502635

Edney, L. C., Haji Ali Afzali, H., Cheng, T. C., & Karnon, J. (2018). Estimating the reference incremental cost-effectiveness ratio for the Australian health system. *PharmacoEconomics*, *36*(2), 239–252. doi:10.100740273-017-0585-2 PMID:29273843

Elayan, H., Aloqaily, M., & Guizani, M. (2021). Digital Twin for Intelligent Context-Aware IoT Healthcare Systems. *IEEE Internet of Things Journal, 8*(23), pp. 16749-16757. doi:10.1109/JIOT.2021.3051158

Elsy, P. (2020). Elderly care in society 5.0 and kaigo rishoku in Japanese hyper-aging society. *Jurnal Studi Komunikasi*, *4*(2), 435–452.

Engst, C., Chhokar, R., Miller, A., Tate, R. B., & Yassi, A. (2005). Effectiveness of overhead lifting devices in reducing the risk of injury to care staff in extended care facilities. *Ergonomics*, *48*(2), 187–199. doi:10.1080/001401304123312 90826 PMID:15764316

Erol, T., Mendi, A. F., & Dogan, D. (2020). The Digital Twin Revolution in Healthcare. *4th International Symposium on Multidisciplinary Studies and Innovative Technologies, Proceedings*. Science Open. doi:10.1109/ISMSIT50672.2020.9255249

Erol, T., Mendi, A. F., & Doğan, D. (2020, October). The digital twin revolution in healthcare. *2020 4th International Symposium on Multidisciplinary Studies and Innovative Technologies (ISMSIT)* (pp. 1-7). IEEE. https://ieeexplore.ieee.org/abstract/document/9255249

Esfandiari, S., Lund, J. P., Penrod, J. R., Savard, A., Mark Thomason, J., & Feine, J. S. (2009). Implant overdentures for edentulous elders: Study of patient preference. *Gerodontology*, *26*(1), 3–10. doi:10.1111/j.1741-2358.2008.00237.x PMID:18498362

Evans, S., Savian, C., Burns, A., & Cooper, C. (2019). Digital Twins for the Built Environment: An Introduction to the Opportunities, Benefits, Challenges and Risks. *Built Environmental News*. https://www.theiet.org/impact-society/ sectors/built-environment/built-environment-news/digital-twins-for-the-built-envi
ronment/.

Fang, T. (2018, August). A novel computer-aided lung cancer detection method based on transfer learning from GoogLeNet and median intensity projections. In *2018 IEEE international conference on computer and communication engineering technology (CCET)* (pp. 286-290). IEEE.

Farsi, M., Daneshkhah, A., Hosseinian-Far, A., & Jahankhani, H. (2020). *Digital twin technologies and smart cities*. Springer. doi:10.1007/978-3-030-18732-3

Ferrag, M. A., Maglaras, L. A., Janicke, H., Jiang, J., & Shu, L. (2017). Authentication Protocols for Internet of Things: A Comprehensive Survey. *Security and Communication Networks*, *2017*, 1–41. doi:10.1155/2017/6562953

Firouzi, F., Farahani, B., Daneshmand, M., Grise, K., Song, J., Saracco, R., Wang, L.L., Lo, K., Angelov, P., Soares, E., Loh, P.-S., Talebpour, Z., Moradi, R., Goodarzi, M., Ashraf, H., Talebpour, M., Talebpour, A., Romeo, L., Das, R., Heidari, H., Pasquale, D., Moody, J., Woods, C., Huang, E.S., Barnaghi, P., Sarrafzadeh, M., Li, R., Beck, K.L., Isayev, O., Sung, N., & Luo, A. (2021). Harnessing the Power of Smart and Connected Health to Tackle COVID-19: IoT, AI, Robotics, and Blockchain for a Better World. *IEEE Internet of Things Journal, 8* (16), pp. 12826-12846. doi:10.1109/ JIOT.2021.3073904

Firouzi, F., Farahani, B., Barzegari, M., & Daneshmand, M. (2020). Ai-driven data monetization: The other face of data in iot-based smart and connected health. *IEEE Internet of Things Journal*.

Flaherty, K. R., Andrei, A. C., King, T. E. Jr, Raghu, G., Colby, T. V., Wells, A., & Martinez, F. J. (2007). Idiopathic interstitial pneumonia: Do community and academic physicians agree on diagnosis? *American Journal of Respiratory and Critical Care Medicine*, *175*(10), 1054–1060.

Foster, L. (2021), Authoritative Geospatial Data and Digital Twins. *techUK*. https://www.techuk.org/resource/authoritive-geospatial-data-and-digital-twins-denmark-in-3d.html

Fradelos, E. C., Papathanasiou, I. V., Mitsi, D., Tsaras, K., Kleisiaris, C. F., & Kourkouta, L. (2014). Health Based Geographic Information Systems (GIS) and their Applications. *Acta Inform Med., 22*(6), 402-405, . doi:10.5455/aim.2014.22.402-405

French, P., Flora, L. F. W., Ping, L. S., Bo, L. K., & Rita, W. H. Y. (1997). The prevalence and cause of occupational back pain in Hong Kong registered nurses. *Journal of Advanced Nursing, 26*(2), 380–388. doi:10.1046/j.1365-2648.1997.1997026380.x PMID:9292374

Fuller, A., Fan, Z., Day, C., & Barlow, C. (2020). Digital twin: Enabling technologies, challenges and open research. *IEEE Access: Practical Innovations, Open Solutions, 8*, 108952–108971.

Fu, X. "Application of Artificial Intelligence Technology in Medical Cell Biology," *2019 International Conference on Robots & Intelligent System (ICRIS)*, 2019, pp. 401-404, 10.1109/ICRIS.2019.00106

Gabrys, B., & Bargiela, A. (2000). General fuzzy min-max neural network for clustering and classification. *IEEE Transactions on Neural Networks, 11*(3), 769–783. doi:10.1109/72.846747 PMID:18249803

Galbán, C. J., Han, M. K., Boes, J. L., Chughtai, K. A., Meyer, C. R., Johnson, T. D., & Ross, B. D. (2012). Computed tomography–based biomarker provides unique signature for diagnosis of COPD phenotypes and disease progression. *Nature Medicine, 18*(11), 1711–1715.

Gallagher, S. M. (2011). Women's health, size and safe patient handling: What are the ethical issues? *Bariatric Nursing and Surgical Patient Care, 6*(2), 69–72. doi:10.1089/bar.2011.9973

Garg, P. K., & Tripathi, N. K., Kappas, M., & Gaur, L. (2022) Geospatial Data Science for Healthcare in Society 5.0. Springer Nature.

Garg, A., & Kapellusch, J. M. (2012). Long-Term Efficacy of an Ergonomics Program That Includes Patient-Handling Devices on Reducing Musculoskeletal Injuries to Nursing Personnel. *Human Factors, 54*(4), 608–625. doi:10.1177/0018720812438614 PMID:22908684

Garg, A., Owen, B. D., & Carlson, B. (1992). An ergonomics evaluation of nursing assistants' job in a nursing home. *Ergonomics, 35*(9), 979–995. doi:10.1080/00140139208967377 PMID:1387079

Garg, H., Sharma, B., Shekhar, S., & Agarwal, R. (2022). Spoofing detection system for e-health digital twin using EfficientNet Convolution Neural Network. *Multimedia Tools and Applications*. doi:10.100711042-021-11578-5

Garg, P. K. (2019). *Theory and Principles of Geoinformatics*. Khanna Book Publishing, Co. Ltd.

Garg, P. K. (2020). *Introduction to UAV*. New Age International Pvt Ltd.

Gaur, L. (2022). Internet of Things in Healthcare. In Geospatial Data Science in Healthcare for Society 5.0 (pp. 131-140). Springer.

Gaur, L., Afaq, A., Solanki, A., Singh, G., & Sharma, S., Jhanjhi, N.Z, My, H. T., & Le, D. N. (2021). Capitalizing on big data and revolutionary 5G technology: Extracting and visualizing ratings and reviews of global chain hotels. *Computers & Electrical Engineering, 95*, 107374. doi:10.1016/j.compeleceng.2021.107374

Gaur, L., Bhatia, U., & Bakshi, S. (2022). Cloud driven framework for skin cancer detection using deep CNN. *Proceedings of 2nd International Conference on Innovative Practices in Technology and Management,* (pp. 460-464). Science Open. doi:10.1109/ICIPTM54933.2022.9754216

Gaur, L., Solanki, A., Wamba, S. F., & Jhanjhi, N. Z. (2021). Advanced AI Techniques and Applications in Bioinformatics (1st ed.). CRC Press. https://doi.org/10.1201/9781003126164.

Gaur, L., Afaq, A., Singh, G., & Dwivedi, Y. K. (2021). Role of artificial intelligence and robotics to foster the touchless travel during a pandemic: A review and research agenda. *International Journal of Contemporary Hospitality Management, 33*(11), 4079–4098. https://doi.org/10.1108/IJCHM-11-2020-1246

Gaur, L., Bhandari, M., Razdan, T., Mallik, S., & Zhao, Z. (2022). Explanation-driven deep learning model for prediction of brain tumour status using MRI image data. *Frontiers in Genetics, 13*. doi:10.3389/fgene.2022.822666

Gaur, L., Bhatia, U., Jhanjhi, N. Z., Muhammad, G., & Masud, M. (2021). Medical image-based detection of COVID-19 using deep convolution neural networks. *Multimedia Systems*, 1–10. doi:10.100700530-021-00794-6

Gaur, L., Singh, G., & Ramakrishnan, R. (2017). Understanding Consumer Preferences using IoT SmartMirrors. *Pertanika Journal of Science & Technology, 25*(3).

Gaur, L., Singh, G., Solanki, A., Jhanjhi, N. Z., Bhatia, U., Sharma, S., & Kim, W. (2021). Disposition of youth in predicting sustainable development goals using the neuro-fuzzy and random forest algorithms. *Human-Centric Computing and Information Sciences, 11*. doi doi:10.22967/HCIS.2021.11.024

Gelernter, D. (1993). *Mirror Worlds: Or the Day Software Puts the Universe in A Shoebox. How It Will Happen and What It Will Mean*. Oxford University Press.

Genzel, M., Macdonald, J., & Marz, M. (2022). Solving inverse problems with deep neural networks-robustness included. *IEEE Transactions on Pattern Analysis and Machine Intelligence*.

Ghazanfari, A. (2022), How digital-twin technology could revolutionise the healthcare industry. *Computer Weekly*. https://www.computerweekly.com/opinion/How-Digital-Twin-Technology-Could-Revolutionise-the-Healthcare-Industry

Gibson, G., Dickinson, C., Brittain, K., & Robinson, L. (2019). Personalisation, customisation and bricolage: How people with dementia and their families make assistive technology work for them. *Aging and Society: An Interdisciplinary Journal, 39*(11), 2502–2519. doi:10.1017/S0144686X18000661

Godager, B.; Onstein, E.; Huang, L. (2021). *The Concept of Enterprise BIM: Current Research Practice and Future Trends*. IEEE

Godager, B.; Onstein, E.; Huang, L. (2021). The Concept of Enterprise BIM: Current Research Practice and Future Trends. *IEEE, 9*, 42265–42290.

Godfrey, C., & Harrison, M. B. (2010). *Systematic Review Resource Package. The Joanna Briggs Institute Method for Systematic Review Research Quick Reference Guide*. Queen's Joanna Briggs Collaboration.

Gong, J., & Navimipour, N. J. (2022). An in-depth and systematic literature review on the blockchain-based approaches for cloud computing. *Cluster Computing, 25*(1), 383–400. doi:10.100710586-021-03412-2

González García, C., Núñez Valdéz, E. R., García Díaz, V., Pelayo García-Bustelo, B. C., & Cueva Lovelle, J. M. (2019). A review of artificial intelligence in the internet of things. International Journal Of Interactive Multimedia And Artificial Intelligence, 5.

Greene, A. J. (2022). Elder financial abuse and electronic financial instruments: Present and future considerations for financial capacity assessments. *The American Journal of Geriatric Psychiatry, 30*(1), 90–106. doi:10.1016/j.jagp.2021.02.045 PMID:33781661

Grieves, M. (2014) *Digital Twin: Manufacturing Excellence through Virtual Factory Replication (Digital Twin White Paper-2014),* https://www.researchgate.net/publication/275211047_Digital_Twin_Manufacturing_

Guan, Z., Yang, W., Zhu, L., Wu, L., & Wang, R. (2021, June). Achieving adaptively secure data access control with privacy protection for lightweight IoT devices. *Science China. Information Sciences*, *64*(6), 1–14. doi:10.100711432-020-2957-5

Gubbi, J., Buyya, R., Murusic, S., & Palaniswami, M. (2013). Internet of Things (IoT): A vision, architectural elements, and future directions. *Future Generation Computer Systems*, *29*(7), 1645–1660. doi:10.1016/j.future.2013.01.010

Guevara, N., Diaz, C., Sguerra, M., Martinez, M., Agudelo, O., Suarez, J., Rodriguez, A., Acuña, G., & Garcia, A. (2019). Towards the design and implementation of a Smart City in Bogotá, Colombia. Rev. Fac. DeIng. [CrossRef]. *Univ. Antioq.*, *93*(93), 41–45. doi:10.17533/udea.redin.20190407

Gupta, A., Tripathi, M., Shaikh, T. J., & Sharma, A. (2019, February). A lightweight anonymous user authentication and key establishment scheme for wearable devices. *Computer Networks*, *149*, 29–42. doi:10.1016/j.comnet.2018.11.021

Gupta, D., Kayode, O., Bhatt, S., & Gupta, M. (2021). Tosun, AS Hierarchical Federated Learning based Anomaly Detection using Digital Twins for Smart Healthcare. Proceedings - 2021 IEEE 7th International Conference on Collaboration and Internet Terms and conditions Privacy policy. *Computing*, *CIC*, 16–25. IEEE. doi:10.1109/CIC52973.2021.00013

Gutierrez-Franco, E., Mejia-Argueta, C., & Rabelo, L. (2021). Data-Driven Methodology to Support Long-Lasting Logistics and Decision Making for Urban Last-Mile Operations. [CrossRef]. *Sustainability*, *13*(11), 6230. doi:10.3390u13116230

Haas, B., Coradi, T., Scholz, M., Kunz, P., Huber, M., Oppitz, U., André, L., Lengkeek, V., Huyskens, D., van Esch, A., & Reddick, R. (2008). Automatic segmentation of thoracic and pelvic CT images for radiotherapy planning using implicit anatomic knowledge and organ-specific segmentation strategies. *Physics in Medicine and Biology*, *53*(6), 1751–1771. doi:10.1088/0031-9155/53/6/017 PMID:18367801

Hagan, M. T., Demuth, H. B., & Beale, M. H. (1996). *Neural network design* (Vol. 20). Pws Pub.

Haiyuan, Y., Dachuan, W., Mengcha, S., & Qi, Y. (2021). Application of Digital Twins in Port System. [CrossRef]. *Journal of Physics: Conference Series*, •••, 1846.

Harber, P., Peña, L., Hsu, P., Billet, E., Greer, D., & Kim, K. (1994). Personal history, training and worksite as predictors of back pain of nurses. *American Journal of Industrial Medicine, 25*(4), 519–526. https://doi. doi:org/10.1002/ajim.4700250406

Harbi, Y., Aliouat, Z., Refoufi, A., Harous, S. A., & Bentaleb, A. (2019). Enhanced authentication and key management scheme for securing data transmission in the Internet of Things. *Ad Hoc Networks*, *94*(Nov), 101948. doi:10.1016/j.adhoc.2019.101948

Hecht-Nielsen, R. (1992). Theory of the backpropagation neural network. In Deep Neural Networks for perception (pp. 65-93).

Heermann, P. D., & Khazenie, N. (1992). Classification of multispectral remote sensing data using a back-propagation neural network. *IEEE Transactions on Geoscience and Remote Sensing*, *30*(1), 81–88.

Hegmann, K. T., & Garg, A. (2004). *Home healthcare: Reducing musculoskeletal hazards.* Final report (NIOSH [CDC] Grant No. U50/CCU 300860). CDC/NIOSH.

Hemingway, P., & Brereton, N. (2009) What is a systematic review? London: Hayward Medical.

Hepner, G., Logan, T., Ritter, N., & Bryant, N. (1990). Artificial neural network classification using a minimal training set- Comparison to conventional supervised classification. *Photogrammetric Engineering and Remote Sensing*, *56*(4), 469–473.

He, X., Qiu, Y., Lai, X., Li, Z., Shu, L., Sun, W., & Song, X. (2021). Towards a shape-performance integrated digital twin for lumbar spine analysis. *Digital Twin.*, *1*, 8. doi:10.12688/digitaltwin.17478.1

Hinch, R., Probert, W., Nurtay, A., Kendall, M., Wymant, C., Hall, M., Fraser, C., Hall, M., Lythgoe, K., Cruz, A. B., Zhao, L., Stewart, A., Ferretti, L., Parker, M., Meroueh, A., Mathias, B., Stevenson, S., Montero, D., Warren, J., Mather, N. K., Finkelstein, A., Abeler-Domer, L., Bonsall, D., & Fraser, C. (2020). *Effective configurations of a digital contact tracing app: A report to NHSX (NHSX Report).* The Conversation Trust (UK).

Hinch, R., Probert, W., Nurtay, A., Kendall, M., Wymant, C., Hall, M., Fraser, C., Lythgoe, K., Cruz, A. B., Zhao, L., Stewart, A., Ferretti, L., Parker, M., Meroueh, A., Mathias, B., Stevenson, S., Montero, D., Warren, J., Mather, N. K., & Fraser, C. (2020). Effective configurations of a digital contact tracing app: A report to NHSX (NHSX Report). *The Conversation Trust (UK).* https://cdn.theconversation.com/static_files/files/1009/Report_-_Effectiv_App_Configurations.pdf

Hirsch, T., Forlizzi, J., Hyder, E., Goetz, J., Kurtz, C., & Stroback, J. (2000, November). The ELDer project: social, emotional, and environmental factors in the design of eldercare technologies. In *Proceedings on the 2000 conference on Universal Usability* (pp. 72-79). ACM. 10.1145/355460.355476

Hoover, R. S., & Koerber, A. L. (2011). Using NVivo to answer the challenges of qualitative research in professional communication: Benefits and best practices tutorial. *IEEE Transactions on Professional Communication*, *54*(1), 68–82. doi:10.1109/TPC.2009.2036896

Hosny, A., Parmar, C., Coroller, T. P., Grossmann, P., Zeleznik, R., Kumar, A., & Aerts, H. J. (2018). Deep learning for lung cancer prognostication: A retrospective multi-cohort radiomics study. *PLoS Medicine*, *15*(11), e1002711.

Hu, Y. C., Perrig, A., & Johnson, D. B. (2003). *Packet leashes: A defense against wormhole attacks in wireless networks.* In *Twenty-Second Annual Joint Conference of the Computer and Communications. INFOCOM*, *3*, 1976–1986. IEEE 10.1109/INFCOM.2003.1209219

Huang, J., Wang, Y., Tan, T., & Cui, J. (2004, August). A new iris segmentation method for recognition. In *Proceedings of the 17th International Conference on Pattern Recognition*, (Vol. 3, pp. 554-557). IEEE.

Huang, S., Yang, J., Fong, S., & Zhao, Q. (2020). Artificial intelligence in cancer diagnosis and prognosis: Opportunities and challenges. *Cancer Letters*, *471*, 61–71. doi:10.1016/j.canlet.2019.12.007 PMID:31830558

Hunter, B., Branson, M., & Davenport, D. (2010). Saving costs, saving health care providers' backs and creating a safe patient environment. *Nursing Economics*, *28*(2), 130. PMID:20446387

Hussein, S., Cao, K., Song, Q., & Bagci, U. (2017, June). Risk stratification of lung nodules using 3D CNN-based multi-task learning. In *International conference on information processing in medical imaging* (pp. 249-260). Springer, Cham.

Hussein, S., Kandel, P., Bolan, C. W., Wallace, M. B., & Bagci, U. (2019). Lung and pancreatic tumor characterization in the deep learning era: Novel supervised and unsupervised learning approaches. *IEEE Transactions on Medical Imaging*, *38*(8), 1777–1787.

Inoue, A., Johnson, T. F., Voss, B. A., Lee, Y. S., Leng, S., Koo, C. W., & Fletcher, J. G. (2021). A Pilot Study to Estimate the Impact of High Matrix Image Reconstruction on Chest Computed Tomography. *Journal of Clinical Imaging Science, 11*. 10.25259/JCIS_143_2021

Islami, S. M. R., Kwak, D., Humaun Kabiri, M .D., Hossain, M., & Kwaki, K. (2015). The Internet of Things for Health Care: A Comprehensive Survey. *IEEE Translations and content mining, 3,* (pp. 678-708). IEEE.

Ivanov, S., Nikolskaya, K., Radchenko, G., Sokolinsky, L., & Zymbler, M. Digital Twin of City: Concept Overview. In *Proceedings of the 2020 Global Smart Industry Conference (GloSIC)*, Chelyabinsk, Russia, 17–19 November 2020. 10.1109/GloSIC50886.2020.9267879

Jain, A., Jain, A., & Jain, S. (2000). *Artificial intelligence techniques in breast cancer diagnosis and prognosis* (Vol. 39). World Scientific. doi:10.1142/4484

Jamshidi, M., Lalbakhsh, A., Talla, J., Peroutka, Z., Hadjilooei, F., Lalbakhsh, P., Jamshidi, M., Spada, L. L., Mirmozafari, M., Dehghani, M., Sabet, A., Roshani, S., Roshani, S., Bayat-Makou, N., Mohamadzade, B., Malek, Z., Jamshidi, A., Kiani, S., Hashemi-Dezaki, H., & Mohyuddin, W. (2020). Artificial Intelligence and COVID-19: Deep Learning Approaches for Diagnosis and Treatment. *IEEE Access: Practical Innovations, Open Solutions*, *8*, 109581–109595. doi:10.1109/ACCESS.2020.3001973 PMID:34192103

Jimenez, J. I., Jahankhani, H., & Kendzierskyj, S. (2020). Health care in the cyberspace: Medical cyber-physical system and digital twin challenges. In *Digital twin technologies and smart cities* (pp. 79–92). Springer.

Johansson-Pajala, R. M., & Gustafsson, C. (2022). Significant challenges when introducing care robots in Swedish eldercare. *Disability and Rehabilitation. Assistive Technology*, *17*(2), 166–176. doi:10.1080/17483107.2020.1773549 PMID:32538206

Juarez, M., Botti, V., & Giret, A. (2021). Digital Twins: Review and Challenges. *Journal of Computing and Information Science in Engineering*, *21*, 030802.

June, K. J., & Cho, S.-H. (2011). Low back pain and work-related factors among nurses in intensive care units. *Journal of Clinical Nursing*, *20*(3-4), 479–487. doi:10.1111/j.1365-2702.2010.03210.x PMID:20673308

Jung, A., Gsell, M. A. F., Augustin, C. M., & Plank, G. (2022). An integrated workflow for building digital twins of cardiac electromechanics-a multi-fidelity approach for personalising active mechanics. *Mathematics*, *10*(5), 823. doi:10.3390/math10050823 PMID:35295404

Kachouie, R., Sedigheh Deli, S., Khosla, R., & Chu, M. T. (2014). Socially assistive robots in elderly care: A mixed-method systematic literature review. *International Journal of Human-Computer Interaction*, *30*(5), 369–393. doi:10.1080/10447318.2013.873278

Kamel Boulos, M. N., & Zhang, P. (2021). Digital Twins: From Personalised Medicine to Precision Public Health. *Journal of Personalized Medicine*, *2021*(11), 745. doi:10.3390/jpm11080745 PMID:34442389

Karbasi, A. H., & Shahpasand, S. (2021). SINGLETON: A lightweight and secure end-to-end encryption protocol for the sensor networks in the Internet of Things based on cryptographic ratchets. *The Journal of Supercomputing*, *77*(4), 3516–3554. doi:10.100711227-020-03411-x

Karhula, K., Ronnholm, T., & Sjogren, T. (2006), Development of observation instrument for assessing work load on personnel involved in patient transfer tasks. *Proceedings of NES 38th Annual Congress*, 148-152. NES.

Karlof, C., & Wagner, D. (2003). Secure routing in wireless sensor networks: Attacks and countermeasures. *Ad Hoc Networks*, *1*(2), 293–315. doi:10.1016/S1570-8705(03)00008-8

Kaswan, K. S., Gaur, L., Dhatterwal, J. S., & Kumar, R. (2021). AI-based natural language processing for the generation of meaningful information electronic health record (EHR) data. In Advanced AI Techniques and Applications in Bioinformatics (pp. 41-86). CRC Press.

Kaswan, K. S., Gaur, L., Dhatterwal, J. S., & Kumar, R. (2021). AI-based natural language processing for the generation of meaningful information electronic health record (EHR) data. In Advanced AI Techniques and Applications in Bioinformatics, 41-86. CRC Press.

Kaushik, K., & Dahiya, S. (2018). Security and Privacy in IoT based EBusiness and Retail, *2018 International Conference on System Modeling & Advancement in Research Trends (SMART)*, (pp. 78–81). 10.1109/SYSMART.2018.8746961

Kaushik, K., & Singh, K. (2020). Security and Trust in IoT Communications: Role and Impact. In S. Choudhury, R. Mishra, R. Mishra, & A. Kumar (Eds.), *Intelligent Communication, Control and Devices. Advances in Intelligent Systems and Computing, 989*. Springer. doi:10.1007/978-981-13-8618-3_81

Khan, K. M., Arshad, J., Iqbal, W., Abdullah, S., & Zaib, H. (2022). Blockchain-enabled real-time SLA monitoring for cloud-hosted services. *Cluster Computing*, *25*(1), 537–559. doi:10.100710586-021-03416-y

Khan, S., Arslan, T., & Ratnarajah, T. (2022). Digital Twin Perspective of Fourth Industrial and Healthcare Revolution. *IEEE Access*, *10*, 25732-25754. doi:10.1109/ACCESS.2022.3156062

Khan, S., Lee, W. K., & Hwang, S. O. (2022, March). AEchain: A lightweight blockchain for IoT applications. *IEEE Consumer Electronics Magazine*, *11*(2), 64–76. doi:10.1109/MCE.2021.3060373

Khubrani, M. M., & Alam, S. (2021, August). A detailed review of blockchain-based applications for protection against pandemic like COVID-19 [Telecommunication Computing Electronics and Control]. *TELKOMNIKA*, *19*(4), 1185–1196. doi:10.12928/telkomnika.v19i4.18465

Kim, H., Dropkin, J., Spaeth, K., Smith, F., & Moline, J. (2012). Patient handling and musculoskeletal disorders among hospital workers: Analysis of 7 years of institutional workers' compensation claims data. *American Journal of Industrial Medicine*, *55*(8), 683–690. doi:10.1002/ajim.22006 PMID:22237853

Kiran, S. R. A., Rajper, S., Shaikh, R. A., Shah, I. A., & Danwar, S. H. (2021). Categorization of CVE Based on Vulnerability Software By Using Machine Learning Techniques. *International Journal (Toronto, Ont.)*, *10*(3).

Knibbe, H. J., Knibbe, N. E., & Klaassen, A. J. (2007). Safe patient handling program in critical care using peer leaders: Lessons learned in the Netherlands. *Critical Care Nursing Clinics*, *19*(2), 205–211. doi:10.1016/j.ccell.2007.02.009 PMID:17512476

Knickerbocker, J. U., ... "Heterogeneous Integration Technology Demonstrations for Future Healthcare, IoT, and AI Computing Solutions," 2018 IEEE 68th Electronic Components and Technology Conference (ECTC), 2018, pp. 15191528, 10.1109/ECTC.2018.00231

Knickerbocker, J. U., Budd, R., Dang, B., Chen, Q., Colgan, E., Hung, L. W., & Wen, B. (2018, May). Heterogeneous integration technology demonstrations for future healthcare, IoT, and AI computing solutions. In 2018 IEEE 68th electronic components and technology conference (ECTC) (pp. 1519-1528). IEEE.

Knickerbocker, J. U., Budd, R., Dang, B., Chen, Q., Colgan, E., Hung, L. W., . . . Wen, B. (2018, May). Heterogeneous integration technology demonstrations for future healthcare, IoT, and AI computing solutions. In 2018 IEEE 68th electronic components and technology conference (ECTC) (pp. 1519-1528). IEEE.

Komalasari, R., Nurhayati, N., & Mustafa, C. (2022). Enhancing the Online Learning Environment for Medical Education: Lessons From COVID-19. In Policies and Procedures for the Implementation of Safe and Healthy Educational Environments: Post-COVID-19 Perspectives (pp. 138-154). IGI Global.

Kumar, A. (2020). Bonus benefit! Satellite data shows significant decrease in NO2 emissions in India due to Covid-19 lockdown. India Today.

Kundel, H. L. (2006). History of research in medical image perception. *Journal of the American College of Radiology, 3*(6), 402–408.

Laaki, H., Miche, Y., & Tammi, K. (2019). Prototyping a Digital Twin for Real Time Remote Control Over Mobile Networks: Application of Remote Surgery. *IEEE Access, 7*, 20325–20336.

Laaki, H.; Miche, Y.; Tammi, K. Prototyping a Digital Twin for Real Time Remote Control Over Mobile Networks: Application of Remote Surgery. IEEE Access 2019, 7, 20325–20336. [CrossRef]

Laamarti, F., Badawi, H., Ding, Y., Arafsha, F., Hafidh, B., & El Saddik, (2021). An ISO/IEEE 11073 Standardized Digital Twin Framework for Health and Well-Being in Smart Cities. *IEEE Access, 8*, 105950–105961.

Laamarti, F.; Badawi, H.; Ding, Y.; Arafsha, F.; Hafidh, B.; El Saddik, A. An ISO/IEEE 11073 Standardized Digital Twin Framework for Health and Well-Being in Smart Cities. IEEE Access 2020, 8, 105950–105961. [CrossRef]

Laamarti, F., Badawi, H. F., Ding, Y., Arafsha, F., Hafidh, B., & El Saddik, A. (2020). An ISO/IEEE 11073 standardized digital twin framework for health and well-being in smart cities. *IEEE Access: Practical Innovations, Open Solutions, 8*, 105950–105961.

Lagerström, M., & Hagberg, M. (1997). Evaluation of a 3-year education and training program for nursing personnel at a Swedish hospital. *AAOHN Journal, 45*(2), 83–92. doi:10.1177/216507999704500207 PMID:9146108

Lagerström, M., Hansson, T., & Hagberg, M. (1998). Work-related low-back problems in nursing. *Scandinavian Journal of Work, Environment & Health, 24*(6), 449–464. doi:10.5271jweh.369 PMID:9988087

Laubenbacher, R., Sluka, J., & Glazier, J. (2021). Using digital twins in viral infection. [CrossRef]. *Science, 371*(6534), 1105–1106. doi:10.1126cience.abf3370 PMID:33707255

Le Nguyen, T., & Do, T. T. H. "Artificial Intelligence in Healthcare: A New Technology Benefit for Both Patients and Doctors," *2019 Portland International Conference on Management of Engineering and Technology (PICMET)*, 2019, pp. 1-15, 10.23919/PICMET.2019.8893884

Lee, S., Jain, S., Zhang, Y., Liu, J., & Son, Y. J. (2020). A Multi-Paradigm Simulation for the Implementation of Digital Twins in Surveillance Applications. In *Proceedings of the 2020 IISE Annual Conference*. IISE.

Lee, Y., Tsung, P., & Wu, M. "Techology trend of edge AI," 2018 International Symposium on VLSI Design, Automation and Test (VLSI-DAT), 2018, pp. 1-2, 10.1109/VLSI-DAT.2018.8373244

Lee, H., Kang, D., Ryu, J., Won, D., Kim, H., & Lee, Y. (2020, June). A three-factor anonymous user authentication scheme for Internet of Things environments. *Journal of Information Security Application., 52*, 102494. doi:10.1016/j.jisa.2020.102494

Lee, S. J., Faucett, J., Gillen, M., Krause, N., & Landry, L. (2010). Factors associated with safe patient handling behaviors among critical care nurses. *American Journal of Industrial Medicine, 53*(9), 886–897. doi:10.1002/ajim.20843 PMID:20698021

Lee, S. J., Faucett, J., Gillen, M., Krause, N., & Landry, L. (2013). Musculoskeletal pain among critical-care nurses by availability and use of patient lifting equipment: An analysis of cross-sectional survey data. *International Journal of Nursing Studies, 50*(12), 1648–1657. doi:10.1016/j.ijnurstu.2013.03.010 PMID:23648391

Lee, S. W., & Sim, K. B. (2021, May). Design and hardware implementation of a simplified dag-based blockchain and new aes-cbc algorithm for iot security. *Electronics (Basel), 10*(9), 1127. doi:10.3390/electronics10091127

Lee, S., Jain, S., Zhang, Y., Liu, J., & Son, Y. J. A Multi-Paradigm Simulation for the Implementation of Digital Twins in Surveillance Applications. In *Proceedings of the 2020 IISE Annual Conference*, New Orleans, LA, USA, 30 May–2 June 2020.

Ley, B., Collard, H. R., & King, T. E. Jr. (2011). Clinical course and prediction of survival in idiopathic pulmonary fibrosis. *American Journal of Respiratory and Critical Care Medicine*, *183*(4), 431–440.

Li, J., Wolf, L., & Evanoff, B. (2004). Use of mechanical patient lifts decreased musculoskeletal symptoms and injuries among health care workers. *Injury Prevention*, *10*(4), 212–216. doi:10.1136/ip.2003.004978 PMID:15314047

Lim, K., Zheng, P., & Chen, C. (2020). A state-of-the-art survey of Digital Twin: Techniques, engineering product lifecycle management and business innovation perspectives. [CrossRef]. *Journal of Intelligent Manufacturing*, *31*(6), 1313–1337. doi:10.100710845-019-01512-w

Lippmann, R. P. (1989). Pattern classification using neural networks. *IEEE Communications Magazine*, *27*(11), 47–50.

Li, S., Zhao, S., Min, G., Qi, L., & Liu, G. (2021). Lightweight privacy-preserving scheme using homomorphic encryption in industrial internet of things. *IEEE Internet of Things Journal*, 2021.

Liu, Y.K., Ong, S.K., Nee, A.Y.C. (2022). State-of-the-art survey on digital twin implementations. *Advances in Manufacturing, 10*(1), . doi:10.1007/s40436-021-00375-w

Liu, L., Xu, J., Huan, Y., Zou, Z., Yeh, S.-C., & Zheng, L.-R. (2020, March). A Smart Dental Health-IoT Platform Based on Intelligent Hardware, Deep Learning, and Mobile Terminal. *IEEE Journal of Biomedical and Health Informatics*, *24*(3), 898–906. doi:10.1109/JBHI.2019.2919916 PMID:31180873

Liu, S., Bao, J., Lu, Y., Li, J. L. S., & Sun, X. (2021). Digital twin modeling method based on biomimicry for machining aerospace components. *Journal of Manufacturing Systems*, *58*, 180–195. doi:10.1016/j.jmsy.2020.04.014

Liu, T., Wang, Y., Li, Y., Tong, X., Qi, L., & Jiang, N. (2020, September). Privacy protection based on stream cipher for spatiotemporal data in IoT. *IEEE Internet of Things Journal*, *7*(9), 7928–7940. doi:10.1109/JIOT.2020.2990428

Liu, X., Chen, K., Wu, T., Weidman, D., Lure, F., & Li, J. (2018). Use of multimodality imaging and artificial intelligence for diagnosis and prognosis of early stages of Alzheimer's disease. *Translational Research; the Journal of Laboratory and Clinical Medicine*, *194*, 56–67. doi:10.1016/j.trsl.2018.01.001 PMID:29352978

Liu, Y., Zhang, L., Yang, Y., Zhou, L., Ren, L., Wang, F., Liu, R., Pang, Z., & Deen, M. J. (2019). A novel cloud-based framework for the elderly healthcare services using digital twin. *IEEE Access: Practical Innovations, Open Solutions*, *7*, 49088–49101.

Li, Y., Zhang, L., Chen, H., & Yang, N. (2019). Lung nodule detection with deep learning in 3D thoracic MR images. *IEEE Access: Practical Innovations, Open Solutions*, *7*, 37822–37832.

Loveleen, G., Mohan, B., Shikhar, BS, Nz, J., Shorfuzzaman, M. & Masud, M. (2022). Explanation-driven HCI Model to Examine the Mini-Mental State for Alzheimer's Disease. *ACM Transactions on Multimedia Computing, Communications, and Applications (TOMM).* doi:10.1145/3527174

Lu, Q., Ye, Z., Fang, Z., Meng, J., Pitt, M., Lin, J., Xie, X., & Chen, L.(2021). Creating an Inter-Hospital Resilient Network for Pandemic Response Based on Blockchain and Dynamic Digital Twins *Proceedings - Winter Simulation Conference*. doi:10.1109/WSC52266.2021.9715517

Luo, X., Yin, L., Li, C., Wang, C., Fang, F., Zhu, C., & Tian, Z. (2020). A lightweight privacy-preserving communication protocol for heterogeneous IoT environment. *IEEE Access: Practical Innovations, Open Solutions*, *8*, 67192–67204. doi:10.1109/ACCESS.2020.2978525

Lyth, J., Lind, L., Persson, H. L., & Wiréhn, A. B. (2021). Can a telemonitoring system lead to decreased hospitalization in elderly patients? *Journal of Telemedicine and Telecare*, *27*(1), 46–53. doi:10.1177/1357633X19858178 PMID:31291794

Maddikunta, P.K.R., & Pham, Q.-V., B, P., Deepa, N., Dev, K., Gadekallu, T.R., Ruby, R., & Liyanage, M. (2022). Industry 5.0: A survey on enabling technologies and potential applications. *Journal of Industrial Information Integration*, *26*, art. no. 100257. doi:10.1016/j.jii.2021.100257

Madni, A. M., Madni, C. C., & Lucero, S. D. (2019). Leveraging digital twin technology in model-based systems engineering. *Systems*, *7*(1), 1–13. doi:10.3390ystems7010007

Mahbub, M. K., Biswas, M., Gaur, L., Alenezi, F., & Santosh, K. C. (2022). Deep features to detect pulmonary abnormalities in chest X-rays due to infectious diseaseX: Covid-19, pneumonia, and tuberculosis. *Information Sciences*, *592*, 389–401. doi:10.1016/j.ins.2022.01.062

Mahmud, N., Schonstein, E., Schaafsma, F., Lehtola, M. M., Fassier, J.-B., Reneman, M. F., & Verbeek, J. H. (2010). Pre-employment examinations for preventing occupational injury and disease in workers. *Cochrane Database of Systematic Reviews*, (12), CD008881. doi:10.1002/14651858.CD008881 PMID:21154401

Mandolla, C., Petruzzelli, A. M., Percoco, G., & Urbinati, A. (2019). Building a digital twin for additive manufacturing through the exploitation of blockchain: A case analysis of the aircraft industry. *Computers in Industry*, *109*, 134–152. doi:10.1016/j.compind.2019.04.011

Manne, R., & Kantheti, S. C. (2021). Application of artificial intelligence in healthcare: Chances and challenges. *Current Journal of Applied Science and Technology*, *40*(6), 78–89. doi:10.9734/cjast/2021/v40i631320

Marcantonio, E. R., Bergmann, M. A., Kiely, D. K., Orav, E. J., & Jones, R. N. (2010). Randomized trial of a delirium abatement program for post-acute skilled nursing facilities. *Journal of the American Geriatrics Society*, *58*(6), 1019–1026. doi:10.1111/j.1532-5415.2010.02871.x PMID:20487083

Marcucci, E., Gatta, V., Le-Pira, M., Hansson, L., & Brathen, S. (2020). Digital Twins: A Critical Discussion on Their Potential for Supporting Policy-Making and Planning in Urban Logistics. *Sustainability*, *12*(24), 623. doi:10.3390u122410623

Marras, W. S. (2000). Occupational low back disorder causation and control. *Ergonomics*, *43*(7), 880–902. doi:10.1080/001401300409080 PMID:10929824

Marras, W. S., Knapik, G. G., & Ferguson, S. (2009). Lumbar spine forces during manoeuvring of ceiling-based and floor-based patient transfer devices. *Ergonomics*, *52*(3), 384–397. doi:10.1080/00140130802376075 PMID:19296324

Mason, S., Craig, D., O'Neill, S., Donnelly, M., & Nugent, C. (2012). Electronic reminding technology for cognitive impairment. *British Journal of Nursing (Mark Allen Publishing)*, *20*(14), 855–861. doi:10.12968/bjon.2012.21.14.855 PMID:23252168

Matz, M. W. (2019). Patient Handling and Mobility Assessments (2nd ed). The Facility Guidelines Institute.

Mbed, O. S. (2022). *Mbed OS Features*. armMedbed. https://www.mbed.com/en/platform/mbed-os/ (accessed on July 2022).

McKenna, G., Allen, P. F., Hayes, M., DaMata, C., Moore, C., & Cronin, M. (2018). Impact of oral rehabilitation on the quality of life of partially dentate elders in a randomized controlled clinical trial: 2 year follow-up. *PLoS One*, *13*(10), e0203349. doi:10.1371/journal.pone.0203349 PMID:30307966

Melnyk, B. M., & Fineout-Overholt, E. (Eds.). (2011). *Evidence-based practice in nursing & healthcare: A guide to best practice*. Lippincott Williams & Wilkins.

Memon, M., Wagner, S. R., Pedersen, C. F., Beevi, F. H. A., & Hansen, F. O. (2014). Ambient assisted living healthcare frameworks, platforms, standards, and quality attributes. *Sensors (Basel)*, *14*(3), 4312–4341. doi:10.3390140304312 PMID:24599192

Meraghni, S., Benaggoune, K., Al Masry, Z., Terrissa, L.S., Devalland, C., & Zerhouni, N. (2021). Towards Digital Twins Driven Breast Cancer Detection. *Lecture Notes in Networks and Systems*, *285*, pp. 87-99. doi:10.1007/978-3-030-80129-8_7

Mihailidis, A., Boger, J. N., Craig, T., & Hoey, J. (2008). The COACH prompting system to assist older adults with dementia through handwashing: An efficacy study. *BMC Geriatrics*, *8*(1), 1–18. doi:10.1186/1471-2318-8-28 PMID:18992135

Mishra, N. (2017). In-network Distributed Analytics on Data-centric IoT Network for BI-service Applications. *International Journal of Scientific Research in Computer Science, Engineering and Information Technology (IJSRCSEIT)*, *2*(5), pp.547-552.

Mishra, N., Lin, C. C., & Chang, H. T. (2014, December). A cognitive-oriented framework for IoT big-data management perspective. In *International Conference on Communication Problem-Solving (ICCP),* (pp. 124-127). IEEE.

Mishra, N. (2011). A Framework for associated pattern mining over Microarray database. *International Journal of Global Research in Computer Science*, *2*(2).

Mishra, N., Chang, H. T., & Lin, C. C. (2014). Data-centric knowledge discovery strategy for a safety-critical sensor application. *International Journal of Antennas and Propagation*, 2014.

Mishra, N., Chang, H. T., & Lin, C. C. (2015). An IoT knowledge reengineering framework for semantic knowledge analytics for BI-services. *Mathematical Problems in Engineering*, 2015.

Mishra, N., Chang, H. T., & Lin, C. C. (2018). Sensor data distribution and knowledge inference framework for a cognitive-based distributed storage sink environment. *International Journal of Sensor Networks*, *26*(1), 26–42.

Mishra, N., Lin, C. C., & Chang, H. T. (2014). Cognitive inference device for activity supervision in the elderly. *The Scientific World Journal*, 2014.

Mishra, N., Lin, C. C., & Chang, H. T. (2015). A cognitive adopted framework for IoT big-data management and knowledge discovery perspective. *International Journal of Distributed Sensor Networks*, *11*(10), 718390.

Misumi, S., & Lynch, D. A. (2006). Idiopathic pulmonary fibrosis/usual interstitial pneumonia: Imaging diagnosis, spectrum of abnormalities, and temporal progression. *Proceedings of the American Thoracic Society*, *3*(4), 307–314. doi:10.1513/pats.200602-018TK PMID:16738194

Mitchell, T., O'Sullivan, P. B., Smith, A., Burnett, A. F., Straker, L., Thornton, J., & Rudd, C. J. (2009). Biopsychosocial factors are associated with low back pain in female nursing students: A cross-sectional study. *International Journal of Nursing Studies*, *46*(5), 678–688. doi:10.1016/j.ijnurstu.2008.11.004 PMID:19118828

Modares, H., Salleh, R., & Moravejosharieh, A. (2011). Overview of security issues in wireless sensor networks. In *Third International Conference on Computational Intelligence, Modelling and Simulation (CIMSiM)*, (pp. 308–311). IEEE. 10.1109/CIMSim.2011.62

Mohanta, B., P. Das and S. Patnaik, "Healthcare 5.0: A Paradigm Shift in Digital Healthcare System Using Artificial Intelligence, IOT and 5G Communication," 2019 International Conference on Applied Machine Learning (ICAML), 2019, pp. 191-196, 10.1109/ICAML48257.2019.00044

Moher, D., Liberati, A., Tetzlaff, J., & Altman, D.PRISMA Group. (2009). Preferred reporting items for systematic reviews and meta-analyses: The PRISMA Statement. *Annals of Internal Medicine*, *151*(4), 264–269. doi:10.7326/0003-4819-151-4-200908180-00135 PMID:19622511

Morato, J., Sanchez-Cuadrado, S., Iglesias, A., Campillo, A., & Fernández-Panadero, C. (2021). Sustainable technologies for older adults. *Sustainability, 13*(15), 8465. doi:10.3390u13158465

Mostaghel, R. (2016). Innovation and technology for the elderly: Systematic literature review. *Journal of Business Research, 69*(11), 4896–4900. doi:10.1016/j.jbusres.2016.04.049

Mostak, T. (2021). The Future of Geospatial Analytics Is In Digital Twins. *Forbes*. https://www.forbes.com/sites/forbestechcouncil/2021/11/18/the-future-of-geospatial-analytics-is-in-digital-twins/?sh=168ffc7dd590

Mozumder, M. A. I., Sheeraz, M. M., Athar, A., Aich, S., & Kim, H.-C. (2022). Overview: Technology Roadmap of the Future Trend of Metaverse based on IoT, Blockchain, AI Technique, and Medical Domain Metaverse Activity. *International Conference on Advanced Communication Technology, ICACT,* (pp. 256-261). doi:10.23919/ICACT53585.2022.9728808

Mujeeb Rahman, K. K., & Subashini, M. M. (2022). Identification of Autism in Children Using Static Facial Features and Deep Neural Networks. *Brain Sciences, 12*(1), 94.

Muzafar, S., & Jhanjhi, N. Z. (2020). Success stories of ICT implementation in Saudi Arabia. In *Employing Recent Technologies for Improved Digital Governance* (pp. 151–163). IGI Global. https://www.igi-global.com/chapter/success-stories-of-ict-implementation-in-saudi-arabia/245980 doi:10.4018/978-1-7998-1851-9.ch008

Myers, D., Silverstein, B., & Nelson, N. A. (2002). Predictors of shoulder and back injuries in nursing home workers: A prospective study. *American Journal of Industrial Medicine, 41*(6), 466–476. doi:10.1002/ajim.10076 PMID:12173371

Nagaraj, A. (2021). Introduction to Sensors in IoT and Cloud Computing Applications. Bentham Science Publishers. doi:10.2174/97898114793591210101

Nagaraj, A. (2022). Adapting Blockchain for Energy Constrained IoT in Healthcare Environment. In Sustainable and Advanced Applications of Blockchain in Smart Computational Technologies (pp. 103-112). Chapman and Hall/CRC.

Nakamoto, S. (2008). *Bitcoin: A peer-to-peer electronic cash system.* Bitcoin.

Nativi, S., Mazzetti, P., & Craglia, M. (2021). Digital Ecosystems for Developing Digital Twins of the Earth: The Destination Earth Case. *Remote Sensing, 13*(11), 2119. doi:10.3390/rs13112119

Nelson, A. L., Lloyd, J. D., Menzel, N., & Gross, C. (2003). Preventing nursing back injuries: Redesigning patient handling tasks. *AAOHN Journal, 51*(3), 126–134. doi:10.1177/216507990305100306 PMID:12670100

Newsome, J., Shi, E., Song, D., & Perrig, A. (2004). The sybil attack in sensor networks: Analysis & defenses. In *Proceedings of the 3rd International Symposium on Information Processing in Sensor Networks*, (pp. 259–268). ACM. 10.1145/984622.984660

Nibali, A., He, Z., & Wollersheim, D. (2017). Pulmonary nodule classification with deep residual networks. *International Journal of Computer Assisted Radiology and Surgery, 12*(10), 1799–1808.

Nishio, M., Sugiyama, O., Yakami, M., Ueno, S., Kubo, T., Kuroda, T., & Togashi, K. (2018). Computer-aided diagnosis of lung nodule classification between benign nodule, primary lung cancer, and metastatic lung cancer at different image size using deep convolutional neural network with transfer learning. *PLoS One, 13*(7), e0200721.

Nørgård, P. M. (1997). *The Neural Network Based System Identification Toolbox: For use with MATLAB.* Matlab.

North, N., Leung, W., Ashton, T., Rasmussen, E., Hughes, F., & Finlayson, M. (2013). Nurse turnover in New Zealand: Costs and relationships with staffing practices and patient outcomes. *Journal of Nursing Management*, *21*(3), 419–428. doi:10.1111/j.1365-2834.2012.01371.x PMID:23405958

Noura, H., Couturier, R., Pham, C., & Chehab, A. (2019). Lightweight stream cipher scheme for resource-constrained IoT devices. In *Proc. Int. Conf. Wireless Mobile Comput., Netw. Commun. (WiMob),* (pp. 1–8).

O'Leary, Z. (2013). *The essential guide to doing your research project. Sage (Atlanta, Ga.).*

Olson, A. L., Swigris, J. J., Sprunger, D. B., Fischer, A., Fernandez-Perez, E. R., Solomon, J., & Brown, K. K. (2011). Rheumatoid arthritis–interstitial lung disease–associated mortality. *American Journal of Respiratory and Critical Care Medicine*, *183*(3), 372–378.

Page, T. (2014). Touchscreen mobile devices and older adults: A usability study. International. *Journal of Human Factors and Ergonomics*, *3*(1), 65–85. doi:10.1504/IJHFE.2014.062550

Pal, K. (2019). Algorithmic Solutions for RFID Tag Anti-Collision Problem in Supply Chain Management. In *the 9th International Symposium on Frontiers in Ambient and Mobile Systems (FAMS 19),* 929-934. Procedia Computer Science.

Pal, K. (2021a). *Privacy, Security and Policies: A Review of Problems and Solutions with Blockchain-Based Internet of Things Applications in Industrial Industry*. In the 18th International Conference on Mobile Systems and Pervasive Computing (MobiSPC), Procedia Computer Science, Leuven, Belgium.

Pal, K. (2021b). A Novel Frame-Slotted ALOHA Algorithm for Radio Frequency Identification System in Supply Chain Management. In *11th International Symposium on Frontiers in Ambient and Mobile Systems (FAMS)*, (pp. 871- 876). Procedia Computer Science. 10.1016/j.procs.2021.03.110

Pal, K. (2022a). Application of Game Theory in Blockchain-Based Healthcare Information System. In Malay Dutta Borah, Peng Zhang, and Ganesh Chandra Deka (eds.), Prospects of Blockchain Technology for Accelerating Scientific Advancement in Healthcare, 84-99. IGI Global Publishing.

Pal, K. (2022b). A Decentralized Privacy Preserving Healthcare Blockchain for IoT, Challenges and Solutions. In Malay Dutta Borah, Peng Zhang, Ganesh Chandra Deka (eds.), Prospects of Blockchain Technology for Accelerating Scientific Advancement in Healthcare, 158-188. IGI Global Publishing.

Pal, K. (2022b). Semantic Interoperability in Internet of Things: Architecture, Protocols, and Research Challenges. In M Pejic-Bach and C Dogru (eds), Management Strategies for Sustainability, New Knowledge Innovation, and Personalized Products and Services, 40-171. The IGI Global Publishing.

Pal, K. (2022d). Cryptography and Blockchain Solutions for Security Protection of Internet of Things Applications. In Biswa Mohan Sahoo and Suman Avdhesh Yadav (eds.), Information Security Practices for the Internet of Things, 5G, and Next-Generation Wireless Networks, 152-178. IGI Global.

Pal, K., & Yasar, A. (2020b). Semantic Approach to Data Integration for an Internet of Things Supporting Apparel Supply Chain Management. In *the 17th International Conference on Mobile Systems and Pervasive Computing (MobiSPC),* 197 - 204. Procedia Computer Science.

Pal, K., & Yasar, K. (2020a). Internet of Things and Blockchain Technology in Apparel Manufacturing Supply Chain Data Management. In *the 11th International Conference on Ambient Systems, Networks, and Technologies (ANT 2020),* 450 – 457. Procedia Computer Science.

Pan, S., Zhou, W., Piramuthu, S., Giannikas, V., & Chen, C. (2021). Smart city for sustainable urban freight logistics. Int. J. Prod. Res. 2021, 59, 2079–2089. [CrossRef] 51. Shengli, W. Is Human Digital Twin possible? *Comput. Methods Programs Biomed. Update*, *1*, 100014.

Pan, S., Zhou, W., Piramuthu, S., Giannikas, V., & Chen, C. (2021). Smart city for sustainable urban freight logistics. Int. J. Prod. Res. 2021, 59, 2079–2089. 51. Shengli, W. Is Human Digital Twin possible? . *Comput. Methods Programs Biomed. Update*, *1*, 100014.

Paranjape, K., Schinkel, M., & Nanayakkara, P. (2020). Short Keynote Paper: Mainstreaming Personalized Healthcare–Transforming Healthcare Through New Era of Artificial Intelligence. *IEEE Journal of Biomedical and Health Informatics*, *24*(7), 1860–1863. doi:10.1109/JBHI.2020.2970807 PMID:32054591

Park, J., & Yang, B. (2020). GIS-Enabled Digital Twin System for Sustainable Evaluation of Carbon Emissions: A Case Study of Jeonju City, South Korea. *Sustainability*, *2020*(12), 9186. doi:10.3390u12219186

Park, Y., Woo, J., & Choi, S. (2020). A cloud-based digital twin manufacturing system based on an interoperable data schema for smart manufacturing. *International Journal of Computer Integrated Manufacturing*, *33*(12), 1259–1276. doi:10.1080/0951192X.2020.1815850

Patnaik, B. C., & Mishra, N. (2016). A Review on Enhancing the Journaling File System. *Imperial Journal of Interdisciplinary Research, 2*(11).

Paul, S. (2018), Digital twins – connecting information and insights through the entire project lifecycle. *Geospatial World.* https://www.geospatialworld.net/blogs/digital-twins-connecting-information-and-insights-through-the-entire-project-lifecycle/

Paul, R., Hawkins, S. H., Balagurunathan, Y., Schabath, M., Gillies, R. J., Hall, L. O., & Goldgof, D. B. (2016). Deep feature transfer learning in combination with traditional features predicts survival among patients with lung adenocarcinoma. *Tomography*, *2*(4), 388–395.

Pawar, U., O'Shea, D., Rea, S., & O'Reilly, R. (2020, June). Explainable ai in healthcare. In *2020 International Conference on Cyber Situational Awareness, Data Analytics and Assessment (CyberSA)* (pp. 1-2). IEEE.

Pedersen, A., Brup, M., Brink-Kjaer, A., Christiansen, L., & Mikkelsen, P. (2021). Living and Prototyping Digital Twins for Urban Water Systems: Towards Multi-Purpose Value Creation Using Models and Sensors. *Water (Basel)*, *13*(5), 592. doi:10.3390/w13050592

Peikert, T., Daniels, C. E., Beebe, T. J., Meyer, K. C., & Ryu, J. H. (2008). Assessment of current practice in the diagnosis and therapy of idiopathic pulmonary fibrosis. *Respiratory Medicine*, *102*(9), 1342–1348. doi:10.1016/j.rmed.2008.03.018 PMID:18621518

Pérez, M. J., & Grande, R. G. (2020). Application of artificial intelligence in the diagnosis and treatment of hepatocellular carcinoma: A review. *World Journal of Gastroenterology*, *26*(37), 5617–5628. doi:10.3748/wjg.v26.i37.5617 PMID:33088156

Pham, Q.-V., Nguyen, D. C., Huynh-The, T., Hwang, W.-J., & Pathirana, P. N. (2020). Artificial Intelligence (AI) and Big Data for Coronavirus (COVID-19) Pandemic: A Survey on the State-of-the-Arts. *IEEE Access: Practical Innovations, Open Solutions*, *8*, 130820–130839. doi:10.1109/ACCESS.2020.3009328 PMID:34812339

Polini, W., & Corrado, A. (2020). Digital twin of composite assembly manufacturing process. *International Journal of Production Research*, *58*(17), 5238–5252. doi:10.1080/00207543.2020.1714091

Pompeii, L. A., Lipscomb, H. J., Schoenfisch, A. L., & Dement, J. M. (2009). Musculoskeletal injuries resulting from patient handling tasks among hospital workers. *American Journal of Industrial Medicine*, *52*(7), 571–578. doi:10.1002/ajim.20704 PMID:19444808

Popay, J., Rogers, A., & Williams, G. (1998). Rationale and standards for the systematic review of qualitative literature in health services research. *Qualitative Health Research*, *8*(3), 341–351. doi:10.1177/104973239800800305 PMID:10558335

Prasad, R. B., & Groop, L. (2019). Precision medicine in type 2 diabetes. *Journal of Internal Medicine*, *285*(1), 40–48. doi:10.1111/joim.12859 PMID:30403316

Qia. Q. F. Y. (2018). Digital Twin Service towards Smart Manufacturing. Elsevier, 237-242.

Qi, Q., Tao, F., Hu, T., Anwer, H., Liu, A., Wei, Y., Wang, L., & Nee, A. (2021). Enabling technologies and tools for digital twin. *Journal of Manufacturing Systems*, *53*, 3–21. doi:10.1016/j.jmsy.2019.10.001

Quirk, D., Lanni, J., & Chauhan, N. (2020). Digital twins: Answering the hard questions. *ASHRAE Journal*, *62*, 22–25.

Quirk, D., Lanni, J., & Chauhan, N. (2020). *Digital Twins: Details of Implementation: Part 2. AHRAE J.*, *62*, 20–24.

Raes, L., Michiels, P., Adolphi, T., Tampere, C., Dalianis, T., Mcaleer, S., & Kogut, P. (2021). DUET: A Framework for Building Secure and Trusted Digital Twins of Smart Cities. *IEEE Internet Computing*.

Rafi, T. H., Shubair, R. M., Farhan, F., Hoque, M. Z., & Quayyum, F. M. (2021). Recent Advances in Computer-Aided Medical Diagnosis Using Machine Learning Algorithms with Optimization Techniques. *IEEE Access: Practical Innovations, Open Solutions*, *9*, 137847–137868. doi:10.1109/ACCESS.2021.3108892

Ragab, A. A. M., Madani, A., Wahdan, A. M., & Selim, G. M. L. (2021, January). Design, analysis, and implementation of a new lightweight block cipher for protecting IoT smart devices. *Journal of Ambient Intelligence and Humanized Computing*, 1–18. doi:10.100712652-020-02782-6

Raghu, G., Collard, H. R., Egan, J. J., Martinez, F. J., Behr, J., Brown, K. K., Colby, T. V., Cordier, J.-F., Flaherty, K. R., Lasky, J. A., Lynch, D. A., Ryu, J. H., Swigris, J. J., Wells, A. U., Ancochea, J., Bouros, D., Carvalho, C., Costabel, U., Ebina, M., & Schunemann, H. J. (2011). An official ATS/ERS/JRS/ALAT statement: idiopathic pulmonary fibrosis: evidence-based guidelines for diagnosis and management. *American Journal of Respiratory and Critical Care Medicine*, *183*(6), 788–824. doi:10.1164/rccm.2009-040GL PMID:21471066

Raghu, G., Weycker, D., Edelsberg, J., Bradford, W. Z., & Oster, G. (2006). Incidence and prevalence of idiopathic pulmonary fibrosis. *American Journal of Respiratory and Critical Care Medicine*, *174*(7), 810–816.

Raju, K., Chinna Rao, B., Saikumar, K., & Lakshman Pratap, N. (2022). An Optimal Hybrid Solution to Local and Global Facial Recognition Through Machine Learning. In P. Kumar, A. J. Obaid, K. Cengiz, A. Khanna, & V. E. Balas (Eds.), A Fusion of Artificial Intelligence and Internet of Things for Emerging Cyber Systems. Intelligent Systems Reference Library (Vol. 210). Springer. https://doi.org/10.1007/978-3-030-76653-5_11.

Ramakrishnan, R., & Gaur, L. (2016). Application of Internet of Things (IoT) for smart process manufacturing in Indian packaging industry. In *Information Systems Design and Intelligent Applications* (pp. 339–346). Springer.

Ramakrishnan, R., & Gaur, L. (2019). *Internet of Things: Approach and Applicability in Manufacturing*. CRC Press.

Ramakrishnan, R., Gaur, L., & Singh, G. (2016). Feasibility and efficacy of BLE beacon IoT devices in inventory management at the shop floor. *Iranian Journal of Electrical and Computer Engineering*, *6*(5), 2362–2368. doi:10.11591/ijece.v6i5.10807

Ramu, S. P., Boopalan, P., Pham, Q.-V., Maddikunta, P. K. R., Huynh-The, T., Alazab, M., Nguyen, T. T., & Gadekallu, T. R. (2022). Federated learning enabled digital twins for smart cities: Concepts, recent advances, and future directions. *Sustainable Cities and Society*, *79*, 103663. doi:10.1016/j.scs.2021.103663

Ran, Y., Lin, P., Zhou, X., & Wen, Y. (2019). A Survey of Predictive Maintenance: Systems, Purposes and Approaches. *Comput. Sci. Eng*. http://xxx.lanl.gov/abs/1912.07383.

Ran, Y., Lin, P., Zhou, X., & Wen, Y. A (2019). Survey of Predictive Maintenance: Systems, Purposes and Approaches. *Comput. Sci. Eng*. http://xxx.lanl.gov/abs/1912.07383 .

Rana, J., Gaur, L., Singh, G., Awan, U., & Rasheed, M. I. (2021). Reinforcing customer journey through artificial intelligence: a review and research agenda. *International Journal of Emerging Markets*. doi:10.1108/IJOEM-08-2021-1214

Randall, S. B., Pories, W. J., Pearson, A., & Drake, D. J. (2009). Expanded Occupational Safety and Health Administration 300 log as metric for bariatric patient-handling staff injuries. *Surgery for Obesity and Related Diseases*, *5*(4), 463–468. doi:10.1016/j.soard.2009.01.002 PMID:19359222

Rathore, M.; Shah, S.; Shukla, D.; Bentafat, E.; Bakiras, S. (2021). The Role of AI, Machine Learning, and Big Data in Digital Twinning: A Systematic Literature Review, Challenges, and Opportunities. *IEEE Access, 9*, 32030–32052.

Rathore, M.; Shah, S.; Shukla, D.; Bentafat, E.; Bakiras, S. (2021). The Role of AI, Machine Learning, and Big Data in Digital Twinning: A Systematic Literature Review, Challenges, and Opportunities. IEEE.

Ready, A. E., Boreskie, S. L., Law, S. A., & Russell, R. (1993). Fitness and lifestyle parameters fail to predict back injuries in nurses. *Canadian Journal of Applied Physiology*, *18*(1), 80–90. doi:10.1139/h93-008 PMID:8471996

Redelinghuys, A. J., Basson, A. H., & Kruger, K. (2020). A six-layer architecture for the digital twin: A manufacturing case study implementation. *Journal of Intelligent Manufacturing*, *31*(6), 1383–1402. doi:10.100710845-019-01516-6

Reyna, A., Martín, C., Chen, J., Soler, E., & Díaz, M. (2018, November). On blockchain and its integration with IoT. Challenges and opportunities. *Future Generation Computer Systems*, *88*, 173–190. doi:10.1016/j.future.2018.05.046

Riemersma-Van Der Lek, R. F., Swaab, D. F., Twisk, J., Hol, E. M., Hoogendijk, W. J., & Van Someren, E. J. (2008). Effect of bright light and melatonin on cognitive and noncognitive function in elderly residents of group care facilities: A randomized controlled trial. *Journal of the American Medical Association*, *299*(22), 2642–2655. doi:10.1001/jama.299.22.2642 PMID:18544724

Rivera, M. J., Teruel, M. A., Maté, A., & Trujillo, J. (2021). Diagnosis and prognosis of mental disorders by means of EEG and deep learning: A systematic mapping study. *Artificial Intelligence Review*, 1–43.

Roberts, C., & Mort, M. (2009). Reshaping what counts as care: Older people, work and new technologies. *Alter*, *3*(2), 138–158. doi:10.1016/j.alter.2009.01.004

Robinson, H., MacDonald, B., & Broadbent, E. (2014). The role of healthcare robots for older people at home: A review. *International Journal of Social Robotics*, *6*(4), 575–591. doi:10.100712369-014-0242-2

Rudie, J. D., Rauschecker, A. M., Bryan, R. N., Davatzikos, C., & Mohan, S. (2019). Emerging applications of artificial intelligence in neuro-oncology. *Radiology*, *290*(3), 607–618. doi:10.1148/radiol.2018181928 PMID:30667332

Russell, H. (2020). Sustainable Urban Governance Networks: Data-driven Planning Technologies and Smart City Software Systems. *Geopolit. Hist. Int. Relations*, *12*, 9–15.

Ryerson, C. J., Urbania, T. H., Richeldi, L., Mooney, J. J., Lee, J. S., Jones, K. D., & Collard, H. R. (2013). Prevalence and prognosis of unclassifiable interstitial lung disease. *The European Respiratory Journal*, *42*(3), 750–757.

Saddik, A. E. (2022). *Digital Twin for Healthcare: Design, Challenges and Solutions*. Elsevier.

Sadhukhan, D., Ray, S., Biswas, G. P., Khan, M. K., & Dasgupta, M. (2021). A lightweight remote user authentication scheme for IoT communication using elliptic curve cryptography. *The Journal of Supercomputing*, *77*(2), 1114–1151. doi:10.100711227-020-03318-7

Saeed, S., Jhanjhi, N. Z., Naqvi, M., Humyun, M., Ahmad, M., & Gaur, L. (2022). Optimized Breast Cancer Premature Detection Method With Computational Segmentation: A Systematic Review Mapping. *Approaches and Applications of Deep Learning in Virtual Medical Care*, 24-51.

Saeed, S., Jhanjhi, N. Z., Naqvi, M., Humyun, M., Ahmad, M., & Gaur, L. (2022). *Optimized Breast Cancer Premature Detection Method With Computational Segmentation: A Systematic Review Mapping*. Approaches and Applications of Deep Learning in Virtual Medical Care.

Sahal, R., Alsamhi, S. H., Brown, K. N., O'Shea, D., & Alouffi, B. (2022). Blockchain-Based Digital Twins Collaboration for Smart Pandemic Alerting: Decentralized COVID-19 Pandemic Alerting Use Case (2022). *Computational Intelligence and Neuroscience*, 7786441. doi:10.1155/2022/7786441

Saikumar, K., & Rajesh, V. (2020). A novel implementation heart diagnosis system based on random forest machine learning technique International. *Journal of Pharmacy Research*, *12*, 3904–3916.

Saikumar, K., & Rajesh, V. (2020). Coronary blockage of artery for Heart diagnosis with DT Artificial Intelligence Algorithm. *Int J Res Pharma Sci*, *11*(1), 471–479.

Sakdirat, K., Rungskunroch, P., & Welsh, J. (2019). A Digital-Twin Evaluation of Net Zero Energy Building for Existing Buildings. *Sustainability*, *11*, 159.

Saketkoo, L. A., Matteson, E. L., Brown, K. K., Seibold, J. R., & Strand, V. (2011). Developing disease activity and response criteria in connective tissue disease-related interstitial lung disease. *The Journal of Rheumatology*, *38*(7), 1514–1518.

Salahuddin, Z., Woodruff, H. C., Chatterjee, A., & Lambin, P. (2022). Transparency of deep neural networks for medical image analysis: A review of interpretability methods. *Computers in Biology and Medicine*, *140*, 105111.

Sandelowski, M. (2000). Focus on research methods-whatever happened to qualitative description? *Research in Nursing & Health*, *23*(4), 334–340. doi:10.1002/1098-240X(200008)23:4<334::AID-NUR9>3.0.CO;2-G PMID:10940958

Sankara Babu, B., Nalajala, S., Sarada, K., Muniraju Naidu, V., Yamsani, N., & Saikumar, K. (2022). Machine Learning Based Online Handwritten Telugu Letters Recognition for Different Domains. In P. Kumar, A. J. Obaid, K. Cengiz, A. Khanna, & V. E. Balas (Eds.), A Fusion of Artificial Intelligence and Internet of Things for Emerging Cyber Systems. Intelligent Systems Reference Library (Vol. 210). Springer. https://doi.org/10.1007/978-3-030-76653-5_12.

Santosh, K. C., & Gaur, L. (2021). Ai in precision medicine. In Artificial Intelligence and Machine Learning in Public Healthcare, 41-47. Springer.

Santosh, K. C., & Gaur, L. (2021). Introduction to ai in public health. In Artificial Intelligence and Machine Learning in Public Healthcare, 1-10. Springer.

Santosh, K., & Gaur, L. (2021). AI in Precision Medicine. In Artificial Intelligence and Machine Learning in Public Healthcare. SpringerBriefs in Applied Sciences and Technology. Springer. https://doi.org/10.1007/978-981-16-6768-8_5.

Santosh, K., & Gaur, L. (2021). Introduction to AI in Public Health. In Artificial Intelligence and Machine Learning in Public Healthcare. SpringerBriefs in Applied Sciences and Technology. Springer. https://doi.org/10.1007/978-981-16-6768-8_1.

Santosh, K. C., & Gaur, L. (2022). *Artificial Intelligence and Machine Learning in Public Healthcare: Opportunities and Societal Impact*. Springer Nature, Sugarhood, P., Wherton, J., Procter, R., Hinder, S., & Greenhalgh, T. (2014). Technology as system innovation: a key informant interview study of the application of the diffusion of innovation model to telecare. *Disability and Rehabilitation. Assistive Technology*, *9*(1), 79–87.

Saravanan, M., Shubha, R., Marks, A. M., & Iyer, V. (2017). SMEAD: A Secured Mobile Enabled Assisting Device for Diabetics Monitoring, *IEEE International Conference on Advanced Networks and Telecommunications Systems (ANTS)*, (pp. 1-6). IEEE.

Sasubilli, G., & Kumar, A. "Machine Learning and Big Data Implementation on Health Care data," 2020 4th International Conference on Intelligent Computing and Control Systems (ICICCS), 2020, pp. 859-864, 10.1109/ICICCS48265.2020.9120906

Sawada, Y., & Kozuka, K. (2015, May). Transfer learning method using multi-prediction deep Boltzmann machines for a small scale dataset. In *14th IAPR International Conference on Machine Vision Applications (MVA)* (pp. 110-113). IEEE.

Schinkel, M., Paranjape, K., Panday, R. N., Skyttberg, N., & Nanayakkara, P. W. (2019). Clinical applications of artificial intelligence in sepsis: A narrative review. *Computers in Biology and Medicine*, *115*, 103488. doi:10.1016/j.compbiomed.2019.103488 PMID:31634699

Schröders, J. (2021). *Diversity, dynamics, and deficits: the role of social networks for the health of aging populations in Indonesia* [Doctoral dissertation, Umeå University, Sweeden].

Schrotter, G., & Hurzeler, C. (2021). The Digital Twin of the City of Zurich for Urban Planning. *J. Photogramm. Remote Sens. Geoinf. Sci.*, *88*, 99–112.

Seelan, L. J., Suresh, L. P., & Veni, S. K. (2016, October). Automatic extraction of Lung lesion by using optimized toboggan based approach with feature normalization and transfer learning methods. In *2016 International Conference on Emerging Technological Trends (ICETT)* (pp. 1-10). IEEE.

Shah, I. A. (2022). Cybersecurity Issues and Challenges for E-Government During COVID-19: A Review. *Cybersecurity Measures for E-Government Frameworks*, 187-222.

Shah, I. A., Wassan, S., & Usmani, M. H. (2022). E-Government Security and Privacy Issues: Challenges and Preventive Approaches. In Cybersecurity Measures for E-Government Frameworks (pp. 61-76). IGI Global.

Shaheen, M. Y. (2021). *Applications of Artificial Intelligence (AI) in healthcare: A review*. ScienceOpen Preprints.

Shah, I. A., Habeeb, R. A. A., Rajper, S., & Laraib, A. (2022). The Influence of Cybersecurity Attacks on E-Governance. In *Cybersecurity Measures for E-Government Frameworks* (pp. 77–95). IGI Global. doi:10.4018/978-1-7998-9624-1.ch005

Shah, I. A., Jhanjhi, N. Z., Amsaad, F., & Razaque, A. (2022). The Role of Cutting-Edge Technologies in Industry 4.0. In *Cyber Security Applications for Industry 4.0* (pp. 97–109). Chapman and Hall/CRC. doi:10.1201/9781003203087-4

Shah, I. A., Jhanjhi, N. Z., Humayun, M., & Ghosh, U. (2022). Health Care Digital Revolution During COVID-19. In *How COVID-19 is Accelerating the Digital Revolution* (pp. 17–30). Springer. doi:10.1007/978-3-030-98167-9_2

Shah, I. A., Jhanjhi, N. Z., Humayun, M., & Ghosh, U. (2022). Impact of COVID-19 on Higher and Post-secondary Education Systems. In *How COVID-19 is Accelerating the Digital Revolution* (pp. 71–83). Springer. doi:10.1007/978-3-030-98167-9_5

Shah, I. A., & Rajper, S., & Zaman-Jhanjhi, N. (2021). Using ML and Data-Mining Techniques in Automatic Vulnerability Software Discovery. *International Journal (Toronto, Ont.)*, *10*(3).

Shahzadi, R., Anwar, S. M., Qamar, F., Ali, M., & Rodrigues, J. P. C. (2019). Chaos based enhanced RC5 algorithm for security and integrity of clinical images in remote health monitoring. *IEEE Access: Practical Innovations, Open Solutions*, *7*, 52858–52870. doi:10.1109/ACCESS.2019.2909554

Shan, H., Wang, G., Kalra, M. K., de Souza, R., & Zhang, J. (2017, June). Enhancing transferability of features from pretrained deep neural networks for lung nodule classification. In *Proceedings of the 2017 International Conference on Fully Three-Dimensional Image Reconstruction in Radiology and Nuclear Medicine*.

Shannon, C. E. (1949). Communication Theory of Secrecy Systems. *The Bell System Technical Journal*, *28*(4), 656–715. doi:10.1002/j.1538-7305.1949.tb00928.x

Sharafi, M., Fotouhi-Ghazvini, F., Shirali, M., & Ghassemian, M. (2019). A low power cryptography solution based on chaos theory in wireless sensor nodes. *IEEE Access: Practical Innovations, Open Solutions*, *7*, 8737–8753. doi:10.1109/ACCESS.2018.2886384

Sharma, C., & Gupta, G. (2021). Innovation insight for healthcare provider digital twins: A review. Mobile Health: Advances in Research and Applications, pp. 97-128.

Sharma, A., Kosasih, E., Zhang, J., Brintrup, A., & Calinescu, A. (2021). Digital Twins: State of the Art Theory and Practice, Challenges, and Open Research Questions. arXiv 2021, arXiv:2011.02833.

Sharma, A., Kosasih, E., Zhang, J., Brintrup, A., & Calinescu, A. (2021). *Digital Twins: State of the Art Theory and Practice*. Challenges, and Open Research Questions.

Sharma, D. K., Gaur, L., & Okunbor, D. (2007). Image compression and feature extraction with neural network. In Allied Academies International Conference. Academy of Management Information and Decision Sciences, *11*(1), 33. Jordan Whitney Enterprises, Inc .

Sharma, M., & George, J. P. (2018). *Digital Twin in the Automotive Industry: Driving Physical-Digital Convergence; TCS White Papers*. Tata Consultancy Services Limited.

Sharma, S., Singh, G., Gaur, L., & Sharma, R. (2022). Does psychological distance and religiosity influence fraudulent customer behaviour? *International Journal of Consumer Studies*. Advance online publication. doi:10.1111/ijcs.12773

Shen, D., Wu, G., & Suk, H. I. (2017). Deep learning in medical image analysis. *Annual Review of Biomedical Engineering*, *19*(1), 221–248. doi:10.1146/annurev-bioeng-071516-044442 PMID:28301734

Shen, W., Zhou, M., Yang, F., Dong, D., Yang, C., Zang, Y., & Tian, J. (2016, October). Learning from experts: developing transferable deep features for patient-level lung cancer prediction. In *International conference on medical image computing and computer-assisted intervention* (pp. 124-131). Springer.

Shi, E., & Perrig, A. (2004). Designing secure sensor networks. *IEEE Wireless Communications*, *11*(6), 38–43. doi:10.1109/MWC.2004.1368895

Shi, N., Tan, L., Yan, C., He, C., Xu, J., Lu, Y., & Xu, H. (2021, September). BacS: A blockchain-based access control scheme in distributed internet of things. *Peer-to-Peer Networking and Applications*, *14*(5), 2585–2599. doi:10.100712083-020-00930-5

Shneiderman, B. (2020). Design lessons from AI's two grand goals: Human emulation and useful applications. *IEEE Transactions on Technology and Society*, *1*(2), 73–82. doi:10.1109/TTS.2020.2992669

Shoji, K., Schudel, S., Onwude, D., Shrivastava, C., & Defraeye, T. (2022). Mapping the postharvest life of imported fruits from packhouse to retail stores using physics-based digital twins. *Resources, Conservation and Recycling*, *176*, 105914. doi:10.1016/j.resconrec.2021.105914

Shouno, H., Suzuki, S., & Kido, S. (2015, November). A transfer learning method with deep convolutional neural network for diffuse lung disease classification. In *International Conference on Neural Information Processing* (pp. 199-207). Springer.

Sierla, S., Azangoo, M., Rainio, K., Papakonstantinou, N., Fay, A., Honkamaa, P., & Vyatkin, V. (2022). Roadmap to semi-automatic generation of digital twins for brownfield process plants. *Journal of Industrial Information Integration*, *27*, 100282. doi:10.1016/j.jii.2021.100282

Simpson, P. K. (1992). Fuzzy min-max neural networks. I. Classification. *IEEE Transactions on Neural Networks*, *3*(5), 776–786.

Singh, K., & Kaushik, K. Ahatsham, & Shahare V. (2020). Role and Impact of Wearables in IoT Healthcare. In: Raju K., Govardhan A., Rani B., Sridevi R., Murty M. (eds) *Proceedings of the Third International Conference on Computational Intelligence and Informatics. Advances in Intelligent Systems and Computing, (vol 1090).* Springer.

Singh, A. P., Pradhan, N. R., Luhach, A. K., Agnihotri, S., Jhanjhi, N. Z., Verma, S., Kavita, Ghosh, U., & Roy, D. S. (2020). A novel patient-centric architectural framework for blockchain-enabled healthcare applications. *IEEE Transactions on Industrial Informatics*, *17*(8), 5779–5789. https://ieeexplore.ieee.org/abstract/document/9259231. doi:10.1109/TII.2020.3037889

Singh, G., Gaur, L., & Ramakrishnan, R. (2017). Internet of things – technology adoption model in india. *Pertanika Journal of Science & Technology*, *25*(3), 835–846.

Singh, M., Fuenmayor, E., Hinchy, E. P., Qiao, Y., Murray, N., & Devine, D. (2021). Digital Twin: Origin to Future. *Appl. Syst. Innov.*, *4*(2), 36. doi:10.3390/asi4020036

Singh, M., Fuenmayor, E., Hinchy, E. P., Qiao, Y., Murray, N., & Devine, D. (2021). Digital Twin: Origin to Future. *Appl. Syst. Innov.*, *4*, 36.

Sleem, L., & Couturier, R. (2021, May). Speck-R: An ultra-light-weight cryptographic scheme for internet of things. *Multimedia Tools and Applications*, *80*(11), 17067–17102. doi:10.100711042-020-09625-8

Solanas, A., Patsakis, C., Conti, M., Vlachos, I. S., Ramos, V., Falcone, F., Postolache, O., Perez-Martinez, P. A., Pietro, R. D., Perrea, D. N., & Martinez-Balleste, A. (2014). Smart health: A context-aware health paradigm within smart cities. *IEEE Communications Magazine*, *52*(8), 74–81.

Solanki, A., Jain, V., & Gaur, L. (Eds.). (2022). *Applications of Blockchain and Big IoT Systems: Digital Solutions for Diverse Industries*. CRC Press.

Soni, R., Guan, J., Avinash, G., & Saripalli, V. R. "HMC: A Hybrid Reinforcement Learning Based Model Compression for Healthcare Applications," 2019 IEEE 15th International Conference on Automation Science and Engineering (CASE), 2019, pp. 146-151, 10.1109/COASE.2019.8843047

Sowjanya, K., Dasgupta, M., & Ray, S. (2021, August). A lightweight key management scheme for key-escrow-free ECC-based CP-ABE for IoT healthcare systems. *Journal of Systems Architecture*, *117*, 102108. doi:10.1016/j.sysarc.2021.102108

Sreelakshmi, D., & Inthiyaz, S. (2021). A pervasive health care device computing application for brain tumors with machine and deep learning techniques. *International Journal of Pervasive Computing and Communications.*

Sreelakshmi, D., & Inthiyaz, S. (2021). Fast and denoise feature extraction based ADMF–CNN with GBML framework for MRI brain image. *International Journal of Speech Technology*, *24*(2), 529–544.

Sruthi, M., & Rajasekaran, R. (2021). Hybrid lightweight signcryption scheme for IoT. *Open Computer Science*, *11*(1), 391–398. doi:10.1515/comp-2020-0105

Stevens, L. (2019), Geospatial Digital Twins. *The Medium.* https://medium.com/@linda_29745/geospatial-digital-twins-a8e2bc886fd4

Stojanovic, L., Usländer, T., Volz, F., Weißenbacher, C., Müller, J., Jacoby, M., & Bischoff, T. (2021). Methodology and Tools for Digital Twin Management—The FA3ST Approach. *IoT*, *2*(4), 717–740. doi:10.3390/iot2040036

Stojanovic, N., & Milenovic, D. (2018, December). Data-driven Digital Twin approach for process optimization: An industry use case. In *2018 IEEE International Conference on Big Data (Big Data)* (pp. 4202-4211). IEEE. 10.1109/BigData.2018.8622412

Stojanovic, N., & Milenovic, D. (2018, December). Data-driven Digital Twin approach for process optimization: An industry use case. In *International Conference on Big Data (Big Data)* (pp. 4202-4211). IEEE.

Stoter, J., Ohori, K. A., & Noardo, F. (2021), Digital Twins: A Comprehensive Solution or Hopeful Vision? *GIM Internationjal*. https://www.gim-international.com/content/article/digital-twins-a-comprehensive-solution-or-hopefulvision?utm_source=new sletter&utm_medium=email&utm_campaign=Newsletter+%7C+GIM+%7C+17-03-2022++&sid=34800

Sujatha, R., Chatterjee, J. M., Jhanjhi, N. Z., & Brohi, S. N. (2021). Performance of deep learning vs machine learning in plant leaf disease detection. *Microprocessors and Microsystems*, *80*, 103615. doi:10.1016/j.micpro.2020.103615

Sun, Y. F., Lo, F. P. W., & Lo, B. (2021). Light-weight internet-of-things device authentication, encryption and key distribution using end-to-end neural cryptosystems. *IEEE Internet of Things Journal*, *14*(8), 1–10. doi:10.1109/JIOT.2021.3123822

Sverzellati, N., Devaraj, A., Desai, S. R., Quigley, M., Wells, A. U., & Hansell, D. M. (2011). Method for minimizing observer variation for the quantitation of high-resolution computed tomographic signs of lung disease. *Journal of Computer Assisted Tomography*, *35*(5), 596–601.

Tagliabue, L., Cecconi, F., Maltese, S., Rinaldi, S., Ciribini, A., & Flammini, A. (2021). Leveraging Digital Twin for Sustainability Assessment of an Educational Building. *Sustainability*, *13*, 480.

Tao, F., Cheng, J., Qi, Q., Zhang, M., Zhang, H., & Sui, F. (2018). Digital twin-driven product design, manufacturing and service with big data. *International Journal of Advanced Manufacturing Technology*, *94*, 3563–3576. doi:10.100700170-017-0233-1

Tao, F., Liu, A., Hu, T., & Nee, A. Y. (2020). *Digital twin driven smart design*. Academic Press.

Tao, F., Zhang, H., Liu, A., & Nee, A. Y. (2018). Digital twin in industry: State-of-the-art. *IEEE Transactions on Industrial Informatics*, *15*(4), 2405–2415. https://ieeexplore.ieee.org/abstract/document/8477101

Tao, F., & Zhang, M. (2017). Digital twin shop-floor: A new shop-floor paradigm towards smart manufacturing. *IEEE Access: Practical Innovations, Open Solutions*, *5*, 20418–20427. doi:10.1109/ACCESS.2017.2756069

Tawalbeh, L. A., & Habeeb, S. "An Integrated Cloud Based Healthcare System," *2018 Fifth International Conference on Internet of Things: Systems, Management and Security*, 2018, pp. 268-273, 10.1109/IoTSMS.2018.8554648

Tewari, S., Yousefi, S., & Webb, A. G. (2022). Deep neural network-based optimization for the design of a multi-element surface magnet for MRI applications. *Inverse Problems*.

Therivel, R., & Paridario, M. R. (2013). *The practice of strategic environmental assessment*. Routledge. doi:10.4324/9781315070865

Thiong'o, G.M., & Rutka, J.T. (2022). Digital Twin Technology: The Future of Predicting Neurological Complications of Pediatric Cancers and Their Treatment. *Frontiers in Oncology*, *11*, 781499

Thomas, B. H., Ciliska, D., Dobbins, M., & Micucci, S. (2004). A process for systematically reviewing the literature: Providing the research evidence for public health nursing interventions. *Worldviews on Evidence-Based Nursing*, *1*(3), 176–184. doi:10.1111/j.1524-475X.2004.04006.x PMID:17163895

Tolga Erol, A. F. (2020). *The Digital Twin Revolution in Healthcare*. Research Gate.

Tomin, N., Kurbatsky, V., Borisov, V., & Musalev, S. (2020). Development of Digital Twin for Load Center on the Example of Distribution Network of an Urban District. *Energy*, *209*, 02029.

Travis, W. D., Costabel, U., Hansell, D. M., King, T. E. Jr, Lynch, D. A., Nicholson, A. G., & Valeyre, D. (2013). An official American Thoracic Society/European Respiratory Society statement: Update of the international multidisciplinary classification of the idiopathic interstitial pneumonias. *American Journal of Respiratory and Critical Care Medicine*, *188*(6), 733–748.

Trinkoff, A. M., Brady, B., & Nielsen, K. (2003). Workplace prevention and musculoskeletal injuries in nurses. *The Journal of Nursing Administration*, *33*(3), 153–158. doi:10.1097/00005110-200303000-00006 PMID:12629302

Trinkoff, A. M., Lipscomb, J. A., Geiger-Brown, J., & Brady, B. (2002). Musculoskeletal problems of the neck, shoulder and back and functional consequences in nurses. *American Journal of Industrial Medicine*, *41*(3), 170–178. doi:10.1002/ajim.10048 PMID:11920961

Tyrväinen, P., Silvennoinen, M., Talvitie-Lamberg, K., Ala-Kitula, A., & Kuoremäki, R. "Identifying opportunities for AI applications in healthcare — Renewing the national healthcare and social services," 2018 IEEE 6th International Conference on Serious Games and Applications for Health (SeGAH), 2018, pp. 1-7, 10.1109/SeGAH.2018.8401381

U.S. Department of Labor, Bureau of Labor Statistics (2018). *Survey of occupational inquiries and illnesses, 2018* [Data set]. Bureau of Labor Statistics.

Umrani, S., Rajper, S., Talpur, S. H., Shah, I. A., & Shujrah, A. (2020). Games based learning: A case of learning Physics using Angry Birds. *Indian Journal of Science and Technology*, *13*(36), 3778–3784.

Usman, M., Ahmed, I., Aslam, M. I., Khan, S., & U. A. Shah U. A. (2017*). SIT: A lightweight encryption algorithm for secure Internet of Things.* arXiv:1704.08688. https://arxiv.org/abs/1704.08688

Van der Roest, H. G., Wenborn, J., Pastink, C., Dröes, R. M., & Orrell, M. (2017). Assistive technology for memory support in dementia. *Cochrane Database of Systematic Reviews*, *2017*(6), 6. doi:10.1002/14651858.CD009627.pub2 PMID:28602027

van derValk, H. H. (03 Dec 2021). *Archetypes of Digital Twins*. Springer.

Vendittelli, D., Penprase, B., & Pittiglio, L. (2016). Musculoskeletal injury prevention for new nurses. *Workplace Health & Safety*, *64*(12), 573–585. doi:10.1177/2165079916654928 PMID:27353509

Videman, T., Ojajärvi, A., Riihimäki, H., & Troup, J. D. (2005). Low back pain among nurses: A follow-up beginning at entry to the nursing school. *Spine*, *30*(20), 2334–2341. doi:10.1097/01.brs.0000182107.14355.ca PMID:16227898

Videman, T., Rauhala, H., Asp, S., Lindström, K., Cedercreutz, G., Kämppi, M., Tola, S., & Troup, J. D. G. (1989). Patient-handling skill, back injuries, and back pain: An intervention study in nursing. *Spine*, *14*(2), 148–156. doi:10.1097/00007632-198902000-00002 PMID:2522242

Vieira, E. R., Kumar, S., Coury, H. J., & Narayan, Y. (2006). Low back problems and possible improvements in nursing jobs. *Journal of Advanced Nursing*, *55*(1), 79–89. doi:10.1111/j.1365-2648.2006.03877.x PMID:16768742

Villamil, S., Hernández, C., & Tarazona, G. (2020, October). An overview of internet of things [Telecommunication Computing Electronics and Control]. *TELKOMNIKA*, *18*(5), 2320–2327. doi:10.12928/telkomnika.v18i5.15911

Voigt, I., Inojosa, H., Dillenseger, A., Haase, R., Akgün, K., & Ziemssen, T. (2021). Digital Twins for Multiple Sclerosis. *Frontiers in Immunology*, *12*, 669811. doi:10.3389/fimmu.2021.669811

Volkov, I. G. A. (2021). Digital Twins, Internet of Things and Mobile Medicine: A Review of Current Platforms to Support Smart Healhcare. Springer.

Volkov, I., Radchenko, G., & Tchernykh, A. (2021). Digital Twins, Internet of Things and Mobile Medicine: A Review of Current Platforms to Support Smart Healthcare. *Programming and Computer Software*, *47* (8), pp. 578-590. doi:10.1134/S0361768821080284

Vuppalapati, C., Ilapakurti, A., Kedari, S., Vuppalapati, R., Vuppalapati, J., & Kedari, S. (2020, December). Stratification of, albeit Mathematical Optimization and Artificial Intelligent (AI) Driven, High-Risk Elderly Outpatients for priority house call visits-a framework to transform healthcare services from reactive to preventive. In 2020 IEEE International Conference on Big Data (Big Data) (pp. 4955-4960). IEEE.

Wang, C., Elazab, A., Wu, J., & Hu, Q. (2017). Lung nodule classification using deep feature fusion in chest radiography. *Computerized Medical Imaging and Graphics*, *57*, 10–18.

Ware, P., Bartlett, S. J., Paré, G., Symeonidis, I., Tannenbaum, C., Bartlett, G., & Ahmed, S. (2017). Using eHealth technologies: Interests, preferences, and concerns of older adults. *Interactive Journal of Medical Research*, *6*(1), e4447. doi:10.2196/ijmr.4447 PMID:28336506

Watadani, T., Sakai, F., Johkoh, T., Noma, S., Akira, M., Fujimoto, K., & Sugiyama, Y. (2013). Interobserver variability in the CT assessment of honeycombing in the lungs. *Radiology*, *266*(3), 936–944.

Waters, T.R. (2007). When is it safe to manually lift a patient? *American Journal of Nursing 107, 6*(1), pp. 40–45.

Waters, T. R. (2008). Science to support specific limits on lifting, pushing, and pulling and static postures. Presentation at the *8th Annual Safe Patient Handling Conference*. Lake Buena Vista, Florida, USA.

Waters, T. R., Collins, J., Galinsky, T., & Caruso, C. (2006). NIOSH research efforts to prevent musculoskeletal disorders in the healthcare industry. *Orthopedic Nursing*, *25*(6), 380–389. doi:10.1097/00006416-200611000-00007 PMID:17130760

Wazid, M., Das, A. K., Odelu, V., Kumar, N., Conti, M., & Jo, M. (2017, February). Design of secure user authenticated key management protocol for generic IoT networks. *IEEE Internet of Things Journal*, *5*(1), 269–282. doi:10.1109/JIOT.2017.2780232

Wehbe, Y., Zaabi, M. A., & Svetinovic, D. "Blockchain AI Framework for Healthcare Records Management: Constrained Goal Model," 2018 26th Telecommunications Forum (TELFOR), 2018, pp. 420-425, 10.1109/TELFOR.2018.8611900

Whaiduzzaman, M., Hossain, M. R., Shovon, A. R., Roy, S., Laszka, A., Buyya, R., & Barros, A. (2020). A Privacy-Preserving Mobile and Fog Computing Framework to Trace and Prevent COVID-19 Community Transmission. *IEEE Journal of Biomedical and Health Informatics*, *24*(12), 3564–3575. doi:10.1109/JBHI.2020.3026060 PMID:32966223

Wickramasinghe, N., Jayaraman, P. P., Zelcer, J., Forkan, A. R. M., Ulapane, N., Kaul, R., & Vaughan, S. (2021). A Vision for Leveraging the Concept of Digital Twins to Support the Provision of Personalised Cancer Care. *Internet Computing*. doi:10.1109/MIC.2021.3065381

Williamson, B. J., Wang, D., Khandwala, V., Scheler, J., & Vagal, A. (2022). Improving Deep Neural Network Interpretation for Neuroimaging Using Multivariate Modeling. *SN Computer Science*, *3*(2), 1–8.

Wolters, M. K., Kelly, F., & Kilgour, J. (2016). Designing a spoken dialogue interface to an intelligent cognitive assistant for people with dementia. *Health Informatics Journal, 22*(4), 854–866. doi:10.1177/1460458215593329 PMID:26276794

Wright, L., & Davidson, S. (2020). How to tell the difference between a model and a digital twin. . *Advanced Modeling and Simulation in Engineering Sciences, 7*(1), 13. doi:10.118640323-020-00147-4

Wright, L., & Davidson, S. (2020). How to tell the difference between a model and a digital twin. *Adv. Model. Simul. Eng. Sci., 7*, 13.

Wu, Y., Zhang, K., & Zhang, Y. (2021). Digital Twin Networks: A Survey. *IEEE Internet of Things Journal, 8* (18), pp. 13789-13804. doi:10.1109/JIOT.2021.3079510

Wu, F., Li, X., Sangaiah, A. K., Xu, L., Kumari, S., Wu, L., & Shen, J. (2018, May). A lightweight and robust two-factor authentication scheme for personalized healthcare systems using wireless medical sensor networks. *Future Generation Computer Systems, 82*, 727–737. doi:10.1016/j.future.2017.08.042

Wu, Y., Giger, M. L., Doi, K., Vyborny, C. J., Schmidt, R. A., & Metz, C. E. (1993). Artificial deep Neural Networks in mammography: Application to decision making in the diagnosis of breast cancer. *Radiology, 187*(1), 81–87.

Xiang, W., & Yuanyuan, Z. (2022). Scalable access control scheme of internet of things based on blockchain based on blockchain. *Procedia Computer Science, 198*, 448–453. doi:10.1016/j.procs.2021.12.268

Xie, S., Zhu, S., & Dai, J. (2021). Feasibility study of intelligent healthcare based on digital twin and data mining. *Proceedings - 2021 International Conference on Computer Information Science and Artificial Intelligence*, (pp. 906-911). IEEE. doi:10.1109/CISAI54367.2021.00182

Xie, X., & Chen, Y. C. (2021, April). Decentralized data aggregation: A new secure framework based on lightweight cryptographic algorithms. *Wireless Communications and Mobile Computing, 2021*(3), 1–12.

Xing, X., Del Ser, J., Wu, Y., Li, Y., Xia, J., Lei, X., Firmin, D., Gatehouse, P., & Yang, G. (2022). HDL: Hybrid Deep Learning for the Synthesis of Myocardial Velocity Maps in Digital Twins for Cardiac Analysis. *IEEE Journal of Biomedical and Health Informatics*. doi:10.1109/JBHI.2022.3158897

Yang Peng, M. Z. (2020). Digital Twin Hospital Buildings: An Exemplary Case Study through Continuous Lifecycle Integration. *Resaerch Gate*.

Yassi, A., Khokhar, J., Tate, R., Cooper, J., Snow, C., & Vallentype, S. (1995). The epidemiology of back injuries in nurses at a large Canadian tertiary care hospital: Implications for prevention. *Occupational Medicine, 45*(4), 215–220. doi:10.1093/occmed/45.4.215 PMID:7662937

Yip, V. Y. B. (2004). New low back pain in nurses: Work activities, work stress and sedentary lifestyle. *Journal of Advanced Nursing, 46*(4), 430–440. doi:10.1111/j.1365-2648.2004.03009.x PMID:15117354

Yitmen, I., Alizadehsalehi, S., Akiner, I., & Akiner, M. (2021). An Adapted Model of Cognitive Digital Twins for Building Lifecycle Management. *Applied Sciences (Basel, Switzerland), 11*(9), 4276. doi:10.3390/app11094276

Yitmen, I., Alizadehsalehi, S., Akiner, I., & Akiner, M. (2021). An Adapted Model of Cognitive Digital Twins for Building Lifecycle Management.. *Appl. Sci., 11*, 4276.

Yu, B., Yang, M., Wang, Z., & Gao, C. S. (2006). Identify Abnormal Packet Loss in Selective Forwarding Attacks. *Chinese Journal of Computers, 9*, 1540–1550.

Yusif, S., Soar, J., & Hafeez-Baig, A. (2016). Older people, assistive technologies, and the barriers to adoption: A systematic review. *International Journal of Medical Informatics, 94*, 112–116. doi:10.1016/j.ijmedinf.2016.07.004 PMID:27573318

Zhang, C., Zhou, G. H. J., Li, Z., & Cheng, W. (2019). A data-and knowledge-driven framework for digital twin manufacturing cell. *11th CIRP Conference on Industrial Product-Service Systems*. 83, (pp. 345-350). ELSEVIER. 10.1016/j.procir.2019.04.084

Zhang, C., Zhou, G., Hu, J., & Li, J. (2020). Deep learning-enabled intelligent process planning for digital twin manufacturing cell. *Knowledge-Based Systems*, *191*, 105247. doi:10.1016/j.knosys.2019.105247

Zhang, C., Zhou, G., Li, H., & Cao, Y. (2020). Manufacturing blockchain of things for the configuration of a data-and knowledge-driven digital twin manufacturing cell. *IEEE Internet of Things Journal*, *7*(12), 11884–11894. doi:10.1109/JIOT.2020.3005729

Zhang, J., & Tai, Y. (2022). Secure medical digital twin via human-centric interaction and cyber vulnerability resilience. *Connection Science*, *34*(1), 895–910. doi:10.1080/09540091.2021.2013443

Zheng, Y., Lu, R., Guan, Y., Zhang, S., & Shao, J. (2021). Towards Private Similarity Query based Healthcare Monitoring over Digital Twin Cloud Platform. *IEEE/ACM 29th International Symposium on Quality of Service*. doi:10.1109/IWQOS52092.2021.9521351

Zheng, Y., Yang, S., & Cheng, H. (2019). An application framework of digital twin and its case study. *Journal of Ambient Intelligence and Humanized Computing*, *10*(3), 1141–1153. doi:10.100712652-018-0911-3

Zhong, X., Babaie Sarijaloo, F., Prakash, A., Park, J., Huang, C., Barwise, A., Herasevich, V., Gajic, O., Pickering, B., & Dong, Y. (2022). A multidisciplinary approach to the development of digital twin models of critical care delivery in intensive care units. *International Journal of Production Research*. doi:10.1080/00207543.2021.2022235

Zhou, G., Zhang, C., Li, Z., Ding, K., & Wang, C. (2020). Knowledge-driven digital twin manufacturing cell towards intelligent manufacturing. *International Journal of Production Research*, *58*(4), 1034–1051. doi:10.1080/00207543.2019.1607978

Zhou, M., Yan, J., & Feng, D. (2019). Digital Twin Framework and Its Application to Power Grid Online Analysis. *CSSE J. Power Energy Syst.*, *5*, 391–398.

Zhuang, C., Miao, T., Liu, J., & Xiong, H. (2021). The connotation of digital twin, and the construction and application method of shop-floor digital twin. *Robotics and Computer-integrated Manufacturing*, *68*, 102075. doi:10.1016/j.rcim.2020.102075

Zhuang, Z., Stobbe, T. J., Collins, J. W., Hsiao, H., & Hobbs, G. R. (2000). Psychophysical assessment of assistive devices for transferring patients/ residents. *Applied Ergonomics*, *31*(1), 35–44. doi:10.1016/S0003-6870(99)00023-X PMID:10709750

Zia, T., & Zomaya, A. (2006). Security issues in wireless sensor networks. In *International Conference on Systems and Networks Communications, ICSNC'06*, (p. 40). IEEE.

Zolli, A. (2020). How Satellite Data Can Help With COVID-19 And Beyond. *Planet*. https://www.planet.com/pulse/how-satellite-data-can-help-with-covid-19-and-beyond/

About the Contributors

Loveleen Gaur is currently working as Professor of Artificial Intelligence and Data Analytics at Amity International Business School, Amity University, India. She is an Adjunct Professor with School of Computer Science, Taylor's University, Malaysia as well as Adjunct Professor in Graduate School of Business at the University of the South Pacific, Fiji. She is in the editorial board of various reputed SCIE journal and reviewer with Q1 journals. She is supervising several PhD scholars, Post Graduate students, mainly in Artificial Intelligence and Data Analytics for business and healthcare. Under her guidance, the AI/Data Analytics research cluster has published extensively in high impact factor journals and has established extensive research collaboration globally with several renowned professionals. She is a senior IEEE member and Series Editor with CRC and Wiley. She has high indexed publications in SCI/ABDC/WoS/Scopus and has several Patents/copyrights on her account, edited/authored many research books published by world-class publishers. She has excellent experience in supervising and co-supervising postgraduate students internationally. An ample number of Ph.D. and master's students graduated under her supervision. She is an external Ph.D./Master thesis examiner/evaluator for several universities globally. She has also served as Keynote speaker for several international conferences, presented several Webinars worldwide, chaired international conference sessions.(f62b0f94-79e9-41ce-b4a3-01d84272442e)

Noor Zaman Jhanjhi is Associate Editor and Editorial Assistant Board for several reputable journals including IEEE Access Journal, PC member for several IEEE conferences around the globe, Active reviewer for a series of Q1 journals. He has authored several research papers in ISI indexed and impact factor research journals\IEEE international conferences, edited 08 international reputed Computer Science area books, supervised a great number of post graduate students, and external thesis examiner to his credit. He has successfully completed more than 19 international funded research grants. He also served as Keynote speaker for several conferences around the globe. He also chaired international conference sessions and presented session talks internationally. He has strong analytical, problem solving, interpersonal and communication skills. His areas of interest include Cyber Security, Wireless Sensor Network (WSN), Internet of Things IoT, Mobile Application Development, Ad hoc Networks, Cloud Computing, Big Data, Mobile Computing, and Software Engineering.(eb32f41f-88dc-4f50-be39-41246cc6ba7d)

***

Sheik Abdullah A., is working as Assistant Professor (Senior), at the School of Computer Science and Engineering, Vellore Institute of Technology, Chennai Campus, Tamil Nadu, India. He received his Doctoral Degree in Computer Science and Engineering from Anna University, Chennai during November 2019. He completed his Post Graduate in M.E (Computer Science and Engineering), from Kongu Engineering College, Erode under Anna University, Chennai. He has been awarded as gold medalist for his excellence in Post Graduate. He is an active member of professional bodies such as ACM, ISTE, IFERP and Internet Society. As an ACM Member he has been rewarded as an ACM coach for ACM World level International Collegiate Programming contest during the year 2013 and 2014. He has handled various E-Governance government projects such as automation system for tracking community certificate, birth and death certificate, DRDA and income tax automation systems. He has received the Honorable chief minister award for excellence in E-Governance for the best project in E-Governance for the academic year 2015-16. He has been serving as an organizing committee member in various National and International conferences. He has published 65+ articles which includes Books, Book chapters, and Journals in SCI, SCIE, and Scopus Indexed publishers. The most renowned publications are from Springer, Inderscience, CRC Press, Intech Open, and IGI publishers. He has been serving as a reviewer in IEEE, IEEE access, Elsevier, Springer, and CRC publishers.

Quartul Aim is in the Emergency Department (UCS) at Aga Khan University Hospital, Karachi (AKUH).

Imdad Ali Shah is at the School of Computer Science SC, Taylor's University, Malaysia.

Sreelakshmi D. is a research scholar in KL university, and assistant professor in Institute of Aeronautical Engineering. Her research interests are image processing and medical image processing.

B. Sunil de Silva works at the Open University of Sri Lanka as a Senior Lecturer in Nursing and the Dean of the Faculty of Health Sciences at present. She has obtained a Bachelor of Science Degree in Nursing from the Open University of Sri Lanka [a program with academic assistance from Athabasca University, Canada] with a Second Class [Upper Division] Honors. de Silva completed a Master's of Nursing by Research degree at Australian Catholic University in Melbourne, Australia in 2009 and PhD in Nursing at University of New Mexico in USA in 2020. de Silva have also had seven years of academic experiences as a lecturer in nursing and ten year experiences as a Registered Staff Nurse after completing three- year General Nursing Training program in Sri Lanka and as a Ward Manager after completing Diploma in Management and Supervision Program of the Ministry of Health in Sri Lanka.

N. Jayantha Dewasiri is a Professor attached to the Department of Accountancy and Finance, Sabaragamuwa University of Sri Lanka. He also serves as the Honorary Secretary/ Chairman – Education and Research at the Sri Lanka Institute of Marketing. He holds a Doctor of Philosophy in Finance from the University of Colombo, MS.c in Applied Finance, and a Postgraduate Diploma from the University of Sri Jayewardenepura, BA (Hons) in Business from Glyndwr University, UK. Further, He is a member of the Sri Lanka Institute of Marketing, and Chartered Institute of Marketing, a Fellow Member of the Chartered Management Institute, and a Certified Management Accountant. After serving 17 years in the industry, he joined academia and he is a pioneer in applying triangulation research approaches in the management discipline. He is currently serving as the Co-Editors-in-Chief of the South Asian Journal of Marketing published by Emerald Publishing, Senior Associate Editor of the FIIB Business Review published by SAGE Publishing, Managing Editor of the South Asian Journal of Tourism and Hospitality published by the Faculty of Management Studies. He has been awarded for research excellence several times, including the University of Michigan International Mixed Methods Scholarship Award, Grand Winner of the IIARI Luminary Award (2021) in Asia for Research Excellence, Grand Winner of the Deans Award for Research Excellence at the Faculty of Management Studies, the Sabaragamuwa University of Sri Lanka for 2021, and several best paper awards at the conferences. He has published extensively in top-tier research journals, including Managerial Finance, Qualitative Research in Financial Markets, Journal of Public Affairs, International Journal of Qualitative Methods, etc. He is the main contributor of the introductory team of the Data Triangulation approach to the finance discipline. Recently, he has been accredited as a Fellow Chartered Manager (FCMI CMgr) by the Chartered Institute of Management, UK. Considering his valuable contribution to research and academia, Emerald Publishing, UK has appointed him as the Brand Ambassador for its South Asian region.

Harshita Gupta is pursuing a B.Tech in Computer Science. Currently, Gupta am in the 3rd year of college. Gupta has done research on how artificial intelligence is emerging in health care sector. Being a Computer science student, Gupta's research interests are in coding and software development. Gupta is good in java development and python language, and is currently employed as an intern at Moody's Analytics.

Sarada K., from the Koneru Lakshmaiah education foundation, has research areas of interest in electric vehicles and image processing.

Rita Komalasari is a lecturer at YARSI University. Her current work is focused on Healthcare for the elderly with digital twins.

W.S.R. Kulasinghe is a nursing professional attached to the Base Hospital, Matara, Sri Lanka.

Mushkan Kumar is a 3rd year Computer science engineering student from the M.S. Ramaiah University of Applied sciences. Kumar has deep interest in coding and designing.

Sowmya M. received a BE degree in Computer Science and Engineering from Visvesvaraya Technological University, Belagavi India in June 2010. She acquired Master's degree in Software Engineering from Visvesvaraya Technological University, Belagavi, India in Jan 2016. She is pursuing Ph D in Computer Science and Engineering from Visvesvaraya Technological University, Belagavi, India since 2020. At present she is working as Assistant Professor at GSSS Institute of Technology for women, Mysuru. Her research interest includes Internet of Things, Computer Networks and wireless Communication.

Suguna M. is an Assistant Professor Senior Grade at the Department of Computer Science and Engineering in Vellore Institute of Technology, Chennai. Her research interests include Data analytics and Agile Project Management. she is completed Ph.D. in Information and Communication Engineering at Anna University, Chennai. She has published more than 20 research articles in international journals and international conferences. She is a member of ISTE, IAENG, IACSIT and CSTA.

Supriya M. S. is an assistant professor in the department of Computer Science and Engineering at M S Ramaiah University of Applied Sciences. AIML, Software Engineering, MSDF, Real-Time Embedded Systems, Wireless Communication Systems, and Healthcare are some of her research interests. She has a few journal articles, conference papers, and book chapters to her credit.

S. Meenakshi Sundaram is currently working as Professor and Head in the Department of Computer Science and Engineering at GSSS Institute of Engineering and Technology for Women, Mysuru. He obtained bachelor's degree in computer science & Engineering from Bharathidasan University, Tiruchirappalli in 1989, M. Tech from National Institute of Technology, Tiruchirappalli in 2006 and Ph.D. in Information and Communication Engineering from Anna University Chennai in 2014. He has published 53 papers in refereed International Journals, presented 3 papers in International Conferences and has delivered more than 40 seminars. He is a reviewer of Springer – SN Computer Science, Soft Computing Journal, International Journal of Ah Hoc Network Systems, Journal of Engineering Science and Technology, Taylor's University, Malaysia and International Journal of Computational Science & Engineering, Inderscience Publishers, UK. He has organized more than 40 seminars / Workshops / FDPs. He has attended more than 45 Workshops / Seminars. His area of interest includes Computer Networks, Wireless Communication, Software Engineering, Optical Networks and Data Mining. He is a Life Member of Indian Society for Technical Education (ISTE) and a member of Computer Society of India (CSI). He has 30+ Years of teaching experience and 13 years of research experience. Two research scholars have completed Ph D and six others are pursuing Ph.D. in VTU Belagavi, India under his guidance.

Nilamadhab Mishra was a Professor in the Post at the School of Computing, Debre Berhan University, Ethiopia. He has around 15 years of rich global exposure in Academic Teaching & Research. He publishes numerous peer-reviewed researches in SCIE & SCOPUS indexed journals & IEEE conference proceedings and serves as a reviewer and editorial member in peer-reviewed Journals and Conferences. Dr. Mishra has received his Doctor of Philosophy (Ph.D.) in Computer Science & Information Engineering from the Graduate Institute of Electrical Engineering, College of Engineering, Chang Gung University (a World Ranking University), Taiwan. He has been involved in academic research by working, as a Journal Editor, an SCIE & Scopus indexed Journals Referee, an ISBN Book Author, and an IEEE Conference Referee. Dr. Mishra has been pro-actively involved with several professional bodies: CSI, ORCID, IAENG, ISROSET, Senior Member of "ASR" (Hong Kong), Senior Member of "IEDRC" (Hong Kong), and Member of "IEEE ". Dr. Mishra's Research areas incorporate Network Centric Data Management, Data Science: Analytics and Applications, CIoT Big-Data System, and Cognitive Apps Design & Explorations.

Tejaswini R. Murgod received a BE degree in Computer Science and Engineering from Visvesvaraya Technological University, Belagavi India on June 2008. She acquired Master's degree in Software Engineering from Visvesvaraya Technological University, Belagavi, India in Jan 2015. She received Ph D in Computer Science and Engineering from Visvesvaraya Technological University, Belagavi, India in February 2022. At present she is working as Associate Professor at Nitte Meenakshi Institute of Technology, Bengaluru. Her research interest includes underwater communication, Optical networks and wireless networks.

Ambika N. is a MCA, MPhil, Ph.D. in computer science. She completed her Ph.D. from Bharathiar university in the year 2015. She has 16 years of teaching experience and presently working for St.Francis College, Bangalore. She has guided BCA, MCA and M.Tech students in their projects. Her expertise includes wireless sensor network, Internet of things, cybersecurity. She gives guest lectures in her expertise. She is a reviewer of books, conferences (national/international), encyclopaedia and journals. She is advisory committee member of some conferences. She has many publications in National & international conferences, international books, national and international journals and encyclopaedias. She has some patent publications (National) in computer science division.

Sahana. P. Shankar completed her B.E in Information Science and Engineering and MTech in Software Engineering from Ramaiah Institute of Technology, Bangalore. She is a third rank holder in B.E and a first rank holder with gold medal in MTech. She has worked with Unisys as Associate Engineer in the Software Product Testing domain for three years. She holds a US Patent bearing patent number US20160034382. She has worked with RIT as a Teaching Assistant for 6 months under the TEQIP-II scholarship program. She has published papers in various national and international journals and conferences. She has also authored several book chapters. She is an ISTQB certified software tester. She is currently working with Ramaiah University of Applied Sciences, Bangalore as an Assistant Professor in the Department of Computer Science and Engineering.

Kamalendu Pal is with the Department of Computer Science, School of Science and Technology, City, University of London. Kamalendu received his BSc (Hons) degree in Physics from Calcutta University, India, Postgraduate Diploma in Computer Science from Pune, India, MSc degree in Software Systems Technology from the University of Sheffield, Postgraduate Diploma in Artificial Intelligence from Kingston University, MPhil degree in Computer Science from the University College London, and MBA degree from the University of Hull, United Kingdom. He has published over eighty international research articles (including book chapters) widely in the scientific community with research papers in the ACM SIGMIS Database, Expert Systems with Applications, Decision Support Systems, and conferences. His research interests include knowledge-based systems, decision support systems, teaching and learning practice, blockchain technology, software engineering, service-oriented computing, sensor network simulation, and supply chain management. He is on the editorial board of an international computer science journal and is a member of the British Computer Society, the Institution of Engineering and Technology, and the IEEE Computer Society.

Priyadarshini R. is working as an Assistant Professor Senior Grade in the School of Computer Science Engineering, Vellore Institute of Technology, Chennai. She has 17+ years of experience in Industry, Teaching and Research. She has a Post-Doctoral fellowship in the Faculty of Computer Science Engineering at Lincoln University Malaysia in the area of IoT and Healthcare. She completed her Ph.D. in Information Technology from UGC recognized by B.S. Abdur Rahman Crescent Institute of Science and Technology and Completed her M. Tech Information Technology at College of Engineering, Anna University, Chennai. She has a national and international patent grant to her credit in IoT Cloud and Data Analytics. She also has six patents published in IoT Cloud, Data Analytics, Cloud Security, and Network Security. She has published more than 50+ papers in reputed international conferences and journals. She has 5 book chapters and 1 Book on amazon to her credit. More recently, she has contributed to interdisciplinary research in blockchain, medical health and IoT. Being a passionate teacher &

topper in all her academic records and a continuous learner, she has 35+ certifications in her research areas to her credit from IBM, NPTEL, SWAYAM, CSC, JPA, Spoken Tutorials IIT Mumbai, Udemy, GVN, etc. and she has been awarded as the best researcher, one of the top reviewers by various national and international bodies. She contributes her interests in various international conferences and serves as a reviewer in IEEE, Elsevier, Springer, and Inderscience publishers. She is an active member of CSI since July 2007 and also a member of ACM, IFERP, etc.

Aditya Raj is a computer science undergrad about to take a new career, with some curious mindset upon the artificial intelligence field.

Jyoti Rana is a full-time research scholar of Amity College of Commerce and Finance, Amity University, Noida. She has worked as an assistant professor in the School of Commerce and Management at Starex University, Gurugram. She has participated and presented papers in many national and international conferences and has publications in high-impact factor journals. Her keen research areas are marketing, retail, artificial intelligence, and customer journey.

Rishika Saha is a computer science engineering student at Ramaiah University who aspires to become a software developer in future.

K. Saikumar is a research scholar in KL university and assistance professor in Malla Reddy University. His research interests are image processing and medical image processing.

Swagat Samantarav is an Asst. Professor at School of Computing Sciences and Engineering, VIT Bhopal University, India.

D. I. K. Sarambage is a medical professional attached to the Base Hospital, Matara, Sri Lanka.

Selvakumar Subramanian received a Doctor of Philosophy in Computer Science and Engineering from the Anna University, Chennai. He received the master's degree in computer science & Engineering from the Madurai Kamaraj University. He has over 25 years experience in various institutions. Currently he is a Professor in Department of Computer Science & Engineering, Visvesvaraya College of Engineering & Technology. His teaching and research interests includes Software Engineering, Data Analytics, Networks. He has published over 150 papers in various Indexed International Journals and Conferences.

Sitharamulu Vedula is an Associate Professor in Department of Computer Science & Engineering, Institute of Aeronautical Engineering. He has 20 years of experience in Teaching. He has published 25 papers in international journals and Conferences and 3 patents in his credit.

Muniraju Naidu Vadlamudi, Assistant Professor, Department of CSE, Institute of Aeronautical Engineering-Hyderabad. Research areas of interest are image and Pattern recognition, and IoT.

Deepak Varadam is working as an Assistant Professor in M.S. Ramaiah University of Applied Sciences. Varadam has experience of 10 years in teaching and research. Varadam has also delivered corporate trainings, seminars and have publications in national, international journals and conferences.

Index

L

M

N

O

P

Q

R

S

T

V

W

Printed in the United States
by Baker & Taylor Publisher Services